The Frontal Lobes

The frontal lobes and their functional properties are recognized as crucial to establishing our identity as autonomous human beings. This book provides a broad introductory overview of this unique brain region. In an accessible and readable style it covers the evolutionary significance of the frontal lobes, typical and atypical development pathways, the role played in normal cognition, memory and emotion, and in damaged states, resulting in a range of neurological syndromes and psychiatric disturbances. The coverage integrates current theoretical knowledge with observation of the both normal and disturbed behavior across the lifespan. The result is an easy-to-read review of this fascinating and involved field suitable for graduate students in neuropsychology and psychology, clinicians from the fields of neurology, neurosurgery or psychiatry, and researchers engaged in neuroscientific investigations.

Jarl Risberg is Professor of Neuropsychology at Lund University and Head of the Neuropsychology Section at the Departments of Clinical Neuroscience and Psychology, Lund University, Lund, Sweden.

Jordan Grafman is the Chief of the Cognitive Neuroscience Section at the National Institute of Neurological Disorders and Stroke in Bethesda, USA.

**Series for the International Neuropsychological Society
Sponsored by the Vivian Smith Foundation**

SERIES EDITOR

Andrew Papanicolaou
Director, Division of Clinical Neurosciences
University of Texas
Houston, Texas
USA

The Frontal Lobes

Development, Function, and Pathology

Edited by

Jarl Risberg and Jordan Grafman

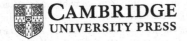
CAMBRIDGE
UNIVERSITY PRESS

CAMBRIDGE UNIVERSITY PRESS
Cambridge, New York, Melbourne, Madrid, Cape Town, Singapore,
São Paulo, Delhi, Dubai, Tokyo

Cambridge University Press
The Edinburgh Building, Cambridge CB2 8RU, UK

Published in the United States of America by Cambridge University Press, New York

www.cambridge.org
Information on this title: www.cambridge.org/9780521672252

First published 2006

A catalogue record for this publication is available from the British Library

Library of Congress Cataloguing in Publication data

The frontal lobes : development, function, and pathology / Jarl Risberg and Jordan
Grafman, editors.
    p. ; cm. – (Series for the International Neuropsychological Society)
Includes bibliographical references and index.
ISBN-13: 978-0-521-67225-2 (pbk.)
ISBN-10: 0-521-67225-2 (pbk.)
1. Frontal lobes. I. Risberg, Jarl. II. Grafman, Jordan. III. Series.
[DNLM: 1. Frontal Lobe–physiology. 2. Frontal Lobe–physiopathology. 3. Mental
Disorders–physiopathology. 4. Mental Processes–physiology. WL 307 F93485 2006]
I. Title. II. Series.
QP382.F7F758 2006
612.8′2–dc22

                                                                        2006028963

ISBN 978-0-521-67225-2 Paperback

Additional resources for this publication at www.cambridge.org/9780521672252

Transferred to digital printing 2009

Contents

Contributors   *page* vii

From the series editor   ix

Introduction   xi

1   Evolutionary aspects on the frontal lobes   1
     Jarl Risberg

2   Organization of the principal pathways of prefrontal lateral,
     medial, and orbitofrontal cortices in primates and implications
     for their collaborative interaction in executive functions   21
     Helen Barbas

3   Human prefrontal cortex: processes and representations   69
     Jordan Grafman

4   A microcircuit model of prefrontal functions: ying and
     yang of reverberatory neurodynamics in cognition   92
     Xiao-Jing Wang

5   Prefrontal cortex: typical and atypical development   128
     Maureen Dennis

6   Case studies of focal prefrontal lesions in man   163
     David W. Loring and Kimford J. Meador

7   Left prefrontal function and semantic organization during
     encoding and retrieval in healthy and psychiatric populations   178
     Daniel Ragland

8   Clinical symptoms and neuropathology in organic dementing
     disorders affecting the frontal lobes   199
     Arne Brun and Lars Gustafson

     Index   222

Contributors

Helen Barbas, Ph.D.
Department of Health Sciences
Boston University
635 Commonwealth Ave., #431
Boston, MA 02215
USA
Phone: 617-353-5036
Fax: 617-353-7567

Arne Brun, MD, Ph.D.
Department of Pathology
University Hospital
SE-221 85 Lund
SWEDEN
Phone: +46-46-120384

Maureen Dennis, Ph.D.
Department of Psychology
The Hospital for Sick Children
555 University Avenue
Toronto, ON M5G 1X8
CANADA
Phone: 416-813-6658
Fax: 416-813-8839

Jordan Grafman, Ph.D.
Cognitive Neuroscience Section
NINDS, NIH
Building 10; Room 5C205
10 Center Drive; MSC 1440
Bethesda, Md. 20892-1440
USA
Phone: 301-496-0220
Fax: 301-480-2909

Lars Gustafson, MD, Ph.D.
Department of Psychogeriatrics
University Hospital
SE-221 85 Lund
SWEDEN
Phone: +46-46-177450

David Loring, Ph.D.
Departments of Neurology and Clinical
    & Health Psychology
Center for Neuropsychological Studies
McKnight Brain Institute
University of Florida
P.O. Box 100236
Gainesville, FL 32610-0236
Phone: 352-273-5550/273-5621

Kimford Meador, Ph.D.
Departments of Neurology and Clinical
  & Health Psychology
Center for Neuropsychological Studies
McKnight Brain Institute University of
  Florida
P.O. Box 100236
Gainesville, FL 32610-0236
USA

J. Daniel Ragland, Ph.D.
Imaging Research Center
University of California at Davis
4701 X Street
Sacramento, CA 95817
USA
Phone: 916-734-3230
Fax: 916-734-8750

Jarl Risberg, Ph.D.
Department of Clinical
  Neurophysiology
University Hospital
SE-221 85 Lund
SWEDEN
Phone: +46-46-177900
Fax: +46-46-177906

Xiao-Jing Wang, Ph.D.
Department of Neurobiology and Kavli
  Institute for Neuroscience
Yale University School of Medicine
333 Cedar Street
New Haven, CT 06510

From the series editor

This volume inaugurates a collection of books on topics of current interest in neuropsychology and systems neuroscience. The series is a natural extension of the annual *Advanced Studies Institute*, which operates under the auspices of the International Neuropsychological Society (INS) with the support of the Vivian L. Smith Foundation of Houston, Texas.

The purposes of the Institute and of the book series are to promote dissemination of knowledge in the fields of systems neurosciences and clinical neuropsychology; to promote the formation of professional bonds among current and future leaders in these fields from across the world; to encourage in-depth study of fundamental issues and evaluation of current advances in these fields, and to seek solutions to unresolved problems under conditions designed to optimize the efficiency of the above named endeavors. This series will, we hope, extend this message to the academic and professional community at large.

In my capacity as organizer and director of the Institute and editor of this series, I wish to express my indebtedness to the president and board of the Vivian L. Smith Foundation of Houston for their abiding support, to the secretary of the INS and to the succession of its board members and presidents since the inception of these projects, for embracing them, to Drs Jarl Risberg and Jordan Grafman who graciously volunteered to edit the present volume and to all the friends and colleagues who contributed its excellent chapters.

I also wish to thank Dr. Marcia Barnes who is editing the second volume of the series focusing on issues of mental retardation, as well as Drs Linas Bieliauskas and Kenneth Adams who have volunteered to prepare the third volume on *Neuropsychology Across the Life Span.*

Andrew C. Papanicolaou
Houston, February 2006

Introduction

The frontal lobes are crucial to understanding our identity as autonomous beings and this significance is now reflected in the number and importance of neuro-psychological, biological, and philosophical papers and books on the functions of the frontal lobes published over the last 40 years. This research effort has identified many of the functional properties of the frontal lobes but there are still numerous unsolved problems and controversies regarding its evolutionary, biological and functional status. Based on the theme of the International Neuropsychological Society's (INS) Summer Institute, this volume reviews this fascinating area of study. The Director of the Vivian Smith Advanced Studies Institute of the INS, Professor Andrew Papanicolaou, presents the background of the Institute in his foreword to this volume. He is also the editor of this new series of INS books starting with the present volume.

As the editors of this first book in the series, we are very proud to introduce you to the contents of the volume with the admittedly broad title *The Frontal Lobes: Development, Function, and Pathology*. While our volume does not cover every detailed aspect of this theme, we hope that the eight chapters will offer everyone interested in the frontal lobes an overview and some new and intriguing insights. The book is intended for graduate students in psychology and neuro-psychology, as well as postdoctoral fellows and faculty members in departments of psychology, psychiatry, neurology, and related fields. The content of the volume should be of value to both practicing clinicians, who see patients with frontal disturbances, and to scientists engaged in neuroscience research.

The first chapter is written by one of the editors (Jarl Risberg) and is entitled *Evolutionary Aspects on the Frontal Lobes*. The chapter gives an introduction to the fascinating story about the evolution of the human brain and especially of its frontal lobes. Special focus is on the development of modern behavior and mental abilities like symbolic language and creative thinking. Disadvantages linked to the dangers and demands of a large size brain are also dealt with and the anatomical differences between the human brain and that of our close relatives, the African great apes, are discussed. Our still very limited knowledge about what changes in the human genome made it possible to develop modern behavior is summarized. The chapter ends by viewing two very old and specifically human mental disturbances, schizophrenia and attention deficit hyperactivity disorder, from an evolutionary perspective.

The second chapter is authored by Helen Barbas and has the title *Organization of the Principal Pathways of Prefrontal Lateral, Medial, and Orbitofrontal Cortices in Primates and Implications for their Collaborative Interaction in Executive Functions*. This chapter describes how the prefrontal cortex in primates guides by selecting relevant information, disregarding irrelevant information, and accessing motor control systems for action. Evidence is explored indicating that highly organized pathways link distinct prefrontal sectors with structures underlying sensory perception, cognition, and emotions. The topographically ordered pathways show consistent patterns in their laminar organization and interface with excitatory and inhibitory brain systems. The chapter ends by discussing how different sectors of the prefrontal cortex communicate with each other, inextricably linking pathways associated with cognition and emotions that guide actions.

The third chapter *Human Prefrontal Cortex: Processes and Representations* is written by the other editor of this volume (Jordan Grafman), and has its focus on what strategies you can use when characterizing the functions of the human prefrontal cortex like language, abstract reasoning, problem solving, social interactions, planning, action generation, and self-recognition. Five criteria that a theory should meet if it is to provide a useful framework for understanding the functions of the prefrontal cortex are described. An overview of the key theories about the function of the prefrontal cortex is given and their ability to stand critical experimental testing is evaluated. The main claims of each key theory are specified and a review of data addressing these claims is given. Theories that take a processing approach as well as theories that take a representational approach are discussed and evaluated.

The fourth chapter, entitled *A Microcircuit Model of Prefrontal Functions: Ying and Yang of Reverberatory Neurodynamics in Cognition*, is written by Xiao-Jing Wang. This chapter introduces the basic concepts and methods in computational neuroscience, develops intuitions about complex and recurrent circuits, and discusses biologically based models for working memory and other cognitive functions of the frontal lobes. Theories of simple and complex networks are described together with the use of these concepts for characterizing the connectivity of the frontal lobes. Behavioral data and mathematical models of working memory and task switching are also covered. The chapter ends by showing how modeling results shed insights into the cellular/circuit basis of cognitive impairments in mental diseases like schizophrenia.

The fifth chapter, written by Maureen Dennis, is entitled *Prefrontal Cortex: Typical and Atypical Development*. This chapter provides a review of the typical development of the frontal lobes with respect to brain microstructure, brain macrostructure, and functions such as working memory, inhibitory control, intentionality, and social cognition. The atypical development of the frontal lobes in children with congenital or acquired neurodevelopmental disturbances is also covered focusing on disturbances of working memory, inhibition, theory of mind, and social comportment and the theoretical implications of these disturbances. The emphasis is on how these early disturbances impact subsequent maturation and development of the frontal lobes.

The sixth chapter is authored by David Loring and Kimford Meador and entitled *Case Studies of Focal Prefrontal Lesions in Man*. The chapter starts with an introduction to the history of clinical neuropsychology and continues with a review of some classical as well as some more recent case studies of frontally damaged patients. A detailed account of the Phineas Gage story is given followed by the case KM, described by Donald Hebb and coworkers. The patent EVR, described by Eslinger and Damasio, is then reviewed as well as patients displaying utilization as described by Lhermitte. Finally the impact of early prefrontal injury is illustrated.

The seventh chapter is authored by Daniel Ragland and has the title *Left Prefrontal Function and Semantic Organization during Encoding and Retrieval in Healthy and Psychiatric Populations*. The chapter begins with definitions of episodic and declarative memory and an overview of the role that the prefrontal cortex plays in these forms of long-term memory. The focus then narrows to the function of semantic organization, with an explication of how semantic organizational processes facilitate word encoding and retrieval in healthy subjects. This explication includes neuropsychological data showing how semantic organization improves performance, and neuroimaging data demonstrating the role of left prefrontal cortex. Schizophrenia is then introduced to illustrate how prefrontal dysfunction caused by a psychiatric illness can impact these same memory functions. Finally, levels-of-processing data are presented to demonstrate that memory performance and left prefrontal function can be normalized when patients are provided with organizational strategies.

The final and eighth chapter is authored by Arne Brun and Lars Gustafson and has the title *Clinical Symptoms and Neuropathology in Organic Dementing Disorders Affecting the Frontal Lobes*. In this chapter the authors offer some possible explanations for why the frontal lobes are such frequent targets for a variety of damaging processes. This is followed by a discussion of some general mechanisms of importance for understanding the relationship between symptoms and brain changes. The authors conclude their chapter with a description of neuropathological findings and clinical symptoms in some of the most common dementing disorders affecting the frontal lobes: frontotemporal dementia forms, Alzheimer's disease with frontal lobe symptoms, Huntington's disease, and vascular dementia with frontal features.

We wish to thank all the chapter authors for participating in the Xylocastro INS Summer Institute and for their dedication to studying the functions of the frontal lobes. We also hope that the book will stimulate your frontal lobes and entice you to join us in exploring its many mysteries.

Jarl Risberg and Jordan Grafman

Evolutionary aspects on the frontal lobes

Jarl Risberg

1 Introduction

The purpose of this chapter is to introduce you to the fascinating story about the evolution of the human brain and especially of its frontal lobes. The story begins in south east Africa some six million years ago and ends with the recent development of modern behavior and mental abilities like symbolic language and creative thinking. Some disadvantages linked to the dangers and demands of a large size brain will be dealt with. A discussion of the anatomical differences between the human brain and that of our close relatives, the African great apes, will follow. Evolutionary advantages linked to the big brain and its advanced frontal lobes will be described, with special focus on the evolution of language and abstract thinking. Our still very limited knowledge about what changes of the human genome, that made it possible to develop modern behavior, is then summarized. The chapter will end by discussing two very old and specifically human mental disturbances, schizophrenia and attention deficit hyperactivity disorder, from an evolutionary perspective.

2 Early history of human evolution and "the creative explosion"

The tremendous success of humanity, regarding population growth and ability to occupy practically all parts of the earth, is not due to any great bodily advantages of our species. Our main advantage is the possession of a brain that makes it possible for us to outsmart and control most of our competitors and enemies on the planet Earth and to change and use the environment to our (short-term) advantage. The chimpanzee is our closest living relative and the still unknown shared ancestor evolved into two lines of development around six million years ago. This separation took place in southeast Africa and was coincidental with marked climate changes — the eastern part of Africa turned into a more open landscape of savanna type including also plenty of wetlands and seashores. The upright position was advantageous for the different forms of hominids (different species of the *Australopithecus* family like *A. afarensis*; "Lucy") that were developed. It is a matter of debate whether the advantages of bipedalism (energy economic movements, easy spotting of food or predators), lack of fur, having sweat glands and body fat were that great on the savanna. There are many supporters of the *water ape* hypothesis claiming that the ancestors of humanity mainly populated the wetlands and the seashore (Leakey & Lewin, 1978). Here the availability of highly nutritious seafood should later be one of the prerequisites for the development of the large size brain. As is shown in Figure 1.1, the brain weight remained at about chimpanzee size for about three million years. Brain growth started with the appearance of the first representative of the *Homo* family, *Homo habilis*, about two-and-a-half million years ago. The first stone tools appear with the evolution of this line of species. No archeological findings indicate that the early hominids behaviorally were more advanced than present day chimpanzees. A steady increase in brain weight has taken place during the last two million years of evolution and peaking with *Homo neanderthalensis* and us, the *Homo sapiens sapiens*. A possible change of the genome responsible for this brain expansion is a successive inactivation of a gene (CMAH) that restricts brain development (Chou *et al.*, 2002). This gene is not active at all in modern humans.

A more precise answer to the question of whether the steady increase in brain weight was accompanied by a parallel development of higher mental functions is still lacking. We can only guess from archeological evidence, primarily from

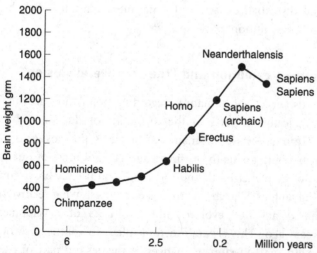

Figure 1.1.   Increase of brain weight during the evolution of different hominid species. (Adapted from Jensen, 1996.)

the stone tools our ancestors left behind, what behavior they displayed. If advances in tool-making techniques are taken as indications of intellectual creativity, the progress was very slow during more than two million years (Calvin, 2004). Bilateral symmetric stone tools were invented about 1.6 million years ago, but after that an additional million years followed without much creative advances, at least regarding tool making. Other abilities, like more accurate throwing and better social and communicative skills might, however, have utilized the increasingly heavy brain. Calvin (2004) suggests that vocal communication skills have evolved from the primate one-call-one meaning to protolanguage abilities perhaps a million years ago. Protolanguage is considered to be close to the language of a normal two-year-old child talking with single words and short sentences (Bickerton, 1990). Protolanguage is not limited to a standard set of situation-dependent calls but can handle novel combinations of words. Calvin and Bickerton (2000) suggest that protolanguage developed gradually over a million years with an increase of vocabulary and mimicry, but still with short sentence length. General intelligence and creativity seem, however, not to have improved that much as indicated by the slow progress in tool-making technology. The simple rule that bigger is smarter might thus not be fully applicable to the evolutionary development of the brain.

Archeological and genetic evidence from variations in mitochondrial DNA indicates that the species *Homo sapiens* (meaning the thinking human) has its origin in southeast Africa some 170 000 years ago (Ingman *et al.*, 2000). This early (archaic) form of *Homo sapiens* had a slightly smaller brain than the Neanderthals and modern humans. Evidence of modern behavior, like symbolic thinking and creativity, is not present until about 80 000 years ago in Africa and about 40 000 years ago in Europe and other parts of the world that were populated by modern humans or *Homo sapiens sapiens* (meaning the human who knows that he/she knows). The rapid appearance of arts, gems, musical instruments, and advanced bone tools was called the *creative explosion* by Pfeiffer (1982) and is by others referred to as the *specialization event*. Recent excavations in the Blombos Cave in South Africa have revealed evidence of personal ornaments such as a sea shell bead and also ochre stones with engravings of most likely symbolic nature (Figure 1.2; Henshilwood *et al.*, 2002, 2004). These artifacts together with advanced bone tools and musical instruments are interpreted as evidence of modern human behavior, including abstract and creative thinking and probably the use of some form of symbolic language with syntax and long and more complicated sentences. The creative explosion does not coincide with any increase in brain weight. The modern cognitive abilities have to be based on a functional reorganization that opened new ways of utilizing the old brain. It is likely that most of the key structures

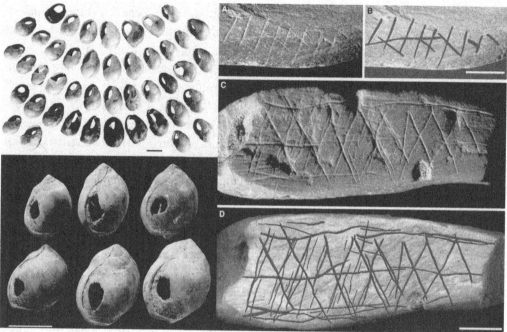

Figure 1.2.   Evidence of modern human behavior from excavations in the Blombos cave in South Africa dated to about 77 000 years before present. A sea shell bead is seen to the left and ochre stones with engravings of probably symbolic nature are shown to the right. (From Henshilwood *et al.*, 2002, 2004, reprinted with permission.)

linked to this new way of thinking were located in the frontal lobes. It has been suggested that the development of modern thinking and language was coincidental with the evolution of a more functionally lateralized brain (Crow, 1998). I will later return to the question of what functional changes that might have occurred during this recent period of human evolution. There are, however, also definite drawbacks and hazards linked to the possession of a big brain.

3   Disadvantages of possessing a big brain

Is the evolutionary development of the large size human brain a unique experiment by nature? Definitely not, we are all familiar with other big-brained species like the dolphins, and also some birds and fishes have relatively large brains (see Allman, 2000 for a review). The brain of one of them, the elephant-nosed fish, was by Nilsson (1996) found to consume 60% of the oxygen used by the entire body of the fish. This fish needed its big brain for an advanced ultrasound system used to locate the prey in muddy water. The very high nutritional demand of a large brain is one of its most significant disadvantages and regarding the human species it has certainly played a significant role for limiting population growth. In the adult human about 20% of the basal metabolism is used for feeding the brain and in the newborn this percentage is about 60 (Holliday, 1971). The brain is thus a very demanding organ that needs much energy for its development, maintenance, and function. The evolutionary change from a low-energy fruit and vegetables diet to one which is rich in energy and nutrients is considered to be a prerequisite for the development of the large brain. The inclusion of animal and fish meat in the diet, that took place several million years ago, has been linked to brain development (Leonard *et al.*, 2003) as well as the introduction of cooking (Wrangham & Conklin-Brittain, 2003). Raw meat and vegetables were not easy enough to chew and digest for the gracile hominids with their small jaws and digestive systems. Supporters of the water ape hypothesis also point to the advantages of seafood over animal meat regarding contents of essential fatty acids and other nutrients that the brain needs. The ability of humans to accumulate body fat during periods of good nutrition has been suggested to protect the brain from the negative effects of periods of starvation. The accumulation of body fat is likely to be of special importance in early childhood. No other land-living species has young ones who, during their first year, have a body fat percentage of about 25 (Leonard, 2002; Leonard *et al.*, 2003). In their review entitled *Survival of the fattest: fat babies were the key to evolution of the large human brain*, Cunnane and Crawford (2003) speculate about the brain protective value that the body fat of the baby has in periods of malnutrition.

A disadvantage of the large size brain is also a markedly increased risk for damage and disease. The population growth of humanity has until very recent times been strongly limited by a commonly brain-related high mortality during delivery, infancy, and childhood. Mortality during delivery is often directly related to the large head of the fetus with great risk for physical damage to mother and child as well as problems with perfusion and nutrition. Also, in adults, the brain is a very vulnerable organ, as is evident from the high prevalence of different forms of often mortal brain diseases, including disorders like Alzheimer's disease, linked to the expanded human life span.

These were some general facts about the big human brain. We will now focus on the subpart of the brain that is the topic of the present volume: the frontal lobes.

4 Do humans have larger frontal lobes than other primates?

The old "truth" that the frontal lobes of humans are exceptionally large and considerably larger than those of any nonhuman primate has recently been challenged by new investigations using modern brain imaging methods (Semendeferi *et al.*, 2002). The classical studies by Brodmann (1912) and Blinkov and Glezer (1968) seemed to show that the surface of the frontal cortex was 20–30% smaller in the chimpanzee (with a brain that is not considered to have changed much from that of our mutual ancestor). These studies used, however, much less precise methods for the delineation of the boundaries between the lobes than available when using present front-line brain imaging methodology. Semendeferi and coworkers (2002) found the following volume relations between the frontal cortex and the total cortex of the cerebral hemispheres: human 37.7%, chimpanzee 35.4%, gorilla 36.9%, orangutan 37.6%. They thus found no or very small differences between humans and the great African apes regarding the relative volume of the frontal lobes. According to these results the enlargement of the human brain has evolved with a generally preserved relationship between its major lobes.

Accepting that the relative size of the frontal lobes is about the same, some investigators have analyzed if any frontal subpart has been enlarged during human evolution. Another study by Semendeferi and collaborators (2001) focused on Brodmann's area 10, positioned in the most polar prefrontal part of the brain with a crucial role for many advanced human mental abilities, like self-control. This area was found to be of about double the relative size in humans compared to that of nonhuman primates. This opens up for speculations about what happened to the brain when modern behavior was developed. Changes of the functional organization and mode of operation are more likely than any major changes of brain anatomy. One such major organizational change is likely to be a relative enlargement of multimodal association areas in both anterior and posterior parts of the brain in combination with an increase of the relative amount of white matter.

The white matter of the brain has been in the focus of some recent studies of differences in brain anatomy between humans and other primates. Schoenemann and collaborators (2005) used magnetic resonance imaging (MRI) in their study of the brains of 11 primate species measuring gray, white, and total volumes of prefrontal regions as well as the entire brain. They found that the prefrontal white matter shows the largest differences between human and nonhuman primates in contrast to a lack of differences regarding gray matter. These results have, however, been questioned by Sherwood and collaborators (2005) based on problems with the method used to delineate the prefrontal part of the brain. The disputed question is whether the frontal white matter is enlarged more than expected from the well-established relationship between total brain size and relative amount of white matter. A larger brain needs more white matter to support the connectivity between its increased number of neurons.

In a recent study, Schenker *et al.* (2005) subdivided the white matter in gyral and core white matter and found that the human gyral white matter was larger than expected in proportion to the core white matter as well as to the cortex. This might indicate that one of the evolutionary changes in humans is a difference in the way information is processed. An elevated proportion of white to gray matter may facilitate neural transmission with positive effects on, for example, fast learning while an increased ratio of gyral to core white matter might facilitate fast and efficient intrahemispheric processing of information. An increased number of axons and dendrites, together with an increased myelination, might thus provide the advanced connectivity needed for human higher cognitive functions. As discussed above, the absolute size of the brain is not the sole factor that determines its functional efficiency. The reorganization of the brain without enlargement seems to be a very important evolutionary mechanism. Within a constant total brain size have some areas been relatively smaller in humans, like the olfactory bulb and the primary visual cortex (Semendeferi *et al.*, 1998), while others have been enlarged with strengthened connectivity like area 10 and Broca's and Wernicke's areas. That the qualitative features of a brain are more important than its size is further illustrated by the fact that Einstein had a rather small brain (Witelson *et al.*, 1999) and that the recently discovered possibly new human species, *Homo floresiensis*, in spite of a small size brain, shows signs of advanced intelligence, like skillful hunting. The main anatomical feature, that is likely to have made this small brain that bright, is its highly convoluted frontal lobes, with a remarkably large Brodmann area 10 (Falk *et al.*, 2005).

At the cellular level there are findings of recently evolved new types of cells like the spindle neurons. These cells are narrow and elongated and mainly present in the anterior cingulate cortex (Nimchinsky *et al.*, 1995). They are unique to humans and the great apes, but much less common in the latter species (Nimchinsky *et al.*, 1999). Allman and collaborators (2002) suggest that the spindle neurons relay to other parts of the brain, especially to area 10, known to be involved in the retrieval of episodic memories and the planning of adaptive responses. The authors suggest that the evolutionary development of a close interaction between the new spindle neurons and area 10 is crucial for the ability to adapt to changing conditions.

5 Evolutionary advantages of the big brain with its advanced frontal lobes

The evolutionary advantages of a big brain have been debated for several decades. There is a general agreement that changes of the behavior of the hominids have been the force beyond brain development. The fossils do not tell us about behavior — behavior can be studied only indirectly by what our ancestors left behind, for example stone tools and signs of culture like burial graves and cave paintings. The earliest theory, popular until the 1950s, suggested that the expanding brain was needed for tool-making. The fact that the progress in tool-making technology was rather slow during millions of years in spite of an increasing brain weight, led, however, to questioning of the theory. In the 1960s the *Man the Tool Maker* theory was replaced by the *Man the Hunter* theory. Successful hunting of game that is physically larger and stronger than a human, does certainly require a bright mind for planning to outsmart the prey in collaboration with fellow hunters. Calvin (2004) has pointed out the fact that killing by throwing a weapon from a distance is a highly demanding activity, not seen in other species. The synchronized ballistic movements when throwing the spear only take about one eighth of a second to complete with no possibility for correction after the initiation of the throw. During the preparation of such a program of movements hundreds of muscles are engaged and their activity released like preprogrammed fireworks. A large and creative brain is likely to be needed, especially for the frequently novel ballistic movements needed for successful hunting.

Others, like Foley (1987), have argued for the importance of nutritional strategy as a force for the development of the brain. The use of tools and cooking increased the amount of energy that was derived from the nutrition-rich meat needed to support the development of the demanding big brain. Food sharing within the group was an important factor for securing nutritional requirements. Such social abilities are today considered to be the main evolutionary force beyond brain development.

Socializing is a very important part of the behavior of primates in general but has reached exceptionally high levels of complexity in humans. Archeological evidence indicates that the change of social activities with work and food sharing is coincidental with the appearance of the *Homo* lineage (Isaac, 1978). This new behavioral pattern could work only in conjunction with the use of tools. The slaughtering of big animals was made possible by the use of proper tools with collaborative efforts also including the transportation of the meat to the homestead for safe sharing. The social demands that are linked to work and food sharing are by Glynn Isaac and others considered to be the most essential factor beyond the development of the human brain and its intelligence. It created a nutritional dependence within the group, a dependence that might have caused a selective pressure favoring collaborative abilities and empathic and altruistic actions. Such abilities strengthened the social bands within the group. There was most likely also a strong selective pressure that favored the ability to plan and calculate and not the least to communicate. Exchanges of experiences are of much more importance for a collaborating group of hominids than for species with more individual methods for providing nutrition. The smoothly collaborating and communicating group had thus a very significant advantage. The strong selective pressure for efficient communication made us develop oral speech.

6　Language evolution

Many mental abilities may be listed when discussing the factors that make us different from other species but our symbolic language stands out as the most important. In its oral and written forms, language is the main tool for exchange and accumulation of knowledge within and in between individuals and generations. The child's innate capacity to learn the sounds, words, sentences, and syntax of the language spoken in its environment is strikingly different from the total inability of a young chimpanzee, even when fostered in a human family, to imitate or utter anything but the simple sounds and calls of wild chimpanzees (Arcadi, 2000). Interestingly, chimpanzees raised in a human environment might learn sign language and both initiate and maintain conversations with their interlocutor using hand movements (Jensvold & Gardner, 2000; Bodamer & Gardner, 2002). The lack of voluntary control of the facial muscles makes it, however, impossible for the chimpanzee to accompany the hand signs with mimicry, which is an important companion of human sign language.

Premack (2004) points out that many species are able to copy someone's choice of an object. A second and more advanced level of imitation is for the observer to copy the model's motor action. To do this a mental representation of the visually perceived action has to be formed and an action conforming to the perceived one must be produced. This is an easy task for young humans but impossible for other species. The unique ability of humans to imitate sounds and motor acts is probably one of the frontally based abilities required for language. The mirror neurons are the likely neuronal basis for this ability. These neurons are active during watching someone moving as well as during the performance (imitation) of the same movement (Rizzolatti & Arbib, 1998). Their presence in the area that is homologous to the Broca's area in nonhuman primates has made these neurons very likely to be linked to the development of human language. There is also evidence that this area is involved in a gestural mirror neuron system in humans (Nishitani & Hari, 2000).

Another unique human ability that Premark (2004) points out is teaching. Teaching is the reverse of imitation. In imitation the novice observes the expert while in teaching the expert observes the novice and also judges the performance and tries to modify it (Premack & Premack, 2003). Imitation thus produces a rough copy, which is subsequently modified and smoothed by the teacher. A chimpanzee mother never teaches her infant anything. The infant observes and imitates but the mother never returns any response to the failure or success of the imitation. This uniquely human ability to teach, likely based on frontal lobe processes, helps to explain why it might take several years for an animal to acquire a new technology, learned by a human child in a short time. When it comes to learning the mother tongue language, adults teach the children words, but not grammar. The evolution of language has thus most likely required the development of the teaching ability.

Human communication is intentional with the goal to inform the listener and to correct the receiver if the information does not result in the action intended. There is no evidence indicating that any nonhuman primates are able to correct errant listeners. Their communication is thus not intentional. Only one-way information is given about, for example, a threat in the immediate environment. Language-trained chimpanzees can learn a few hundred words but all words are based on their sensory experiences. Metaphors or abstract words, like time, cannot be sensed, and cannot be learned by a chimpanzee (Premack, 2004). Human language is thus recursive while other species use nonrecursive ways of communication. Recursive communication requires the frontally based ability to get insight into the mental life of others. Social abilities like mentalizing or theory of mind are thus closely linked to the development of the human language.

7   When and how did human higher intellectual functions evolve?

Traditionally it is assumed that syntax and other features of our ability to communicate evolved through an interaction between culture and genes. Syntax made long and complicated thoughts possible, which were the basis for creativity and innovations appearing at the time of the creative explosion some 50 000 years ago. It made it possible for us to structure our experiences. As pointed out by Calvin (2004) we have a remarkable ability to discover patterns and rules embedded in what we experience, to see hidden patterns in seeming chaos. This is most likely one of the keystone abilities that makes the child able to grasp the words and syntax of the language spoken in its environment. Structuring made it possible to think a long train of connected thoughts, to think about the past and to speculate about the future. How was the mental life of *Homo sapiens* before the creative explosion? It is very difficult for us to imagine a less rich mental life than what we have. We can, however, learn a lot from cases like the 11-year-old boy described by Oliver Sacks (1989), who was considered to be mentally retarded but turned out to be deaf. He was able to learn sign language, which made it possible for Sacks to interview and test him. The boy had no problems with perceptual categorizations or generalizations but seemed unable to hold abstract ideas in mind or reflect or plan. He was stuck in the present and his immediate perceptions, unable to enter an imaginative or abstract world. It is likely that humanity at a certain stage of development functioned in a similar way as the deaf boy. A juvenile *Homo sapiens* living 100 000 years ago most likely used protolanguage for communication. This language of single words and short sentences was probably very useful and constituted still a significant advantage over other species.

As mentioned above, the ability to mimic is not very developed in the apes and has thus most likely been strengthened in our ancestors in parallel to language development. The importance of mimicry and gestures for the development of language has been much discussed by Corballis (2002). The mimicry abilities of modern humans are very extensive — we cross our legs, scratch our face or smile when watching others do the same thing. Some present-day communities like the deaf communicate entirely by means of manual gestures and mimicry. Sign language has been found to have a syntax that is as complex as that of any spoken language (Neidle *et al.*, 2000). Corballis argues that human autonomous speech evolved from manual and facial gestures, which were increasingly accompanied by vocalizations. The utterances became more refined when the Broca's area was further developed with its mirror neurons making it possible for vocalizations to be used as vocal "signs" for real objects and events. Later during the hominin evolution, probably within the last 100 000 years and possibly at the time of the creative explosion, language became autonomously vocal to the point that it was fully intelligible when listened to without visual contact with the speaker.

8 Genetic changes during the evolution of the human brain

Our knowledge about genetic changes that are linked to the development of the brain is at present only rudimentary. The successive inactivation of the CMAH gene has already been mentioned as a possible factor beyond the increase in brain weight (Chou *et al.*, 2002). One of the major evolutionary changes compared to the African great apes is the prolonged brain development during the exceptionally long childhood period of humans. This period is extended about three times compared to that of other primates and is followed by a prolonged adolescence with further maturation, especially of the frontal lobes. Recent studies indicate that the frontal lobes are not fully developed structurally or functionally until around 20 years of age (see Maureen Dennis' Chapter 5 in this volume). The evolutionary changes of brain size and functional organization are generally considered to be due to mutations of the major regulatory, so-called *homeotic*, genes (see Allman *et al.*, 2002 for details). These are genes that control the timing, localization, and sequence of development and not the basic structural building blocks of the organism. One very important family of such regulatory genes is called the forkhead (FOX) genes. These genes produce forkhead proteins that work as transcription factors controlling a wide variety of functions during the growth of an organism. One of these genes, the FOXC1, is, for example, known to control the building of the eye (Nishimura et al., 2001).

Another member of this gene family, the forkhead box P2 (FOXP2) gene, has turned out to be a success story in behavioral genetics (Marcus & Fischer, 2003; Corballis, 2004a). The story started with the discovery that about half of the members of a family named KE suffered from a developmental disorder that severely affected their speech. The speech deficit was primarily one of articulation and nonverbal praxis (Vargha-Khadem et al., 1995). The disorder was inherited with autosomal dominance and could subsequently be linked to a mutation of the FOXP2 gene (Lai et al., 2001). This gene has been sequenced in several species and found to be highly conservative. Two of the mutations found have occurred on the human lineage after the split from the line leading to present-day chimpanzees (Enard et al., 2002). The most recent mutation probably happened during the last 200 000 years that makes it possible that it has played a role in the evolution of Homo sapiens. The precise role of the gene is still unknown but it has been suggested (Corballis, 2004b) that it could be of importance for the evolution of the mirror neuron system in Broca's area, assumed to be critical for language. Support for this idea comes from a recent functional magnetic resonance study by Liégeois and coworkers (2003), who made recordings in affected and unaffected members of the KE family. During generation of verbs in response to nouns did the unaffected family members show the expected activation of Broca's area in the left hemisphere, while the affected members showed absence of activation in this area as well as in other cortical language areas. Interestingly the affected subjects activated a number of areas not normally associated with language while their mean performance was at the same level as that of the unaffected family members. It is definitely an oversimplification to call FOXP2 a gene for language, since it is expressed in many organs in the body outside the brain, like gut, heart, and lung (Shu et al., 2001). It is, however, possible that a mutation of this gene was the most recent event when vocalization was incorporated in the mirror neuron system of Broca's area (Corballis, 2004a).

Little is known about genes that are especially relevant for the evolution of the prefrontal cortex. One of the major candidates is the catechol-O-methyltransferase (COMT) gene found to be involved in cortical dopamine regulation (see Winterer & Goldman, 2003 for a review). Statistically significant associations between COMT genotype variations and prefrontal cognitive function on the behavioral as well as the neurophysiological level have been reported (Egan *et al.*, 2001; Joober *et al.*, 2002; Malhotra *et al.*, 2002; Gallinat *et al.*, 2003).

9 Evolutionary aspects on schizophrenia and ADHD

The advanced human mental abilities are unfortunately also accompanied by mental disorders seemingly unique to humanity. The most discussed one is schizophrenia. This disorder has been named "an evolutionary enigma" by Brüne (2004). The disease is ubiquitous and occurs in virtually all human societies. In a recent review by Jablensky (2000) it was concluded that the incidence rate of about 1% is cross-culturally similar provided the same diagnostic criteria are used. Schizophrenia might thus be considered a "disease of humanity" appearing with a similar incidence irrespective of environmental variations and in populations that have been genetically separated for many thousands of years. The illness is thus very old and might be traced back to the origin of our species or at least to the time of the creative explosion some 50 000 years ago. The evolutionary riddle is caused by the fact that the illness is linked to reduced fecundity especially in males (approximately 70% in males and 30% in females; Berlim *et al.*, 2003). The reduced fecundity is likely to be caused by the difficulties that the ill persons have in establishing pair bonds. Why then were not the genetic changes that are responsible for the disorder rapidly eliminated from the human gene pool due to the natural selection? The cross-cultural persistence of schizophrenia over thousands of years of high selection pressure indicates that the genes related to the illness also convey advantages regarding survival that counterbalance the low fecundity or that the genes are linked to other genes that have advantages. Numerous evolutionary hypotheses regarding schizophrenia have been published during the last four decades (see Brüne, 2004 for a review). Some early suggestions focused on selection advantages outside the nervous system. Huxley and coworkers (1964) proposed that schizophrenic subjects were more resistant to infections than the general population. Findings of decreased mortality in offspring of schizophrenic patients have been reported by Erlenmeyer-Kimling, (1968) and Carter and Watts (1971), who showed a lower rate of accidents and virus infections and increased fertility in first-degree relatives of patients with schizophrenia. These early findings of counterbalancing survival advantages were later criticized due to statistical flaws and the fact that it was not ruled out that the decreased risk of accidents and viral infections was caused by the less social and more withdrawn lifestyle of schizophrenic patients and their families. There is a great need for replication of these findings in larger patient samples for further evaluation of this possible explanation of the riddle of schizophrenia.

Other evolutionary theories have suggested that the disturbances of brain development in schizophrenic patients could be due to dysfunctional genes that regulate the speed of maturation. Millar (1987) argued that schizophrenia represented a condition of insufficient recapitulation of the final steps of the development during adolescence resulting in an insufficient suppression of the old limbic (reptilian) parts of the brain. Another view was based on the *neoteny* (holding on to youth) hypothesis of human evolution suggested already in the 1920s (Brüne, 2000). This theory was based on the observation that juvenile apes superficially resemble adult humans regarding head shape and features like hairlessness. Behaviorally the human resemblance to young apes was suggested to be our curiosity and playfulness. Bemporad (1991) proposed that the lack of curiosity and some other schizophrenic symptoms were caused by a failure of neoteny. Saugstad (1989) reasoned that psychiatric disorders in general are related to abnormalities in the maturational rate and that schizophrenia in particular is caused by a delay in maturation. This idea is certainly not a new one since Ewald Hecker already in 1871 described hebephrenia as a "pathologically permanent state of puberty." The maturational delay leads to reduced connectivity and dendritic branching and possibly also prolongation of the pruning process. The suggestion of dysfunctional intra- and interhemispheric connectivity in schizophrenia has been amply supported by numerous studies using functional brain imaging and electrophysiological methods (see Burns, 2004 for a recent review). Burns accounts schizophrenia as a trade-off of the evolution of the social brain. Many of the cognitive, emotional, and behavioral capacities that are crucial for human socialization (like theory of mind) are impaired in schizophrenia. Our social abilities are closely linked to the utilization of symbolic language, a fact that is in the focus of Crow's evolutionary theory.

Crow (1997) asks if schizophrenia is the price that *Homo sapiens* pays for language and his elaborate theory has recently been the subject of an overview by Berlim and coworkers (2003), arguing that the specialization event was linked to a genetic change that made the brain much more functionally lateralized than in other species. This mutation introduced a new principle to the function of the nervous system, allowing the two hemispheres to develop independently and especially to develop functions critical to language in the speech-dominant hemisphere. By freeing a portion of the association cortex from the reciprocal influence from a contralateral homologue, an escalation of the brain capacity allowed behavior and social abilities to be more complex. Crow's evolutionary theory of schizophrenia thus belongs to the group of theories that focuses on abnormalities in the neurodevelopmental process. It puts, however, a special emphasis on a delay or absence of development of hemispheric functional asymmetries related to language functions. Several studies have, in support of the theory, reported decreased or absent anatomical as well as functional asymmetries in schizophrenic patients (Sommer *et al.*, 2001, 2004). Crow also argues that some core symptoms in schizophrenia like hallucinations and formal thought disorders are related to insufficiently lateralized language functions. He also suggests that the genetic predisposition for schizophrenia overlaps with genes responsible for the development of the cerebral functional asymmetries (Crow, 1988). The asymmetry gene (or genes) is proposed to be situated in the sex chromosomes, possibly in their homologue parts, a suggestion which has been very much debated and for which definite support from genetic studies still is lacking (DeLisi *et al.*, 2000). Thus schizophrenia continues to be an unsolved evolutionary enigma.

The attention deficit hyperactivity disorder (ADHD) has also been discussed in evolutionary terms. Like schizophrenia it is considered to be a disorder caused by dysfunction of the frontal lobes and its connections to posterior brain regions (Hallowell & Ratey, 1994). ADHD is common in the human society affecting 5–6% of school-aged children (Barkley, 1990) and with convincing evidence for a genetic component (Stevenson, 1991). How does the disposition for such a damaging disorder exist in such a large number of individuals? Like for schizophrenia it has been suggested that the disorder had some positive survival value during our evolutionary history. Hartmann (1993) proposed that ADHD traits were preserved because they were of value for the survival of the preagricultural humans. The traits of distractibility, impulsiveness and aggression were suggested to be of positive value for hunting. People with ADHD are the "left over hunters." This theory has, however, been questioned by Shelley-Tremblay and Rosen (1996) on the basis of archeological evidence, indicating that early humans were at worst marginal scroungers and at best supplement hunters (Leakey & Lewin, 1992). They also questioned the advantages of ADHD symptoms for successful hunting. Other survival advantages suggested involve the higher than normal frequency of aggressive and criminal behavior displayed by people with ADHD that could have had survival value in the competition with other human species like the Neanderthals. Finally, the fact that children with ADHD get more attention from their mothers (Barkley, 1990) and initiate more verbal contact and clinging behavior might have been vital to survival in hostile environments.

Final comments on the evolution of the prefrontal cortex

The successive refinement of prefrontal functions is without doubt one of the key changes beyond modern human mental abilities and behavior. As we have seen, the development of successively more refined ways of communication has been central. The development started a few million years ago with abilities that made it possible to organize hunting and other forms of food gathering. Prefrontal functions probably also supported food and work sharing, activities which tightened the social bonds within the group. These abilities might have involved the use of protolanguage and rudimentary forms of what we today label mentalizing or theory of mind. Modern behavior, like the use of symbolic languages, the creation of arts and the emergence of scientific explorations, are all very recent events in the human history. The explosion of knowledge and communicative abilities that we experience today is a totally new phenomenon on the planet Earth. It is far too rapid to possibly be caused by any genetic mutations affecting the functions of the prefrontal cortex or any other parts of the brain. Since modern society has changed and overruled evolutionary mechanisms linked to the "survival of the fittest," any future genetically based brain evolution is very unlikely. Future progress of the human society is more likely to be the result of an extremely efficient collaboration between numerous bright brains, adding together information and creativity, resulting in a community "super brain." The authors of this book each add their special knowledge about the frontal lobes to the present volume. This hopefully will give the reader a "super brain" type of overview and understanding of the magical advantages that these lobes offer when functioning properly and the devastating problems they cause when dysfunctional.

REFERENCES

Allman, J. M. (2000). *Evolving Brains*. New York: Freeman.

Allman, J., Hakeem, A. & Watson, K. (2002). Two phylogenetic specializations in the human brain. *Neuroscientist*, **8**, 335–46.

Arcadi, A. C. (2000). Vocal responsiveness in male wild chimpanzees: implications for the evolution of language. *Journal of Human Evolution*, **39**, 205–23.

Barkley, R. (1990). *Attention Deficit Hyperactivity Disorder: A Handbook for Diagnosis and Treatment*. New York: Guilford Press.

Bemporad, J. R. (1991). Dementia praecox as a failure of neoteny. *Theoretical Medicine*, **12**, 45–51.

Berlim, M. T., Mattevi, B. S., Belmonte-de-Abreu, P. & Crow, T. J. (2003). The etiology of schizophrenia and the origin of language: Overview of a theory. *Comprehensive Psychiatry*, **44**, 7–14.

Bickerton, D. (1990). *Language and Species*. Chicago: University of Chicago Press.

Blinkov, S. M. & Glezer, I. I. (1968). *Das Zentralnervensystem in Zahlen und Tabellen*. Jena: Fischer.

Bodamer, M. D. & Gardner, R. A. (2002). How cross-fostered chimpanzees (*Pan troglodytes*) initiate and maintain conversations. *Journal of Comparative Psychology*, **116**, 12–26.

Brodmann, K. (1912). Neue Ergebnisse über die vergleichende histologische Lokalisation der Grosshirnrinde mit besondere Berücksichrigung des Stirnhirns. *Anatomische Anzeiger*, **41**, 157–216.

Brüne, M. (2000). Neoteny, psychiatric disorders and the social brain hypothesis. *Anthropological Medicine*, **7**, 301–18.

Brüne, M. (2004). Schizophrenia – an evolutionary enigma? *Neuroscience and Biobehavioural Reviews*, **28**, 41–53.

Burns, J. K. (2004). An evolutionary theory of schizophrenia. Cortical connectivity, metarepresentation, and the social brain. *The Behavioral and Brain Sciences*, **27**, 831–55.

Calvin, W. H. (2004). *A Brief History of the Mind: From Apes to Intellect and Beyond*. New York: Oxford University Press.

Calvin, W. H. & Bickerton, D. (2000). *Lingua ex Machina: Reconciling Darwin and Chomsky with the Human Brain*. Cambridge, MA: MIT Press.

Carter, M. & Watts, C. A. H. (1971). Possible biological advantages among schizophrenics relatives. *British Journal of Psychiatry*, **118**, 453–60.

Chou, H. H., Hayakawa, T., Diaz, S., *et al.* (2002). Inactivation of CMP-N-acetylneuraminic acid hydroxylase occurred prior to brain expansion during human evolution. *Proceedings of the National Academy of Science U.S.A.*, **99**, 11736–41.

Corballis, M. C. (2002). *From Hand to Mouth: The Origins of Language*. Princeton, NJ: Princeton University Press.

Corballis, M. C. (2004a). *FOXP2* and the mirror system. *Trends in Cognitive Sciences*, **8**, 95–6.

Corballis, M. C. (2004b). The origins of modernity: Was autonomous speech the critical factor? *Psychological Review*, **111**, 543–52.

Crow, T. J. (1988). Sex chromosomes and psychosis. The case for a pseudoautosomal locus. *British Journal of Psychiatry*, **153**, 675–83.

Crow, T. J. (1997). Is schizophrenia the price that *Homo sapiens* pays for language? *Schizophrenia Research*, **28**, 127–41.

Crow, T. J. (1998). Sexual selection, timing and the descent of man: a theory of the genetic origins of language. *Current Psychology of Cognition*, **17**, 1079–114.

Cunnane, S. C. & Crawford, M. A. (2003). Survival of the fattest: fat babies were the key to evolution of the large human brain. *Comparative Biochemistry and Physiology* Part A, **136**, 17–26.

DeLisi, L. E., Shaw, S., Sherrington, R., *et al.* (2000). Failure to establish linkage on the X chromosome in 301 families with schizophrenia or schizoaffective disorder. *American Journal of Medical Genetics*, **96**, 335–41.

Egan, M. F., Goldberg, T. E., Kolachana, B. S., *et al.* (2001). Effect of COMT val108/158 Met genotype on frontal lobe function and risk for schizophrenia. *Proceedings of the National Academy of Science U.S.A.*, **98**, 6917–22.

Enard, W., Przeworski, M., Fisher, S. E., *et al.* (2002). Molecular evolution of *FOXP2*, a gene involved in speech and language. *Nature*, **418**, 869–72.

Erlenmeyer-Kimling, L. (1968). Mortality rates in the offspring of schizophrenic patients and a physiological advantage hypothesis. *Nature*, **220**, 798–800.

Falk, D., Hildebolt, C., Smith, K., *et al.* (2005). The brain of LB1, *Homo floresiensis. Science*, **308**, 242–5.

Foley, R. (1987). *Another Unique Species. Patterns in Human Evolutionary Ecology.* Harlow, UK: Longman Scientific & Technical.

Gallinat, J., Sander, T., Schlattmann, P., *et al.* (2003). Association of the G1947A COMT (Val$^{108/158}$Met) gene polymorphism with prefrontal P300 during information processing. *Biological Psychiatry*, **54**, 40–8.

Hallowell, E. & Ratey, J. (1994). *Driven to Distraction.* New York: Touchstone.

Hartmann, T. (1993). *Attention Deficit Disorder: A Different Perception.* Lancaster, UK: Underwood-Miller.

Hecker, E. (1871). Die Hebephrenie. *Archiv für Pathologie und Anatomie (Berlin)*, **52**, 394–429. (American translation 1985, *American Journal of Psychiatry*, **142**, 1265–71.)

Henshilwood, C. S., d'Errico, F., Yates, R., *et al.* (2002). Emergence of modern human behavior: Middle stone age engravings from South Africa. *Science*, **295**, 1278–80.

Henshilwood, C., d'Errico, F., Vanhaeren, M, van Niekerk, K. & Jacobs, Z. (2004). Middle stone age shell beads from South Africa. *Science*, **304**, 404.

Holliday, M. (1971). Metabolic rate and organ size during growth from infancy to maturity. *Pediatrics*, **50**, 590.

Huxley, J., Mayr, E., Osmond, H. & Hoffer, A. (1964). Schizophrenia as a genetic morphism. *Nature*, **204**, 220–1.

Ingman, M., Kaessemann, H., Pääbo, S. & Gyllensten, U. (2000). Mitochondrial genome variation and the origin of modern humans. *Nature*, **408**, 708–13.

Isaac, G. (1978). The food-sharing behavior of protohuman hominids. *Scientific American*, **238**, 90–108.

Jablensky, A. (2000). Epidemiology of schizophrenia: the global burden of disease and disability. *European Archives of Psychiatry and Clinical Neuroscience*, **250**, 274–85.

Jensen, P. K. A. (1996). *Menneskets Oprindelse og Udvikling.* Copenhagen: G.E.C. Gad.

Jensvold, M. L. A. & Gardner, R. A. (2000). Interactive use of sign language by cross-fostered chimpanzees (Pan troglodytes). *Journal of Comparative Psychology*, **114**, 335–46.

Joober, R., Gauthier, J., Lal, S., *et al.* (2002). Catechol-O-methyltransferase Val 108/158-Met gene variants associated with performance on the Wisconsin Card Sorting Test. *Archives of General Psychiatry*, **59**, 662–3.

Lai, C. S., Fisher, S. E., Hurst, J. A., Vargha-Khadem, F. & Monaco, A. P. (2001). A forkhead-domain gene is mutated in a severe speech and language disorder. *Nature*, **413**, 519–23.

Leakey, R. & Lewin, R. (1978). *People at the Lake.* New York: Anchor Press/Doubleday.

Leakey, R. & Lewin, R. (1992). *Origins Reconsidered. In Search of What Makes Us Human.* New York: Doubleday.

Leonard, W. R. (2002). Food for thought. Dietary change was a driving force in human evolution. *Scientific American*, **287**, 106–15.

Leonard, W. R., Robertson, M. L., Snodgrass, J. J. & Kuzawa, C. W. (2003). Metabolic correlates of hominid brain evolution. *Comparative Biochemistry and Physiology* Part A, **136**, 5–15.

Liégeois, F., Baldeweg, T., Connelly, A., *et al.* (2003). Language fMRI abnormalities associated with *FOXP2* gene mutation. *Nature Neuroscience*, **6**, 1230–7.

Malhotra, A. K., Kestler, L. J., Mazzanti, C., *et al.* (2002). A functional polymorphism in the COMT gene and performance on a test of prefrontal function. *American Journal of Psychiatry*, **159**, 652–4.

Marcus, G. F. & Fischer, S. E. (2003). *FOXP2* in focus: what can genes tell us about speech and language? *Trends in Cognitive Sciences*, **7**, 257–62.

Millar, T. P. (1987). Schizophrenia: an etiological speculation. *Perspectives in Biology and Medicine*, **30**, 597–607.

Neidle, C., Kegl, J., MacLaughlin, D., Bahan, B. & Lee, R. G. (2000). *The Syntax of American Sign Language*. Cambridge, MA: MIT Press.

Nilsson, G. (1996). Brain and body requirements of *Gnathonemus petersii*, a fish with an exceptionally large brain. *Journal of Experimental Biology*, **199**, 603–7.

Nimchinsky, E. A., Gilissen, E., Allman, J. M., *et al.* (1999). A neuronal morphologic type unique to humans and great apes. *Proceedings of the National Academy of Science U.S.A.*, **96**, 5268–73.

Nimchinsky, E., Vogt, B. A., Morrison, J. & Hof, P. R. (1995). Spindle neurones of the human anterior cingulate cortex. *Journal of Comparative Neurology*, **355**, 27–37.

Nishimura, D. Y., Searby, C. C., Alward, W. L., *et al.* (2001). A spectrum of FOXC1 mutations suggests gene dosage as a mechanism for developmental deficits of the anterior chamber of the eye. *American Journal of Human Genetics*, **68**, 364–72.

Nishitani, N. & Hari, R. (2000). Temporal dynamics of cortical representation for action. *Proceedings of the National Academy of Science U.S.A.*, **97**, 913–18.

Pfeiffer, J. E. (1982). *The Creative Explosion*. New York: Harper and Row.

Premack, D. (2004). Is language the key to human intelligence? *Science*, **303**, 318–20.

Premack, D. & Premack, A. (2003). *Original Intelligence*. New York: McGraw-Hill.

Rizzolatti, G. & Arbib, M. A. (1998). Language within our grasp. *Trends in Neuroscience*, **21**, 188–94.

Sacks, O. (1989). *Seeing Voices: A Journey into the World of the Deaf*. Berkeley: University of California Press.

Saugstad, L. F. (1989). Age and puberty and mental illness. Towards a neurodevelopmental aetiology of Kraepelin's endogenous psychoses. *British Journal of Psychiatry*, **155**, 536–44.

Schenker, N. M., Desgoutte, A.-M. & Semendeferi, K. (2005). Neural connectivity and cortical substrates of cognition in hominoids. *Journal of Human Evolution*, **49**, 547–69.

Schoenemann, P. T., Sheehan, M. J. & Glotzer, L. D. (2005). Prefrontal white matter volume is disproportionately larger in humans than in other primates. *Nature Neuroscience*, **8**, 242–52.

Semendeferi, K., Armstrong, E., Schleicher, A., Zilles, K. & Van Hoesen, G. W. (1998). Limbic frontal cortex in hominoids: a comparative study of area 13. *American Journal of Physical Anthropology*, **106**, 129–55.

Semendeferi, K., Armstrong, E., Schleicher, A., Zilles, K. & Van Hoesen, G.W. (2001). Prefrontal cortex in humans and apes: a comparative study of area 10. *American Journal of Physical Anthropology*, **114**, 224–41.

Semendeferi, K., Lu, A., Schenker, N. & Damasio, H. (2002). Humans and great apes share a large frontal cortex. *Nature Neuroscience*, **5**, 272–6.

Shelley-Tremblay, J. F. & Rosen, L. A. (1996). Attention deficit hyperactivity disorder: An evolutionary perspective. *The Journal of Genetic Psychology*, **157**, 443–54.

Sherwood, C. C., Holloway, R. L., Semendeferi, K. & Hof, P. R. (2005). Is prefrontal white matter enlargement a human evolutionary specialization? *Nature Neuroscience*, **8**, 537–8.

Shu, W., Yang, H., Zhang, L., Lu, M. M. & Morrisey, E. E. (2001). Characterization of a new subfamily of winged-helix/forkhead (Fox) genes that are expressed in the lung and act as transcriptional repressors. *The Journal of Biological Chemistry*, **276**, 27488–97.

Sommer, I., Aleman, A., Ramsey, N., Bouma, A. & Kahn, R. (2001). Handedness, language lateralisation and anatomical asymmetry in schizophrenia. Meta-analysis. *British Journal of Psychiatry*, **178**, 344–51.

Sommer, I. E. C., Ramsey, N. F., Mandl, R. C. W., van Oel, C. J. & Kahn, R. S. (2004). Language activation in monozygotic twins discordant for schizophrenia. *British Journal of Psychiatry*, **184**, 128–35.

Stevenson, J. (1991). Evidence for a genetic etiology in hyperactive children. *Behavior Genetics*, **22**, 337–44.

Vargha-Khadem, F., Watkins, K., Alcock, K., Fletcher, P. & Passingham, R. (1995). Praxis and non-verbal deficits in a large family with genetically transmitted speech and language disorder. *Proceedings of the National Academy of Science U.S.A.*, **92**, 930–3.

Winterer, G. & Goldman, D. (2003). Genetics of human prefrontal function. *Brain Research Reviews*, **43**, 134–63.

Witelson, S., Kigar, D. L. & Harvey, T. (1999). The exceptional brain of Albert Einstein. *Lancet*, **353**, 2149–53.

Wrangham, R. & Conklin-Brittain, N (2003). Cooking as a biological trait. *Comparative Biochemistry and Physiology* Part A, **136**, 35–46.

Organization of the principal pathways of prefrontal lateral, medial, and orbitofrontal cortices in primates and implications for their collaborative interaction in executive functions

Helen Barbas

1   Overview

Ideas about the prefrontal cortex have changed drastically during the past century. Situated at the rostral pole of the brain, the prefrontal cortex was traditionally considered to be the seat of intelligence. Damage to the prefrontal cortex, however, does not affect overall intelligence in humans, but has detrimental effects on executive function. Converging lines of evidence indicate that the prefrontal cortex is an action-oriented region, guiding behavior by selecting relevant signals to accomplish the task at hand.

The prefrontal cortex is in a strategic position to exercise executive control. It receives information from most other cortical areas and subcortical structures and is connected with specialized oculomotor centers for searching the environment, and with motor control systems for action. These functions have been associated with the caudal parts of the lateral prefrontal cortex, namely areas 8 and the caudal part of area 46. These caudal lateral areas are connected with neighboring premotor as well as early-processing sensory association areas and with intraparietal visuomotor areas. However, the lateral prefrontal cortex is considerably more extensive, and includes, in addition, the more anteriorly situated areas around the principal sulcus (rostral area 46), area 9 on the dorsolateral surface, area 12 on the ventrolateral surface, and area 10 at the frontal pole, all of which have been associated with cognitive functions and executive control. Figure 2.1B shows the lateral prefrontal cortex and its relationship to the adjacent premotor/motor cortical system.

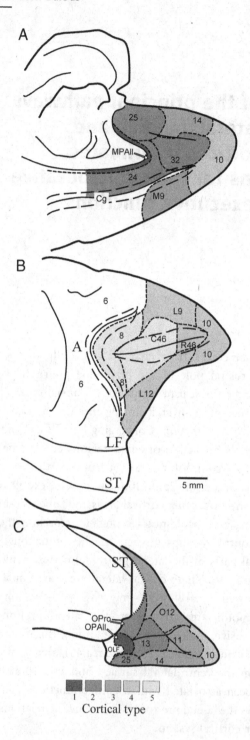

A
25   14
MPAll
32   10
24
Cg   M9

B
6
L9
8   10
A   C46   R46
6   8   10
8   L12
LF
ST
5 mm

C
ST
OPro   O12
OPAll
OLF   13   11
25   14   10

1 2 3 4 5
Cortical type

Lateral prefrontal areas do not function in isolation in these complex functions, but rather in concert with the medial and orbitofrontal components of the prefrontal cortex. The caudal parts of medial (Figure 2.1A) and orbitofrontal (Figure 2.1C) areas belong to the cortical component of the limbic system by virtue of their strong connections with subcortical limbic structures (Broca, 1878; Papez, 1937; Yakovlev, 1948; Nauta, 1979). The prefrontal limbic areas have a role in emotional behavior and social interactions in both human and nonhuman primates (for reviews see Damasio *et al.*, 1994; Damasio, 1994; Barbas, 1997). Medial and orbitofrontal cortices are robustly connected with the rest of the prefrontal cortex, providing the anatomic basis for the synthesis of cognitive and emotional processes in the cortex (for discussion see Barbas, 1995). Dissociation of these pathways disrupts both cognitive and emotional processes with profound effects on behavior, as seen in several psychiatric and neurologic diseases, underscoring the biologic importance of this interaction (for review see Damasio, 1994).

To exercise executive functions the prefrontal cortex must use information from structures associated with sensory perception, memory, and emotion in a way that is specific for the task at hand. The following sections include evidence on the complementary nature of connections of distinct prefrontal areas with cortical and subcortical structures that may underlie their specialization in cognition, emotion and memory, and their capacity to activate distinct motor control channels for action. The roles of different prefrontal sectors are complementary and collaborative in complex behavioral settings. Collaboration among prefrontal areas occurs through a highly organized laminar pattern of connections. In turn, the consistent patterns of connections depend on the structural architecture of the linked areas. These consistent patterns of connections have great potential to reveal the interface of prefrontal areas with distinct excitatory and inhibitory systems in other areas to allow elaboration or halting of signals, and the recruitment of neural structures in behavior.

Figure 2.1   A map of the prefrontal cortex. (A) Medial surface; (B) lateral surface; (C) orbital (basal) surface. Grey shades depict different cortical types as follows: 1 (darkest grey), agranular areas with three distinguishable layers; 2, dysgranular areas with four distinguishable layers, including a poorly developed layer 4; 3–5, eulaminate areas with increasing cellular density and thickness of layer 4 from types 3–5. In A–C, small dashed lines demarcate architectonic areas indicated by numbers; large dashed lines depict the cortex buried in sulci. MPAll, OPAll, OPro, OLF indicate architectonic areas. Letters before architectonic areas designated by letters or numbers denote: C, caudal; L, lateral; M, medial; O, orbital; R, rostral. Abbreviations: A, arcuate sulcus; Cg, cingulate sulcus; LF, lateral fissure; ST, superior temporal sulcus. (The map is from Barbas & Pandya [1989].)

2 Modality specificity of projections to distinct prefrontal cortices

In order to select relevant signals for behavior the prefrontal cortex must have access to the sensory environment. Originally probed under general anesthesia, the prefrontal cortex was considered to be "the silent" cortex. However, physiologic studies in awake animals and functional imaging studies in humans have demonstrated that the prefrontal cortex is actively engaged in behavior. Ideas about the prefrontal cortex consequently shifted from "silent" cortex to polymodal cortex. Indeed, input from cortices representing each of the sensory modalities reaches the prefrontal cortex, originating from a large variety of sensory association cortices, though not the primary sensory koniocortices (visual area V1, somatosensory area 3b, and auditory area A1). The idea that the prefrontal cortex is polymodal carried with it the erroneous implication that sensory input is global and undifferentiated. However, projections from sensory association areas show a distinct organization within the prefrontal cortex. Specific areas of the prefrontal cortex are preferential targets of input from cortices processing signals within specific sensory modalities (for reviews see Pandya *et al.*, 1988; Barbas, 1992; Barbas, 2000).

Lateral prefrontal areas receive visual, auditory and somatosensory projections. This input arises from sensory association cortices and shows a distinct organization within the lateral prefrontal cortex. The posterior part of lateral prefrontal cortex in the periarcuate region receives robust projections from visual association cortices. The principal visual-recipient lateral prefrontal areas include the anterior bank of the arcuate sulcus, the caudal extent of the principal sulcus (area 46), and the caudal part of lateral area 12 (Jones & Powell, 1970; Chavis & Pandya, 1976; Jacobson & Trojanowski, 1977; Barbas & Mesulam, 1981; Maioli *et al.*, 1983; Barbas & Mesulam, 1985; Huerta *et al.*, 1987; Barbas, 1988; Boussaoud *et al.*, 1990; Webster *et al.*, 1994; Schall *et al.*, 1995). The part that is most heavily targeted by visual cortices is area 8, particularly at the confluence of the anterior bank of the upper and lower limbs of the arcuate sulcus. Area 8 is distinguished for its strong projections from every visual association area (Figure 2.2), resembling in this sense the visual association areas in the occipital and inferior temporal regions (Barbas & Mesulam, 1981; Barbas, 1988).

At the other extreme of the lateral prefrontal cortex, frontal polar area 10 is unique among lateral prefrontal areas for its robust connections with auditory association cortices, to the virtual exclusion of direct projections from other unimodal sensory association cortices (Barbas & Mesulam, 1985; Barbas *et al.*, 1999). This remarkable emphasis for auditory projections is shown in Figure 2.3. Besides projections to frontal polar area 10, auditory association areas project

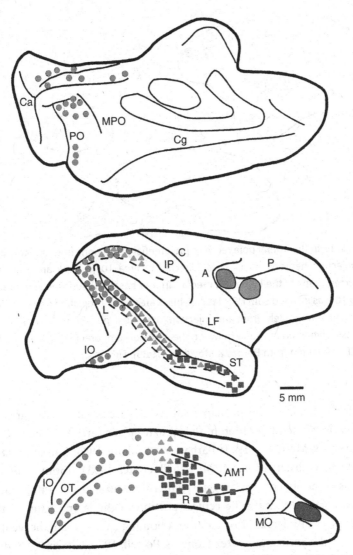

Figure 2.2   Projections from visual cortices to some lateral and orbitofrontal cortices. Neurons projecting to area 8 at the confluence of the upper and lower limbs of the arcuate sulcus (center, red area) originate in posterior visual association cortices (red dots); neurons projecting to the posterior part of ventral area 46 (center, green area) originate in posterior inferior temporal cortices (green triangles); neurons projecting to orbitofrontal area 11 (bottom, blue area) originate in anterior inferior temporal cortices (blue squares). Abbreviations: A, arcuate sulcus; AMT, anterior middle temporal dimple; C, central sulcus; Ca, calcarine fissure; Cg, cingulate sulcus; IO, inferior occipital sulcus; IP, intraparietal sulcus; LF, lateral fissure; MO, medial orbital sulcus; MPO, medial parietooccipital sulcus; P, principal sulcus; PO, parietooccipital sulcus. (For a color version of this figure, please see the color plate section.)

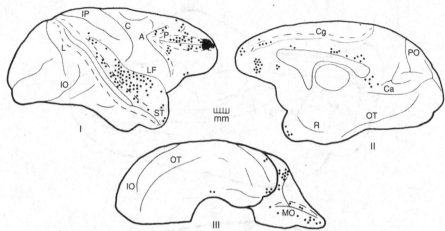

Figure 2.3   Lateral area 10 in the frontal pole receives preferential projections from auditory association areas. Projection neurons (black dots) directed to area 10 (I, black area) are shown on reconstructed maps of the lateral (I), medial (II) and basal (III) surfaces of the brain. In this case area 10 was injected with HRP-WGA (I, black area), and projection neurons (black dots) were labeled retrogradely from the injection site. Most projection neurons originate in auditory association areas found between the superior temporal (ST) sulcus and the lateral fissure (LF). (Adapted from Barbas & Mesulam [1985], Figure 7.)

to the dorsal bank of the principal sulcus at its central extent (area 46) and the rostral tip of the upper limb of the arcuate sulcus (area 8) (Chavis & Pandya, 1976; Barbas & Mesulam, 1981; Barbas & Mesulam, 1985; Barbas, 1988; Distler *et al.*, 1993; Webster *et al.*, 1994; Schall *et al.*, 1995). Input from somatosensory association cortices targets primarily ventral areas within the lateral prefrontal cortex, reaching the central portion of the lateral bank of the principal sulcus (ventral area 46) and the adjoining area 12 on the ventrolateral convexity of the prefrontal cortex (Jones & Powell, 1970; Chavis & Pandya, 1976; Barbas & Mesulam, 1985; Barbas, 1988; Preuss & Goldman-Rakic, 1989).

Medial prefrontal cortices have comparatively limited access to direct input from most sensory association cortices, though they are distinguished for their connections with auditory association areas (Vogt & Pandya, 1987; Barbas, 1988; Petrides & Pandya, 1988; Barbas *et al.*, 1999), as shown in Figure 2.4. In contrast with lateral areas, medial prefrontal areas do not receive significant input from cortices associated with visual or somatosensory modalities. On the other hand, some projections from olfactory areas reach areas 32 and 24, and more substantial projections reach the medial part of area 14 (Barbas *et al.*, 1999).

The orbitofrontal cortex, on the other hand, is by far the most multimodal among prefrontal cortices. Its posterior sector has direct connections with

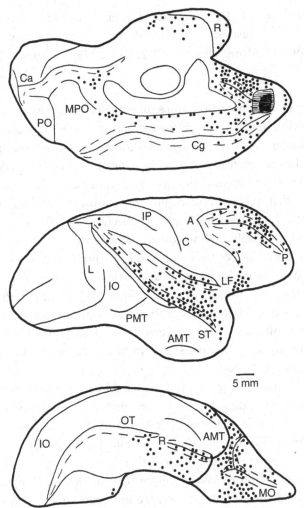

Figure 2.4   Medial prefrontal areas receive preferential projections from auditory association areas. This example shows the distribution of labeled projection neurons (black dots) directed to medial area 32 (top, black area), and mainly in superior temporal auditory association areas, seen on the lateral surface (center). Most projection neurons originate in auditory association areas found between the superior temporal (ST) sulcus and the lateral fissure (LF). Other projection neurons are seen in medial temporal areas around the rhinal sulcus (R) on the basal surface (bottom), which are associated with long-term memory. Abbreviations: A, arcuate sulcus; AMT, anterior middle temporal dimple; C, central sulcus; Ca, calcarine fissure; Cg, cingulate sulcus; IO, inferior occipital sulcus; IP, intraparietal sulcus; LF, lateral fissure; MO, medial orbital sulcus; MPO, medial parietooccipital sulcus; P, principal sulcus; PO, parietooccipital sulcus; R, rhinal sulcus. (Adapted from Barbas, 1988.)

primary olfactory cortices (for review see Takagi, 1986). In addition, orbito-frontal cortices have robust connections with visual, auditory, somatosensory, and gustatory cortices (Morecraft *et al.*, 1992; Barbas, 1993; Carmichael & Price, 1995b).

2.1 Topographic specificity of sensory cortical projections to prefrontal cortex

Beyond the selective targeting of prefrontal cortices by areas associated with each sensory modality, there are overall differences in the specific origin of projections. Lateral prefrontal areas, in general, receive projections from earlier processing sensory areas than either medial or orbitofrontal cortices. In prefrontal areas that receive projections from sensory association cortices devoted predominantly to one modality, the projections arise from a large variety of areas within that modality. A notable example is the core frontal eye field (FEF) area at the confluence of the upper and lower limbs of the arcuate sulcus, which receives projections from visual association areas extending from V2 to the inferior temporal cortex (area TE). Figure 2.2 illustrates the distinct topographic origin of projections from visual association areas to three pre-frontal areas. Orbitofrontal area 11 receives projections from late-processing visual association areas, in comparison with ventral area 46, and especially the core FEF area within area 8.

Similarly, sensory input to area 10 is dominated by projections from auditory association cortices, extending from posterior high-order auditory association areas to the temporal pole (e.g. Barbas & Mesulam, 1985; Barbas *et al.*, 1999, 2005b), as shown in Figure 2.3. Medial prefrontal cortices also receive rich projections from a variety of auditory association cortices, though most originate from late-processing auditory association cortices in the anterior part of the superior temporal gyrus and the adjacent dorsal part of the temporal pole (Barbas *et al.*, 1999, 2005b), as shown in Figure 2.4. Similarly, projections from visual, auditory and somatosensory association cortices to orbitofrontal cortex originate from late-processing sensory areas within the respective modalities. The only exception is a projection from early-processing olfactory areas to orbitofrontal cortex (Barbas, 1993; Carmichael *et al.*, 1994), which is the principal cortical association area for the processing of olfactory signals.

3 The different sectors of the prefrontal cortex have distinct roles in memory

3.1 Lateral prefrontal cortices have a role in working memory

Prefrontal areas are neither sensory nor motor, but rather use sensory and other information as necessary in behavior. Lateral prefrontal areas participate in cognitive tasks requiring the selection, retrieval and holding of information in working memory long enough to accomplish a task with several sequential parts (for reviews see Goldman-Rakic, 1988; Fuster, 1993; Petrides, 1996). There is considerable controversy about the details of the role of particular prefrontal areas within the broad domain of working memory. However, there is general agreement that lateral prefrontal areas are active when a rule must be remembered, consistent with their involvement in plotting out strategy to solve the problem at hand (for review see Miller & Cohen, 2001).

Recent studies suggest that there is a degree of specificity among lateral prefrontal areas within the broad domain of cognition. With regard to working memory, for example, area 46 has classically been implicated in delayed response tasks (Jacobsen, 1936), a finding that was corroborated in subsequent physiologic studies in behaving primates. Physiologic studies have demonstrated that a subset of neurons around the principal sulcus fire during the delay period in delayed response tasks, bridging the gap between the time of presentation of stimuli and the time when they must be remembered to solve the problem at hand (for reviews see Goldman-Rakic, 1988; Fuster, 1989). On the other hand, frontal polar area 10 has a different role, specializing for holding information on line when a secondary goal is introduced in the behavioral task (Koechlin et al., 1999). Area 9 appears to have a role in monitoring sequential self-generated responses (Petrides, 1995), a finding supported in physiologic studies in behaving monkeys (e.g. Hasegawa et al., 2004). Areas at the caudal extent of lateral prefrontal cortex in the periarcuate region are particularly active in the oculomotor version of the delayed response task (e.g. Funahashi et al., 1990, 1991).

3.2 Medial prefrontal cortices are affiliated with structures with a role in long-term memory

As noted above, lateral prefrontal cortices have been associated with a role in the general domain of working memory. Medial and orbitofrontal cortices, on the other hand, are aligned with structures associated with long-term memory. Medial prefrontal areas, in particular, are distinguished for their strong connections with both cortical and subcortical structures associated with long-term memory (Barbas et al., 1999). This connectional feature applies to posterior medial areas, around the anterior cingulate, including the architectonic areas 32 and 25 and the rostral part of area 24. These areas are connected both with medial temporal cortices (entorhinal area 28 and perirhinal areas 35 and 36) (Vogt & Pandya, 1987; Barbas, 1988; Carmichael & Price, 1995a; Bachevalier et al., 1997; Barbas et al., 1999), as shown in Figure 2.4. Among prefrontal cortices, anterior cingulate areas also receive the strongest projections from

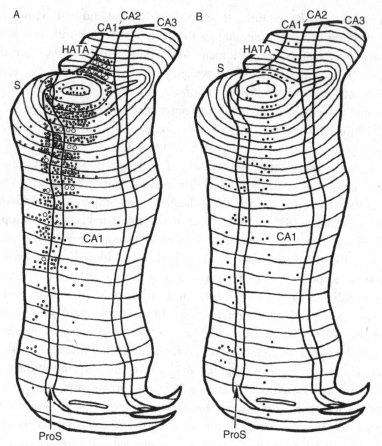

Figure 2.5   Summary of projections from the hippocampal formation to medial (A) and orbitofrontal (B) cortices. Each small symbol represents two neurons; each large symbol represents 40 neurons. Each contour of the reconstructed hippocampal formation shows one section, with rostral sections on top, and caudal sections at the bottom. Note the prevalence of projection neurons in the rostral part of the hippocampal formation, and the comparatively higher density of projections directed to medial prefrontal cortices in the anterior cingulate region (A) than in orbitofrontal cortices (B). Abbreviations: CA1–3, ammonic fields CA1–3; HATA, hippocampal amygdala transition area; ProS, prosubiculum; S, subiculum. (From Barbas & Blatt [1995].)

the hippocampal formation (Barbas & Blatt, 1995). This input originates not only from the subicular and presubicular sectors, but also from area CA1 of the hippocampal formation (Barbas & Blatt, 1995; Insausti & Munoz, 2001), as shown in Figure 2.5. Moreover, anterior cingulate areas receive significant projections from the thalamic midline nuclei, the magnocellular sector of the mediodorsal nucleus (MDmc), and the caudal part of parvicellular MD (MDpc)

(Baleydier & Mauguiere, 1980; Goldman-Rakic & Porrino, 1985; Barbas *et al.*, 1991; Morecraft *et al.*, 1992; Ray & Price, 1993; Dermon & Barbas, 1994), all of which have a role in long-term memory (for reviews see Markowitsch, 1982; Squire & Zola-Morgan, 1988; Amaral *et al.*, 1990; Squire, 1992; Zola-Morgan & Squire, 1993).

3.3 Orbitofrontal areas are connected with the amygdala associated with emotional memory

Orbitofrontal cortices have a different set of connections than either lateral or medial prefrontal cortices. Although both medial and, to a lesser extent, lateral prefrontal areas are connected with the amygdala, the orbitofrontal cortex is distinguished for its strong and specialized connections with the amygdala (e.g. Nauta, 1961; Pandya *et al.*, 1973; Jacobson & Trojanowski, 1975; Aggleton *et al.*, 1980; Porrino *et al.*, 1981; Van Hoesen, 1981; Amaral & Price, 1984; Barbas & De Olmos, 1990; Morecraft *et al.*, 1992; Carmichael & Price, 1995a; Chiba *et al.*, 2001). Situated in the rostral part of the temporal lobe, close to the orbitofrontal cortex, the amygdala has a key role in emotions (Nishijo *et al.*, 1988; Davis, 1992; Damasio, 1994; LeDoux, 1996). The connections between these structures have a specific topography, with the strongest found between the posterior sector of the orbitofrontal cortex and the posterior half of the amygdala (Ghashghaei & Barbas, 2002; for discussion and earlier literature see Stefanacci & Amaral, 2002). In addition, there is partial segregation of input and output zones that link the amygdala with posterior orbitofrontal cortex. Axons from caudal orbitofrontal cortex project to several nuclei of the basal complex of the amygdala, but their most robust projections terminate in the intercalated masses of the amygdala, a group of small GABAergic neurons interposed between nuclei of the basal complex of the amygdala. Projection neurons from the amygdala directed to posterior orbitofrontal cortex are found mostly within the basolateral, basomedial (also known as accessory basal) and lateral nuclei, and to a lesser extent in the cortical nuclei of the amygdala (Barbas & De Olmos, 1990; Ghashghaei & Barbas, 2002).

There is a striking resemblance in the cortical sensory projections to orbitofrontal cortex and the amygdala, both in terms of the modalities represented, as well as in the topography of connections (e.g. Herzog & Van Hoesen, 1976; Turner *et al.*, 1980). Both structures receive rich multimodal input from cortices representing each of the sensory modalities, as well as from polymodal areas. With regard to topography, both structures receive projections from late-processing sensory cortices, which have a role in the analysis of features of stimuli and their memory, as summarized in Figure 2.6.

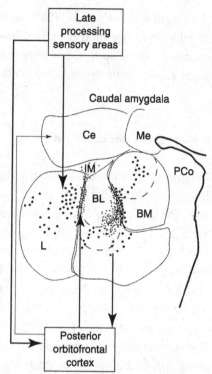

Figure 2.6   Specificity of connections of posterior orbitofrontal cortex with the amygdala and with high-order sensory association areas. Within the amygdala (center), input (small dots) and output (big dots) connection zones that link the amygdala with posterior orbitofrontal cortex are partially segregated, as shown in a coronal section through the posterior part of the amygdala. Axons from orbitofrontal areas terminate heavily in the intercalated masses (IM), interposed between the basal nuclei of the amygdala. A lighter pathway from posterior orbitofrontal cortex terminates in the central (Ce) nucleus of the amygdala. Projection neurons are positioned around the axonal terminations within the lateral (L), basolateral (BL) and basomedial (BM, also known as accessory basal) nuclei of the amygdala. Late-processing sensory areas project to the amygdala as well as to the orbitofrontal cortex, indicating direct and potentially indirect pathways for sensory information to orbitofrontal cortex. Other abbreviations: Me, medial nucleus; PCo, posterior cortical nucleus of the amygdala (Ghashghaei and Barbas, 2002).

3.4   Connections underlie the specialization of prefrontal cortices in behavior

The principal connections of distinct prefrontal areas are consistent with their role in behavioral tasks. For lateral prefrontal areas, searching the environment and orienting to behaviorally relevant signals in the environment is essential for cognitive tasks within working memory. Lateral prefrontal cortices are well suited for orienting to relevant stimuli by their robust connections with brainstem oculomotor systems as well as intralaminar thalamic nuclei and the multiform and parvicellular parts of the mediodorsal thalamic nucleus, associated with eye movements and working memory (e.g. Alexander & Fuster, 1973; Bauer & Fuster, 1976; Lynch & Graybiel, 1983; Heckers, 1997). At the level of the cortex, lateral prefrontal cortices are robustly and bidirectionally connected with the lateral intraparietal cortex (Figure 2.2), and both of these regions have a role in attentional processes and visuomotor functions (for reviews see Colby & Goldberg, 1999; Schiller & Tehovnik, 2001; Bisley & Goldberg, 2003). One key and very robust connection of periarcuate prefrontal cortices is with the lateral bank of the intraparietal sulcus, area 7a, also known as area LIP, as shown in earlier studies (e.g. Barbas & Mesulam, 1981; Barbas, 1988). These interconnected areas have visuomotor functions, engaged in tasks that require directed attention (for reviews see Mesulam, 1999; Barbas et al., 2002).

Sensory input to medial prefrontal areas originates preferentially from auditory association areas, arriving from late-processing areas where neurons are broadly tuned to auditory stimuli (Rauschecker et al., 1995; Kosaki et al., 1997; Rauschecker, 1998), and respond best to complex species-specific vocalizations. These vocalizations can be described as emotional communication, such as distress calls emitted in fear when, for example, infant monkeys are separated from their mothers (for review see Vogt & Barbas, 1988). In humans, caudal medial prefrontal areas around the anterior cingulate have a role in speech production and their damage results in the akinetic mute syndrome (e.g. Nielsen & Jacobs, 1951; Barris & Schuman, 1953; Buge et al., 1975). In monkeys, there is a close functional interaction between anterior cingulate areas and auditory cortices (Jürgens & Müller-Preuss, 1977; Müller-Preuss et al., 1980; Müller-Preuss & Ploog, 1981; Heffner & Heffner, 1986). When the cingulate vocalization cortices are stimulated electrically there is a decrease in auditory-evoked activity in superior temporal auditory areas (Müller-Preuss et al., 1980; Müller-Preuss & Ploog, 1981).

The polymodal projections to the posterior orbitofrontal cortex are closely matched by the polymodal input to the amygdala (Figure 2.6). We previously suggested that this pattern of connection allows the orbitofrontal cortex to receive sensory information through dual pathways: direct input from sensory association cortices, and indirect input through the amygdala (Barbas & De Olmos, 1990; Barbas, 1995). A recent study provided direct evidence, in the same experiments, that pathways from anterior temporal visual and auditory association cortices and caudal orbitofrontal areas have overlapping territories in the basal complex of the amygdala (Ghashghaei & Barbas, 2002). This evidence supports the idea that sensory input reaches orbitofrontal cortices directly through corticocortical pathways (Barbas, 1993; Rempel-Clower

& Barbas, 2000), and indirectly through the amygdala (Barbas, 1995). This intricate network may underlie processing of the emotional significance of events and reward contingencies (Malkova *et al.*, 1997; Schoenbaum *et al.*, 1999; Baxter *et al.*, 2000; Hikosaka & Watanabe, 2000; Wallis & Miller, 2003).

The bidirectional connections between the orbitofrontal cortex and the amygdala may allow prolongation of exchange of signals between these structures, as sensory information is assessed to evaluate the significance of the environment. This connectional architecture may facilitate persistent activity that may be necessary for the conscious appreciation of events. Classic studies indicate that the cortex is necessary for the conscious perception of emotions (Kennard, 1945). On the other hand, the amygdala in humans is activated even when emotional stimuli are presented below the level of conscious awareness (Whalen *et al.*, 1998). In rats, for example, a short subcortical loop connecting the amygdala with the thalamus can support fear conditioning (Romanski & LeDoux, 1992), suggesting that there is a fairly fast pathway for emotional vigilance. In this sense the amygdala may act as a reflex center for quick responses in potentially dangerous situations. The direct and indirect connections of orbitofrontal cortices with sensory cortices may have a critical role in the conscious appreciation of events, making it possible to carry out informed actions beyond the initial alerting response. Direct cortical sensory input to the orbitofrontal cortex may provide a global overview of the external environment, and indirect sensory input through the amygdala may provide the emotional context necessary to interpret the significance of events (Barbas, 1995).

4   The laminar organization of connections is linked to cortical structure

Thus far we have considered the general topography and key connections of prefrontal areas. An additional and important consideration is the pattern of these connections. Patterns reveal rules, and rules help organize the vast number of possible connections in the cerebral cortex, which underwent tremendous growth in evolution. However there is division of labor within the cortex, so that for any one area only a few neurons, within specific layers, are involved in each set of connections. For example, in the sensory cortices, projections from early-processing sensory areas originate in layers 2–3 and their axons terminate mostly in the middle layers of later-processing areas. These connections have been variously described as feedforward, ascending or bottom-up, to reflect the flow of information in sensory systems. Projections proceeding in the reverse direction originate in the deep layers (5–6) and their axons terminate mostly in layer 1, and have been called feedback, descending or top-down (for review see Felleman & Van Essen, 1991). However, the sequence of processing cannot be readily determined beyond the early-processing sensory areas. Moreover, most cortical areas are not strictly sensory, raising the question of what rules apply in the connections of association areas, which comprise a large part of the cerebral cortex, particularly in primates. Interestingly, the best clue that led to a general principle of corticocortical connections emerged from the connections of limbic cortices, which issue projections primarily from their deep layers when they project to association cortices (Barbas & Mesulam, 1981; Barbas, 1986). By analogy with the sensory systems, the limbic cortices behave like feedback or top-down systems.

But what attribute of limbic areas underlies their pattern of connections? Among many possibilities, the feature that most readily and reliably distinguishes limbic from other areas is structure (Barbas & Pandya, 1989). Prefrontal limbic areas can be readily identified as areas with fewer than six layers. This fundamental structural feature differentiates limbic cortices from areas that have six layers, the eulaminate areas. In the prefrontal cortex, anterior orbital, anterior medial and all lateral prefrontal cortices have six layers and are, therefore, eulaminate. These structural differences, which were initially described qualitatively (Barbas & Pandya, 1989), were later formalized quantitatively, when it was established that limbic prefrontal cortices have a lower neuronal density than the eulaminate (Dombrowski et al., 2001), as shown in Figure 2.7. Moreover, these cortices differ by a number of molecular markers, including the prevalence of distinct classes of inhibitory neurons labeled with the calcium binding proteins (CBP) calbindin and parvalbumin (Dombrowski and Barbas, 1998).

It is important to emphasize that structure in this sense refers to global features of cortical layers, including the number of identifiable layers and the cellular density of specific layers. This definition of structure does not refer to unique architectonic features used to parcellate the cortex into architectonic areas, such as the shape and size of neurons and their clustering in columns. Global structure captures similarities among cortical areas and groups them by cortical type, such as agranular, dysgranular or eulaminate. In contrast, specific architectonic features are unique to individual cortical areas, and can be used to distinguish, for example, area 32 from area 24 or area 25. By cortical type all of these areas are dysgranular.

As defined above, structure at the level of layers has been extremely useful in differentiating not only limbic from eulaminate cortices, but also in identifying different types of cortices. The first distinction is within the limbic cortices themselves. Those limbic prefrontal areas that lack layer 4 are called agranular, and adjacent limbic areas that have a rudimentary granular layer 4 are called dysgranular (Barbas & Pandya, 1989). Moreover, eulaminate areas can be further

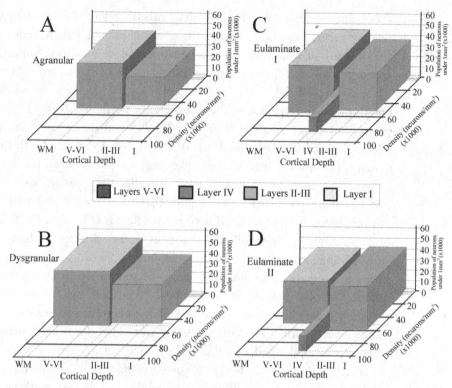

Figure 2.7   Neuronal density profile in different types of prefrontal cortices. Three-dimensional graphs showing differences in neuronal density (Y axis), laminar thickness by layer (X axis), and number of neurons under 1 mm^2 of cortical surface (Z axis) in: (A), agranular; (B), dysgranular; (C), eulaminate I; (D), eulaminate II cortices. Dotted lines for x axis demarcate extent of cortical layers, and solid lines indicate 500-mm intervals of cortical thickness. The density of neurons in the upper layers (IV–II) increases progressively from agranular to eulaminate II areas. (From Dombrowski *et al.* [2001].) (For a color version of this figure, please see the color plate section.)

grouped into different types based on the density of layer 4 and the upper layers (Dombrowski *et al.*, 2001), as shown in Figure 2.1.

In biological systems structure often underlies function and, in the cortex, the systematic differences in structure underlie the laminar pattern of areal interconnections (Barbas, 1986; Barbas & Rempel-Clower, 1997; Rempel-Clower & Barbas, 2000). The reasoning for grouping areas into the broader categories of cortical types is based on strong evidence that cortical type is more fundamental than specific architectonic features in understanding the organization of connections. As discussed above, dysgranular areas are limbic cortices, which behave like feedback systems when they are connected with eulaminate areas.

Type, therefore, identifies the fundamental structure of areas, and is important because it underlies the laminar patterns in corticocortical connections.

Grouping areas by type revealed that in corticocortical connections, when the area of origin is eulaminate, projection neurons are found mostly in the upper layers (2–3), and their axons terminate predominantly in the deep layers (4–6) of areas with fewer layers or lower neuronal density than the origin. The reciprocal connections originate mostly in the deep layers (5–6) of areas with fewer layers or lower cell density, and their axons terminate mostly in the upper layers (1–3) of areas with more layers or higher neuronal density.

We have termed the relationship of structure to the pattern of cortico-cortical connections "the structural model for connections" (for reviews see [Barbas & Hilgetag, 2002; Barbas et al., 2002]). The structural model predicts the prevalence of connections within the superficial and deep layers. Moreover, the model predicts the relative distribution of connections within cortical layers, and indicates that the relative distribution of connections varies as a function of the structural difference of the linked areas (Barbas & Rempel-Clower, 1997). Differences in structure can be compared formally by assigning ordinal values to areas according to their type. As discussed above, type is defined quanti-tatively by the number of layers and the neuronal density of areas. In this scheme, agranular areas with three distinguishable layers are given a rating of 1. Dysgranular areas have an additional layer, a poorly developed granular layer 4, and a rating of 2. Eulaminate areas have six layers and we have previously rated them 3–5, reflecting the lowest (3) to highest (5) overall cell density, seen particularly in layer 4 and in layers 2–3 (Barbas & Rempel-Clower, 1997; Dombrowski et al., 2001). Using the ordinal ratings we can find the type difference of linked areas, Δ (Δ = type [origin] - type [termination]), and determine to what extent the value of Δ predicts the relative distribution of connections in cortical layers.

The structural model predicts that the laminar pattern of connections will be exaggerated when structurally dissimilar areas are connected (e.g. caudal medial, types 1–2, with dorsolateral areas, types 4–5), than when structurally similar areas are interconnected (e.g. caudal medial, type 2 with rostral medial, type 3 prefrontal areas), as summarized in Figure 2.8. Along the same lines, the structural model predicts that when areas of similar type are interconnected, projection neurons will originate in approximately equal numbers in the upper (2–3) and deep (5–6) layers, and their axons will terminate in a columnar pattern, spanning the width of the cortex from pia to white matter.

We have shown that the structural model successfully predicts the laminar pattern of connections not only between pairs of prefrontal areas (Barbas & Rempel-Clower, 1997), but also for other corticocortical connections.

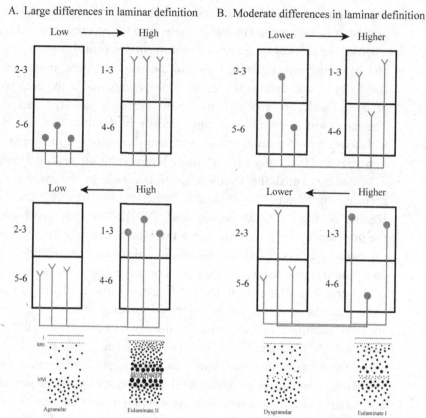

Figure 2.8   The pattern of connections predicted by the structural model. A, top: projections between areas that differ markedly in laminar structure originate predominantly in the deep layers of areas with fewer layers or lower cell density, and their axons terminate mostly in the upper layers of areas with more layers of higher cell density. A, bottom: the opposite pattern is seen for the reciprocal projections. B, top: a less extreme version of the above pattern is predicted in the interconnections of areas that differ moderately in laminar structure, such as when a cortex with lower cell density projects to a cortex with higher cell density. B, bottom: when a cortex with higher cell density projects to a cortex with lower cell density. The bottom panels show a cartoon of laminar features that form the basis for grouping areas into cortical types. The number of types used for parcelling schemes can vary, as areas show gradual changes in neuronal density within layers. (Adapted from Barbas & Rempel-Clower [1997].) (For a color version of this figure, please see the color plate section.)

The extension of the structural model to other areas is based on evidence that parcelling by cortical type can be made in all cortical systems, including each of the sensory cortical systems, as well as high-order association areas. Examples of connections whose laminar pattern can be explained in broad structural terms include connections between prefrontal areas and inferior and medial temporal areas (Rempel-Clower & Barbas, 2000), prefrontal and superior temporal areas (Barbas *et al.*, 1999), and visual cortical projections to prefrontal areas (Barbas, 1986). Thus, projections originating from one cortical area terminate in different laminar patterns in structurally distinct temporal or prefrontal areas. Conversely, projections arising from several structurally different areas terminate in distinct laminar patterns within a single target area. For example, axons from posterior orbitofrontal (dysgranular) cortex, terminate mostly in the middle-deep layers of medial temporal area 28 (agranular cortex), in all layers of dysgranular area 36, and predominantly in the upper layers of visual association area TE (granular cortex), as shown in Figure 2.9. The same patterns are seen in the connections of medial prefrontal areas with superior

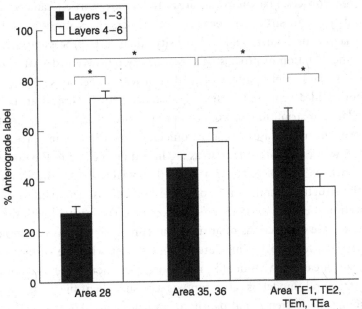

Figure 2.9   Differences in the laminar terminations of axons from posterior orbitofrontal cortex in three groups of anterior temporal cortices. Axonal terminations were heavier in the deep layers of agranular area 28, equally distributed in the upper and deep layers of dysgranular areas 35, 36, and more dense in the upper layers of eulaminate inferior temporal areas (TE1, TE2, TEm, TEa). Bars indicate the mean percentage of total anterograde label in the upper (1–3; black bars) and deep (4–6; white bars) layers of three cases with injections in caudal orbitofrontal area OPro. Vertical lines on the bars indicate the standard error. Horizontal lines above bar graphs show statistically significant differences (∗) between the percentage of anterograde label in the upper and deep layers in a single group of areas or between the percentage of label in the upper layers of two different groups of areas. (From Rempel-Clower & Barbas [2000].)

temporal auditory association areas (Barbas *et al.*, 1999, 2005b). Moreover, structure explains the connections in another species, the cat visual cortex (e.g. Grant & Hilgetag, 2004). This evidence supports the idea that cortical structure underlies the pattern of corticocortical connections in a variety of systems and species.

4.1 Comparison with other models

As discussed above, the laminar pattern of connections was used to construct a hierarchy in sensory cortices, particularly the visual (for reviews see Felleman & Van Essen, 1991; Shipp, 2000), albeit with limited success (Hilgetag *et al.*, 1996). On the other hand, the structural model can be used to understand connections in sensory systems as well as among prefrontal or between prefrontal and other cortices. Like prefrontal areas, the sensory cortices can be grouped into cortical types. In structural terms, earlier-processing sensory areas have either more layers, or higher neuronal density, than later-processing sensory areas. Thus, the direction of processing in sensory systems coincides with, rather than underlies, the laminar pattern of corticocortical connections.

Another idea proposed is that the distance between linked areas determines the relative distribution of connections in cortical layers (e.g. Young, 1992). However, in many cases distance coincides with changes in cortical structure. In cases where pairs of distant areas are linked but belong to the same structural type, such as orbitofrontal area 13 and medial area 32, the distance model and the structural model make opposite predictions. The pattern of ipsilateral connections between areas 13 and 32 is columnar, consistent with the structural model for the connections of areas of the same type (Barbas & Rempel-Clower, 1997). However, the findings are not consistent with the distance model, as the linked areas behave more like neighbors, even though they are not neighbors. The structural model is also more successful than the distance model in predicting the existence and density of ipsilateral and contralateral projections, as well as the laminar origin of contralateral projections (Barbas *et al.*, 2005a).

The structural model thus indicates that a given prefrontal area does not have a single pattern of connection, but rather issues projections and interacts in different laminar microenvironments at the site of termination, following a pattern that depends on the structural relationship of the interconnected areas. Thus the pattern of connections is not fixed or hierarchical, but relational. The significance of the structural model is based on the potential to predict patterns of connections in the human cortex, where it is not possible to use invasive procedures to study connections, but it is possible to study structure (Barbas & Rempel-Clower, 1997).

4.2 Excitatory and inhibitory interactions within the laminar microenvironment of connections

The laminar pattern of connections has profound implications for function, since axons terminating in the upper layers influence different populations of neurons and segments of processes than axons terminating in the deep layers. There is substantial evidence that different cortical layers vary in cell morphology, receptors, and neurochemical properties (e.g. De Lima *et al.*, 1990; Goldman-Rakic *et al.*, 1990; Hof *et al.*, 1995).

An important feature of the laminar microenvironment of connections in different layers is in the type of inhibitory control. Inhibition is particularly relevant for the function of the prefrontal cortex in suppressing the myriad of irrelevant signals impinging on one constantly. In the cortex, synaptic inhibition is mediated through GABAergic interneurons. Other types of inhibition are important as well, such as the complex modulatory influences mediated at the level of G-coupled receptors activated by neurotransmitters or other messengers, but these are beyond the scope of the present discussion.

GABAergic neurons comprise a highly heterogeneous class of neurons acting both through ionotropic and metabotropic receptors. A convenient and useful way of classifying GABAergic neurons is by their neurochemical features, specifically by the expression of distinct calcium binding proteins (CBP). One of these groups is positive for the CBP parvalbumin, which labels the morphologically distinct basket and chandelier cells in the cortex (DeFelipe *et al.*, 1989b; Kawaguchi & Kubota, 1997). An important feature of parvalbumin neurons is their preferential distribution in the middle layers of the cortex, and their synaptic interaction locally with pyramidal cells, targeting preferentially proximal dendrites and axon initial segments (DeFelipe *et al.*, 1989b; Shao & Burkhalter, 1999). A second group of neurochemically identified interneurons is distinguished for their expression of the CBP calbindin. This category includes the morphologically distinct class of bitufted (or double bouquet) inhibitory cells in the cortex. CB-positive neurons have a different laminar distribution than parvalbumin neurons, found mostly in cortical layers 2 and upper layer 3. CB neurons also have a distinct pattern of innervation, targeting mostly the distal dendrites and spines of other neurons (e.g. Peters & Sethares, 1997).

The above discussion suggests that neurons originating and terminating in distinct layers encounter a distinct microenvironment with respect to the type of inhibitory control, as summarized in Figure 2.10. Physiologic studies are consistent with this idea, based on evidence from the sensory systems. In the visual system, for example, stimulation of pathways that terminate in the middle cortical layers, such as the pathway from LGn to V1, or from primary to

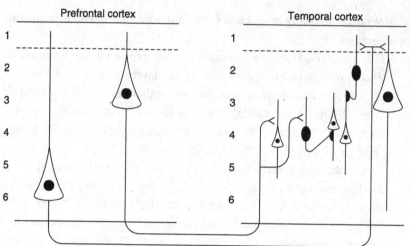

Figure 2.10 Pathways originating and terminating in different layers encounter a different microenvironment with respect to inhibitory control. Hypothetical scheme for prefrontal to temporal
pathways based on rules of corticocortical connections. Pyramidal projection neurons
originating in layer 3 of prefrontal cortex (dark blue) terminate in the middle layers of
temporal cortex among excitatory neurons (green), but also among inhibitory neurons that
are positive for parvalbumin (solid black), which are most prevalent in the middle layers of
the cortex. Parvalbumin neurons innervate the proximal dendrites or axon initial segment of
pyramidal neurons locally. Pyramidal projection neurons from the deep layers of prefrontal
cortex (light blue) terminate in layer 1 of temporal cortex among the distal dendrites of
other pyramidal neurons, but also around calbindin inhibitory neurons which are most
prevalent in layers 2–upper 3 of the cortex. Calbindin neurons innervate the distal
dendrites of pyramidal neurons locally. The model is based on the structural model for
connections (Barbas & Rempel-Clower, 1997), the pattern of connections between
prefrontal & medial and inferior (Rempel-Clower & Barbas, 2000) and superior temporal
(Barbas et al., 1999) cortices, and the prevalence of PV and CB neurons in superior
temporal cortices (Barbas et al., 2005b). (For a color version of this figure, please see the
color plate section.)

association areas in the cortex, results in monosynaptic excitation followed
by disynaptic inhibition (Douglas et al., 1991; Shao & Burkhalter, 1999). In
contrast, stimulation of pathways that terminate in layer 1, lead predominantly
to excitatory effects (Sandell & Schiller, 1982; Shao & Burkhalter, 1999). This
evidence is consistent with the idea that the laminar pattern of terminations may
critically affect the balance of excitatory and inhibitory influences exerted
by prefrontal areas on other cortices.

The laminar distribution of parvalbumin and calbindin neurons is consistent in all cortical areas examined (e.g. Hendry et al., 1989; DeFelipe et al., 1989a;
DeFelipe et al., 1990; Conde et al., 1994; Gabbott & Bacon, 1996; for review

see Hof *et al.*, 1999). However, the relative prevalence of each type of neurochemically distinct class of inhibitory neurons varies widely and in opposite directions in cortical areas (for review see Hof *et al.*, 1999). The differential distribution of these neurochemical classes of inhibitory neurons is seen prominently in the prefrontal cortex, where they vary systematically within cortical types, differing markedly from agranular/dysgranular (limbic) to eulaminate areas (Dombrowski *et al.*, 2001). In limbic areas, calbindin neurons outnumber the parvalbumin by several fold, whereas in eulaminate areas the density of each class is comparable. Moreover, the pattern of distribution of each class is graded, following closely and predictably the graded changes in cortical structure.

When the complement of neurons that express parvalbumin and calbindin is considered, there are more inhibitory neurons in the upper than in the deep layers. It should be noted that a third class of inhibitory neurons expressing the CBP calretinin is also more prevalent in the superficial than in the deep layers (Conde *et al.*, 1994; Gabbott *et al.*, 1997). The significance of this pattern can be further shown when the laminar pattern of connections is super-imposed on the laminar distribution of inhibitory neurons. As described above, in limbic areas the deep layers are the principal sources and targets of corticocortical connections, whereas in eulaminate areas it is the upper layers that primarily issue and receive cortical connections (Barbas & Rempel-Clower, 1997). Thus in prefrontal limbic areas the focus of connections and the prevalence of CBP is mismatched, but in eulaminate areas it is matched. We recently found a similar mismatch in the prevalence of neurons positive for CB and PV and prefrontal connections in the agranular/dysgranular (limbic) parts of the temporal pole (Barbas *et al.*, 2005b). This mismatch in limbic areas may have functional consequences, since neurons with CBP have the capacity to buffer and sequester calcium (for reviews see Baimbridge *et al.*, 1992; Heizmann, 1992). These molecular/connectional relationships likely affect neural dynamics and may provide a clue as to why limbic areas have a predilection for epileptiform activity (Penfield & Jasper, 1954).

5   Distinct prefrontal areas are connected with specialized effector systems for action

5.1   All prefrontal areas have a special connectional association with the basal ganglia

As discussed above, the prefrontal cortex is an action-oriented center through common as well as specialized connections with motor control systems. All prefrontal areas have a common, though topographically organized, association with the basal ganglia. The relationship of prefrontal cortex with the basal ganglia through the thalamus is unique among association cortices, a relationship they share with neighboring premotor and motor cortices (for reviews see Alexander et al., 1986; Alheid et al., 1990; Graybiel et al., 1994). Specifically, the ventral anterior and mediodorsal nuclei, which are bidirectionally connected with prefrontal cortices, are also the targets of input from the internal segment of the globus pallidus (Xiao & Barbas, 2004). The VA nucleus, in particular, is connected with prefrontal as well as premotor areas (Kievit & Kuypers, 1977; Jacobson et al., 1978; Kunzle, 1978; Baleydier & Mauguiere, 1980; Asanuma et al., 1985; Goldman-Rakic & Porrino, 1985; Ilinsky et al., 1985; Preuss & Goldman-Rakic, 1987; Yeterian & Pandya, 1988; Barbas et al., 1991; Chiba et al., 2001; McFarland & Haber, 2002; Middleton & Strick, 2002; for review see Cavada et al., 2000). These circuits were classically thought to be important for motor functions (for reviews see Goldman-Rakic, 1987; Graybiel, 2000; Anderson, 2001; Haber & McFarland, 2001), but recent studies have shown that circuits through the basal ganglia have a role in cognition, motivated behavior, learning, and memory as well (Middleton & Strick, 1994; Hikosaka et al., 1999; Mitchell et al., 1999; Graybiel, 2000; Hollerman et al., 2000; Middleton & Strick, 2000; Schultz et al., 2000; Sato & Hikosaka, 2002; Toni et al., 2002). These cognitive-emotional functions may have their root in pathways through the prefrontal cortex, including its lateral, medial and orbitofrontal sectors.

The VA nucleus is connected through bidirectional pathways with all prefrontal cortices, but its connections are particularly robust with areas 9 and 8 on the lateral surface, medial area 32 and caudal orbitofrontal area OPro (Xiao & Barbas, 2004). Further, the laminar origin of prefrontal projections to the VA is unique among prefrontal projections to other thalamic nuclei, as they originate in nearly equal numbers from layers 5 and 6 (Xiao & Barbas, 2004). Layer 6 gives rise to the vast majority of cortical projections to the thalamus in most systems (Gilbert & Kelly, 1975; Robson & Hall, 1975; Lund et al., 1976; Jones & Wise, 1977; for reviews see Jones, 1985; Steriade et al., 1997), while layer 5 contributes a considerably lower proportion of corticothalamic projections ($\sim$10–20%), including those from prefrontal association areas (Xiao & Barbas, 2002; Xiao & Barbas, 2004).

5.2 Distinct prefrontal areas are connected with specialized motor systems

Beyond the above specific interconnections of all prefrontal cortices with the basal ganglia through the thalamus, there are other connections with motor systems that are specific for the specialized sectors of the prefrontal cortex. Lateral prefrontal areas, and in particular the caudal lateral areas in the peri-arcuate region, are situated immediately anterior to premotor cortices and are connected with them (e.g. Barbas & Pandya, 1987). The premotor cortices are then connected with the motor cortex, and both give rise to pathways that ultimately lead to the final common pathway for action, the motoneurons in the spinal cord (e.g. Hutchins *et al.*, 1988; Dum & Strick, 1991; Galea & Darian-Smith, 1994). Periarcuate areas also project to the superior colliculus, an important oculomotor center, a pathway that is likely critical in the specialization of this region for searching the environment. In fact, the frontal eye field in the periarcuate region received its name by the disturbances in eye movements noted after its damage in classic studies (for review of early literature see Barbas & Mesulam, 1981).

The orbitofrontal and medial prefrontal cortices, on the other hand, have a different set of connections with motor effector systems, specifically the autonomic motor system which innervates autonomic organs and activates them during emotional arousal. Medial prefrontal cortices in the anterior cingulate, including areas 32, 25 and the anterior part of area 32 make up a region that has been associated with vocalization (for review see Vogt & Barbas, 1988). Specifically, these areas have a role in vocalization emitted by primates in distress as a form of emotional communication, in order to signal the presence of danger in the environment, such as a predator. These functions are likely mediated through the direct connections of these anterior cingulate areas with brainstem vocalization centers (for review see Vogt & Barbas, 1988).

Interestingly, medial prefrontal cortices have access to autonomic centers through multiple pathways: they have strong and direct projections to hypothalamic and brainstem autonomic centers (Öngur *et al.*, 1998; Rempel-Clower & Barbas, 1998; Freedman *et al.*, 2000) and the spinal cord (Rempel-Clower & Barbas, 1998), as shown in Figure 2.11. A direct and robust pathway from anterior cingulate area 32 innervates preferentially excitatory neurons in the hypothalamus, and forms asymmetric, and presumed excitatory synapses, mostly on spines in the hypothalamus (Barbas *et al.*, 2003), which are found predominantly on dendrites of excitatory neurons (Peters *et al.*, 1991). There are also other, though less direct, pathways from anterior cingulate areas to autonomic structures. One of these pathways courses through medially situated nuclei of the amygdala, which are connected preferentially with medial prefrontal cortices, as well as the hypothalamus (for review see Petrovich *et al.*, 2001). Another indirect pathway courses from medial prefrontal cortices to the basolateral nucleus of the amygdala, which is known to project to hypothalamic and brainstem autonomic centers. There is evidence that the latter pathway has a role in the process of learning the significance of motivationally relevant cues (Petrovich *et al.*, 2002). Yet another pathway from caudal medial prefrontal areas innervates preferentially the extended amygdala, a striatal-related structure in the basal forebrain, which also innervates autonomic structures downstream

(Ghashghaei & Barbas, 2001). The above circuits suggest that the medial prefrontal cortex has multiple ways to access autonomic centers, in pathways underlying autonomic functions in response to complex emotional situations.

The posterior orbitofrontal cortex appears to have a different and specialized role in emotional expression. As noted above, axons from posterior orbitofrontal cortex terminate not only in the basal nuclei of the amygdala, but target considerably more robustly narrow corridors interposed between nuclei of the basal complex. These corridors are composed of densely packed small neurons, known as the intercalated masses (IM) (for review see De Olmos, 1990). Recent studies have provided evidence that neurons in most IM nuclei in macaques monkeys and other species are GABAergic, and project to the central nucleus of the amygdala, the basal forebrain, and the brainstem (Moga & Gray, 1985; Nitecka & Ben Ari, 1987; Pare & Smith, 1993a, 1993b, 1994; Pitkanen & Amaral, 1994). The central nucleus, in turn, is enriched in inhibitory neurons, and is the main output of the amygdala to hypothalamic and brainstem autonomic structures (Jongen-Relo & Amaral, 1998; Saha et al., 2000; Ghashghaei & Barbas, 2002).

The targeting of GABAergic neurons in IM has special implications about the influence of posterior orbitofrontal cortex on the amygdala. Through these specialized connections, posterior orbitofrontal cortex exercises a direct influence on the internal system of the amygdala. The circuitry from caudal orbitofrontal cortex to IM suggests that orbitofrontal projections have a net effect of suppressing activity in the central nucleus and down-regulating its inhibitory output to hypothalamic and brainstem autonomic centers. This orbitofrontal pathway essentially has a permissive effect on autonomic centers, allowing activation of hypothalamic autonomic centers depending on the behavioral situation. Hypothalamic autonomic centers, in turn, increase their activity by direct excitatory projections from orbitofrontal and medial prefrontal areas (Ongur et al., 1998; Rempel-Clower & Barbas, 1998; Barbas et al., 2003). Pathways with disinhibitory or excitatory effects on the hypothalamus may be activated when pathways linking the amygdala and orbitofrontal cortex signal the need for emotional vigilance arising when a potential danger lurks in the environment (Figure 2.11). It should be emphasized that this special interaction through the IM nuclei is evident only for axons originating in posterior orbitofrontal cortex, and neither rostral orbitofrontal, nor medial or other prefrontal areas show this special pattern of connection with the amygdala.

Moreover, the caudal orbitofrontal cortex has another specific, though lighter, pathway that terminates directly on the central nucleus of the amygdala (Carmichael & Price, 1995a; Ghashghaei & Barbas, 2002), as seen in Figure 2.6. Activation of this pathway would have the opposite effect than the pathway

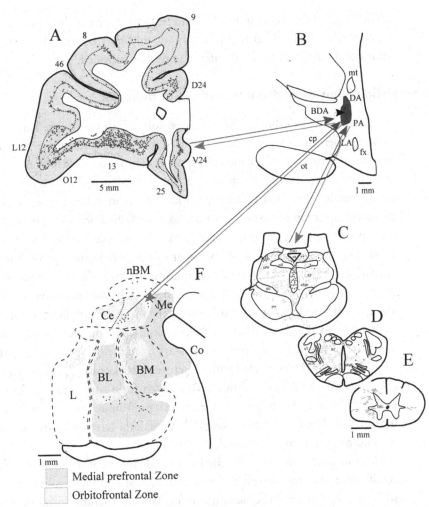

Figure 2.11 Serial pathways from the prefrontal cortex reach central autonomic structures. Pathways were mapped after injection of the bidirectional tracer BDA in the lateral (LA) hypothalamic area. (A) The first pathway is marked by projection neurons (blue dots) originating most densely from medial prefrontal and orbitofrontal cortices leading to the injection site (brown area in B); (B) the second pathway is marked by labeled axons emanating from the injection site and terminating in several autonomic nuclei (brown lines); (C, D) brainstem nuclei; (E) the thoracic spinal cord; (F) a bidirectional pathway links the amygdala with the same hypothalamic nuclei. The shaded areas in the amygdala show the specific termination zones of axons from orbitofrontal cortex (yellow), which originate from the deep layers (mainly layer 5), and the diffuse termination zone by axons from medial prefrontal cortex (light brown), as described by Ghashghaei & Barbas (2002). (Reproduced from Barbas *et al.* [2003].) (For a color version of this figure, please see the color plate section.)

to IM, by inhibiting autonomic centers. This pathway has the potential to suppress hypothalamic autonomic activity, and may be recruited when further information arrives that a potential danger has subsided.

6   Synergistic action of prefrontal cortices in behavior

As we have seen above, there is division of labor in prefrontal cortices, both in their set of connections with sensory and memory systems, as well as with effector systems for motor responses. The pattern of connections suggests that there is specialization within the lateral, medial and orbitofrontal cortices. Let's consider the role of lateral prefrontal areas in distinct aspects of working memory, for example when it's necessary to keep track of steps in following a recipe. But even for a simple task, it may be necessary to retrieve information from long-term memory, such as remembering where the kitchen utensils and specific ingredients are stored for preparing the meal. Moreover, decisions and actions in behavior are inextricably embedded in an emotional context. The choice of the recipe, for example, may depend on several factors, including its desirability to the cook, time for preparation, etc. The motivational aspects of a task are likely mediated through pathways from medial and orbitofrontal areas, which are robustly connected with structures associated with long-term memory and emotions, as discussed above. Thus, even for a simple task within working memory, it may be necessary for lateral prefrontal areas to gain access to information from structures associated with long-term memory, and place an impending action in an emotional context.

Orbitofrontal areas are well suited to provide information about the emotional significance of events through their direct, robust and bidirectional connections with the amygdala. The sensory information reaching orbitofrontal areas originates from late-processing sensory areas, and may provide an overview of the environment. This sensory information, however, may lack the level of resolution needed to evaluate the sensory detail of the environment. This system, alone, may be inadequate to decide whether an ambiguous figure in a dark alley is a limb from a tree, an animal or a human. Lateral prefrontal areas, on the other hand, especially the caudal parts of area 8, are connected with a large variety of visual areas, going as far back as V2, much like other visual association cortices (Barbas & Mesulam, 1981; Barbas, 1988; Schall et al., 1995), and may be capable of extracting the necessary detail from the environment.

Posterior orbitofrontal cortices, which are robustly connected with the amygdala, are not directly connected with posterior lateral prefrontal areas for the direct transfer of information between these cortices. However, posterior orbitofrontal cortices have strong connections with anterior orbitofrontal areas

(Barbas & Pandya, 1989; Carmichael & Price, 1996), which, in turn, are robustly connected with lateral prefrontal areas. Information about the emotional significance of events may thus follow a sequential path from posterior orbitofrontal cortex to anterior orbitofrontal cortex and then to lateral prefrontal areas. Lateral prefrontal cortices, which are connected with early-processing visual areas, may retrieve information necessary to identify the ambiguous object in the dark. This information may then be transmitted from lateral prefrontal areas to orbitofrontal cortices, through the reverse sequence. Projections to posterior orbitofrontal cortex, as we have seen, may either activate autonomic centers through a projection to IM and mobilization of autonomic structures, if the ambiguous object in the dark alley is a threatening person, or posterior orbitofrontal cortex may activate directly the central nucleus of the amygdala, which would dampen autonomic activity and allow return to autonomic homeostasis, if the figure is a tree branch.

An important consideration in the sequence of information processing for emotions is that the laminar pattern of connections, as specified by the rules of the structural model, is consistent with the sequential flow of information necessary to evaluate the emotional significance of the environment for action. Caudal orbitofrontal areas issue projections mostly from their deep layers, and to a lesser extent from the upper layers, to anterior orbitofrontal areas, and target the superficial and deep layers of anterior orbitofrontal cortices, in the pattern depicted in Figure 2.8B. In turn, anterior orbitofrontal areas project predominantly from their deep layers and their axons terminate in the upper layers (1–3a) of lateral prefrontal areas. As noted above, posterior lateral prefrontal areas in the periarcuate region receive robust projections from early-processing visual areas (Figure 2.2) and may extract signals on the fine detail of the sensory environment. Lateral prefrontal areas project from their upper layers and their axons terminate in the middle to deep layers of orbitofrontal cortex, including layer 5, which projects robustly to the amygdala. The laminar relationships of these sequential connections provide a feasible path for speedy transfer of information necessary for decision and action in behavior.

Lateral prefrontal areas, especially areas 8 and caudal area 46, which receive projections from early-processing sensory areas, also have the strongest connections with the neighboring premotor areas (for review see Barbas, 1992). Thus, information may flow from orbitofrontal to lateral prefrontal areas and to premotor areas, demonstrating the collaborative communication of different prefrontal sectors for decision and action in behavior. If the ambiguous figure is a menacing person, it would be necessary to get out of the way quickly.

The other component of the motor control system is information coursing through the basal ganglia, via the VA nucleus of the thalamus, which has bidirectional connections with the prefrontal cortex (e.g. Barbas *et al.*, 1991; Dermon & Barbas, 1994; Xiao & Barbas, 2004), as discussed above. A prominent feature of this system is the high prevalence of prefrontal projections to the VA from layer 5. This is different from sensory and other association areas which issue projections to thalamic nuclei mostly from layer 6. In sensory systems, there is evidence that corticothalamic projections from layer 5 differ markedly from projections originating in layer 6 (for review see Rouiller & Welker, 2000). The details of this circuitry in any cortical system are largely unknown, but there is some evidence that axons from neurons in layer 6 of sensory association areas terminate as small and diffuse terminals in the thalamus and innervate the distal dendrites of thalamic neurons that project focally to cortical layer 4 (Rouiller & Welker, 1991; Ojima, 1994; Rockland, 1996). In contrast, axons from corticothalamic neurons in layer 5 terminate as large and clustered boutons and innervate the proximal dendrites of thalamocortical projection neurons which innervate wide territories within cortical layer 1 (for reviews see Jones, 1985; Steriade *et al.*, 1997; Rouiller & Welker, 2000; Haber & McFarland, 2001; Jones, 2002). The pattern of termination of laminar-specific pathways from prefrontal areas to the VA is not known, but substantial projections from the VA terminate in layer 1 of the frontal cortex (McFarland & Haber, 2002; for review see Castro-Alamancos & Connors, 1997; and personal observations). Projections terminating in layer 1 extend over long distances, impinging on the apical dendrites of neurons from layer 5. In turn, neurons in layer 5 project to the thalamus and other subcortical structures, including the neostriatum. A projection to layer 1 could thus help recruit additional areas by synapsing over long distances on the dendrites of neurons from layer 5, activating wider territories of the thalamus and back to the cortex.

7   Differential vulnerability of distinct prefrontal sectors in neurologic and psychiatric diseases

The deficits associated with damage to distinct prefrontal cortices can be understood in the context of disconnection of anatomic pathways. Damage to the periarcuate or lateral intraparietal cortex, two areas that are strongly interconnected, results in the classic syndrome of neglect, characterized by inattention of the contralateral side (reviewed in Mesulam, 1981, 1990). Human and nonhuman primates with damage to each of these areas are not blind, but they ignore the sensory environment on the side opposite the lesion. This deficit is consistent with disconnection of pathways linking areas with a role in directing attention to relevant stimuli in the environment in order to perform a specific task.

We have also seen that the similarly strong pathways from prefrontal to temporal areas have a role in cognitive tasks. Area 10 at the frontal pole, specifically, is engaged when humans must hold a main task on line while juggling secondary tasks (Koechlin *et al.*, 1999), and this pathway may support auditory working memory. Damage of lateral prefrontal areas impairs the ability of humans to extract relevant auditory signals from noise (Chao & Knight, 1997b, 1998). A frequent complaint in humans with damage to the frontal lobe is that they are unable to follow conversations in noisy environments. As we have seen above, connections originating and terminating in different layers encounter a distinct microenvironment with respect to distinct classes of neurochemically identified inhibitory interneurons. These interactions likely affect neural dynamics, and may allow recruitment of laminar-specific components of pathways in behavior. In the superior temporal cortex the calbindin class of inhibitory neurons is most prevalent in the superficial layers, particularly layer 2, while parvalbumin neurons are most densely distributed in a central band at the bottom of layer 3 to upper layer 5 (Barbas *et al.*, 2005b). Dense connections from prefrontal cortices terminate in spatially extensive bands within layers 1 and 2 of superior temporal auditory association areas, mingling within a dense band of calbindin-positive neurons. This class of inhibitory neurons appears to have a role in focusing on relevant features of stimuli and suppressing distractors, according to a theoretical model based on neuronal responses during a working memory task in lateral prefrontal cortex (Wang *et al.*, 2004). Disruption of this pathway may help explain the detrimental effect of distractors in auditory association tasks in patients with frontal lobe damage, demonstrating the critical role of prefrontal areas in selecting relevant signals and ignoring irrelevant signals in behavior (Chao & Knight, 1997a, 1997b; Knight *et al.*, 1999; Gehring & Knight, 2002).

On the other hand, projections from prefrontal cortices target the middle and deep layers of the temporal pole, an area that has dysgranular architecture and is thus considered structurally limbic by its architecture as well as its connections with other cortical and subcortical limbic structures (Gower, 1989; Kondo *et al.*, 2003). This type of connection is considered to be feedforward and "driving," and may provide signals related to the emotional significance of auditory stimuli, such as species-specific vocalization associated with the temporal pole (Poremba *et al.*, 2004).

The pathway from medial prefrontal to superior temporal auditory association cortex has a role in emotional communication in nonhuman primates (for review see Vogt & Barbas, 1988). The functional interaction between anterior cingulate and auditory areas is evident in humans when engaged in verbal speech, and when imagining speech in someone else's voice. In humans, the pathway from the anterior cingulate to superior temporal auditory association cortex is functionally impaired in those schizophrenic patients who experience auditory hallucinations (McGuire *et al.*, 1995; McGuire *et al.*, 1996; reviewed in Barbas *et al.*, 2002). Interestingly, hippocampal pathology in schizophrenia (for review see Nelson *et al.*, 1998; Heckers & Konradi, 2002), is most prominent in the anterior half of the hippocampus (Szeszko *et al.*, 2003; Narr *et al.*, 2004); but see also Weiss *et al.* (2005), the part that sends robust projections to medial prefrontal cortices in the anterior cingulate (Barbas & Blatt, 1995), as seen in Figure 2.5.

The medial prefrontal areas in the anterior cingulate are also connected with cortical and subcortical structures associated with long-term memory (Figures 2.4 and 2.5). The strong affiliation of the anterior cingulate with these structures is exemplified by the repercussions on memory when it is damaged. In humans strokes affecting the anterior communicating artery that feeds the anterior cingulate (Crowell & Morawetz, 1977; D'Esposito *et al.*, 1996), including Brodmann's areas 25, 24 and 32, around the rostrum of the corpus callosum (Brodmann, 1905) lead to anterograde amnesia, similar to the amnesic syndrome seen after hippocampal lesions (Talland *et al.*, 1967; Alexander & Freedman, 1984; for review see Barbas, 1997). In monkeys, lesions of the anterior cingulate result in deficits in visual recognition (Voytko, 1985; Bachevalier & Mishkin, 1986). The memory deficits are seen after damage to caudal medial areas. Anterior medial areas 9 and 10, have comparatively few connections with memory-related medial temporal and hippocampal structures. Area 14 occupies an intermediate position with respect to its connections with medial temporal and hippocampal structures, receiving a significant projection from them (Barbas & Blatt, 1995; Barbas *et al.*, 1999).

As discussed above, a notable connectional feature of the orbitofrontal cortex is its polymodal nature and its strong connections with the equally polymodal amygdala. Direct cortical sensory input to the orbitofrontal cortex may provide a global overview of the external environment, and indirect sensory input through the amygdala may provide the emotional context necessary to appreciate the significance of events. This interpretation is consistent with the consequences of damage to orbitofrontal cortex in nonhuman primates, which include impairment in the ability to show appropriate emotional responses or social interactions (for review see Kling & Steklis, 1976). Damage of the amygdala results in the classic Klüver-Bucy syndrome, including hyperorality and indiscriminate mouthing of objects, suggesting inability to appreciate the significance of objects as edible or inedible. The behavioral consequences though differ depending on the time of damage of the amygdala, so that monkeys with lesions in adulthood show a reduction in social stress and engage in uninhibited social interactions

(Amaral, 2002), while damage in infancy results in abnormal fear and avoidance of social interactions (Bauman *et al.*, 2004).

Humans with orbitofrontal lesions appear to be unaware of the social consequences of their actions, which appears to be related to difficulty in appreciating and integrating social and emotional cues necessary for appropriate interpretation of events (e.g. Cicerone & Tanenbaum, 1997; Wood, 2003; Mah *et al.*, 2004). Lesions of the amygdala impair the ability of humans to judge facial expressions, especially fear (Adolphs *et al.*, 1994, 1998; Bechara *et al.*, 1999). These findings are consistent with the idea that the amygdala monitors the environment for potential threats, and the orbitofrontal cortex has a role in assessing the emotional significance of events prior to making a decision.

Consistent with its specialized connections, pathology in orbitofrontal cortex shows specific behavioral symptomatology. Psychiatric diseases that are characterized by abnormal fear, including panic disorder, anxiety, phobias and obsessive-compulsive disorder (e.g. Zald & Kim, 1996; Simpson *et al.*, 2001; Mayberg, 2003), may have in common overactivity in orbitofrontal cortex. As noted above, activation of the highly specialized projection from caudal orbitofrontal cortex to the IM of the amygdala would allow activation of hypothalamic and brainstem autonomic centers. Activity in this pathway may be sustained in pathologic conditions dominated by anxiety, resulting in overactivity of the autonomic nervous system associated with emotional arousal. In contrast, in sociopathic personality disorder there is underactivation of the orbitofrontal cortex and concomitant underactivation of autonomic responses in emotional situations (e.g. Bechara *et al.*, 1996).

8 Specification of cortical types in development

In the sections above we have seen that the structural type of cortical areas is critical in understanding the overall connections, their laminar patterns, interface with distinct excitatory and inhibitory systems, and sequential engagement in behavior. But how do these consistent patterns in areal structure arise? Differences in cortical structure among prefrontal areas are consistent with differences in the timing of their development (Dombrowski *et al.*, 2001). According to this hypothesis, limbic prefrontal areas, which have a lower cell density than eulaminate areas, complete their development before eulaminate areas. Moreover, the differences in density can be explained by a higher density in eulaminate areas in the upper layers, including layers 4, 3 and 2, which develop after the deep layers, according to the inside-out development of the cerebral cortex. If the development of cortical areas starts at about the same time in gestation for different areas according to experimental findings in nonhuman primates (Rakic, 1988), then development in limbic areas may be completed earlier than in eulaminate areas. This would account for the sparser population of neurons in the upper layers in limbic cortices than in eulaminate areas. Evidence that areas of different cortical types complete their development at different rates emerged recently for a limited number of prefrontal areas, demonstrating that dysgranular area 24 completes its development before area 11, and area 11 before area 46 (Rakic, 2002). Although further data are necessary, the findings are consistent with the "developmental" hypothesis of cortical types based on their laminar structure and overall neuronal density (Dombrowski et al., 2001). There is evidence that projections arise as different layers are generated, suggesting that a punctuated course of development of prefrontal areas can explain the graded laminar distribution of projections for ipsilateral (Barbas & Rempel-Clower, 1997) as well as contralateral projections (Barbas et al., 2005a). At the behavioral level, cognitive abilities that rely on the orbitofrontal cortex develop earlier than those dependent on lateral prefrontal areas (Goldman-Rakic et al., 1983). Developmental differences among the structurally distinct prefrontal areas could help explain the varied symptomatology of diseases of developmental origin, including schizophrenia, some forms of epilepsy and autism.

9 Conclusion

The prefrontal cortex has lateral, medial, and orbitofrontal sectors characterized by differences in their principal connections, their topography and laminar patterns. These cortices also differ in structure, a feature that is key in understanding their connections and laminar distributions, their interface with excitatory and inhibitory systems, and sequence of processing in their collaborative functions in behavior. Through their robust connections with early-processing sensory cortices, eulaminate areas may extract the essential features of the environment, whereas the limbic areas provide information about the emotional context. Limbic and eulaminate prefrontal areas are intricately linked according to rules based on their structure, and their interaction appears to be necessary to accomplish even simple tasks. Disconnection of pathways linking eulaminate areas associated with cognitive processes from limbic areas associated with motivation and emotion may be at the root of a number of psychiatric diseases. The structure of different types of prefrontal cortices likely emerges as a consequence of punctuated developmental events, an idea that has specific implications for diseases of developmental origin and wide implications for the development of structurally distinct cortices in evolution.

Acknowledgments

I thank my collaborators who contributed to the original papers cited in this review, Piro Lera for help with the figures, and Lainie Posecion, Ola Alade, Marcia Feinberg and Karen Trait for technical assistance. This work was supported by NIH grants from NINDS and NIMH.

REFERENCES

Adolphs, R., Tranel, D. & Damasio, A. R. (1998). The human amygdala in social judgment. *Nature*, **393**, 470–4.

Adolphs, R., Tranel, D., Damasio, H. & Damasio, A. (1994). Impaired recognition of emotion in facial expressions following bilateral damage to the human amygdala. *Nature*, **372**, 669–72.

Aggleton, J. P., Burton, M. J. & Passingham, R. E. (1980). Cortical and subcortical afferents to the amygdala of the rhesus monkey (*Macaca mulatta*). *Brain Research*, **190**, 347–68.

Alexander, G. E., Delong, M. R. & Strick, P. L. (1986). Parallel organization of functionally segregated circuits linking basal ganglia and cortex. *Annual Review of Neuroscience*, **9**, 357–81.

Alexander, M. P. & Freedman, M. (1984). Amnesia after anterior communicating artery aneurysm rupture. *Neurology*, **34**, 752–7.

Alexander, G. E. & Fuster, J. M. (1973). Effects of cooling prefrontal cortex on cell firing in the nucleus medialis dorsalis. *Brain Research*, **61**, 93–105.

Alheid, G. F., Heimer, L. & Switzer, R. C. III. (1990). Basal ganglia. In *The Human Nervous System*, ed. G. Paxinos. San Diego: Academic Press, pp. 483–582.

Amaral, D. G. (2002). The primate amygdala and the neurobiology of social behavior: implications for understanding social anxiety. *Biological Psychiatry*, **51**, 11–17.

Amaral, D. G., Insausti, R., Zola-Morgan, S., Squire, L. R. & Suzuki, W. A. (1990). The perirhinal and parahippocampal cortices and medial temporal lobe memory function. In *Vision, Memory, and the Temporal Lobe* eds. E. Iwai and M. Mishkin. New York: Elsevier Science Publishing Co., Inc., pp. 149–161.

Amaral, D. G. & Price, J. L. (1984). Amygdalo-cortical projections in the monkey (Macaca fascicularis). *The Journal of Comparative Neurology*, **230**, 465–96.

Anderson, M. E. (2001). Pallidal and cortical detriments of thalamic activity. In *Basal Ganglia and Thalamus in Health and Movement Disorders*, ed. K. Kultas-Ilinsky and I. A. Ilinsky. New York: Kluwer Academic/Plenum Publishers, pp. 93–104.

Asanuma, C., Andersen, R. A. & Cowan, W. M. (1985). The thalamic relations of the caudal inferior parietal lobule and the lateral prefrontal cortex in monkeys: Divergent cortical projections from cell clusters in the medial pulvinar nucleus. *The Journal of Comparative Neurology*, **241**, 357–81.

Bachevalier, J., Meunier, M., Lu, M. X. & Ungerleider, L. G. (1997). Thalamic and temporal cortex input to medial prefrontal cortex in rhesus monkeys. *Experimental Brain Research*, **115**, 430–44.

Bachevalie, J. & Mishkin, M. (1986). Visual recognition impairment follows ventromedial but not dorsolateral prefrontal lesions in monkeys. *Behavioral Brain Research*, **20**, 249–61.

Baimbridge, K.G., Celio, M.R. & Rogers, J.H. (1992). Calcium-binding proteins in the nervous system. *Trends in Neuroscience*, **15**, 303–8.

Baleydier, C. & Mauguiere, F. (1980). The duality of the cingulate gyrus in monkey. Neuroanatomical study and functional hypothesis. *Brain*, **103**, 525–54.

Barbas, H. (1986). Pattern in the laminar origin of corticocortical connections. *The Journal of Comparative Neurology*, **252**, 415–22.

Barbas, H. (1988). Anatomic organization of basoventral and mediodorsal visual recipient prefrontal regions in the rhesus monkey. *The Journal of Comparative Neurology*, **276**, 313–42.

Barbas, H. (1992). Architecture and cortical connections of the prefrontal cortex in the rhesus monkey. In *Advances in Neurology*, Vol. 57, ed. P. Chauvel, A.V. Delgado-Escueta, E. Halgren and J. Bancaud. New York: Raven Press, Ltd., pp. 91–115.

Barbas, H. (1993). Organization of cortical afferent input to orbitofrontal areas in the rhesus monkey. *Neuroscience*, **56**, 841–64.

Barbas, H. (1995). Anatomic basis of cognitive-emotional interactions in the primate prefrontal cortex. *Neuroscience and Biobehavioral Reviews*, **19**, 499–510.

Barbas, H. (1997). Two prefrontal limbic systems: Their common and unique features. In *The Association Cortex: Structure and Function*, ed. H. Sakata, A. Mikami and J.M. Fuster. Amsterdam: Harwood Academic Publ, pp. 99–115.

Barbas, H. (2000). Complementary role of prefrontal cortical regions in cognition, memory and emotion in primates. *Advances in Neurology*, **84**, 87–110.

Barbas, H. & Blatt, G.J. (1995). Topographically specific hippocampal projections target functionally distinct prefrontal areas in the rhesus monkey. *Hippocampus*, **5**, 511–33.

Barbas, H. & De Olmos, J. (1990). Projections from the amygdala to basoventral and mediodorsal prefrontal regions in the rhesus monkey. *The Journal of Comparative Neurology*, **301**, 1–23.

Barbas, H., Ghashghaei, H., Dombrowsk, S.M. & Rempel-Clower, N.L. (1999). Medial prefrontal cortices are unified by common connections with superior temporal cortices and distinguished by input from memory-related areas in the rhesus monkey. *The Journal of Comparative Neurology*, **410**, 343–67.

Barbas, H., Ghashghaei, H., Rempel-Clower, N. & Xiao, D. (2002). Anatomic basis of functional specialization in prefrontal cortices in primates. In *Handbook of Neuropsychology*, ed. J. Grafman. Amsterdam: Elsevier Science B.V., pp. 1–27.

Barbas, H., Henion, T.H. & Dermon, C.R. (1991). Diverse thalamic projections to the prefrontal cortex in the rhesus monkey. *The Journal of Comparative Neurology*, **313**, 65–94.

Barbas, H. & Hilgetag, C.C. (2002). Rules relating connections to cortical structure in primate prefrontal cortex. *Neurocomputing*, **44–46**, 301–8.

Barbas, H., Hilgetag, C.C., Saha, S., Dermon, C.R. & Suski, J.L. (2005a). Parallel organization of contralateral and ipsilateral prefrontal cortical projections in the rhesus monkey. *BioMed Central Neuroscience*, **6**, 32.

Barbas, H., Medalla, M., Alade, O., *et al.* (2005b). Relationship of prefrontal connections to inhibitory systems in superior temporal areas in the rhesus monkey. *Cerebral Cortex,* **15**, 1356–70.

Barbas, H. & Mesulam, M.M. (1981). Organization of afferent input to subdivisions of area 8 in the rhesus monkey. *The Journal of Comparative Neurology,* **200**, 407–31.

Barbas, H. & Mesulam, M.M. (1985). Cortical afferent input to the principalis region of the rhesus monkey. *Neuroscience,* **15**, 619–37.

Barbas, H. & Pandya, D.N. (1987). Architecture and frontal cortical connections of the premotor cortex (area 6) in the rhesus monkey. *The Journal of Comparative Neurology,* **256**, 211–18.

Barbas, H. & Pandya, D.N. (1989). Architecture and intrinsic connections of the prefrontal cortex in the rhesus monkey. *The Journal of Comparative Neurology,* **286**, 353–75.

Barbas, H. & Rempel-Clower, N. (1997). Cortical structure predicts the pattern of corticocortical connections. *Cerebral Cortex,* **7**, 635–46.

Barbas, H., Saha, S., Rempel-Clower, N. & Ghashghaei, T. (2003). Serial pathways from primate prefrontal cortex to autonomic areas may influence emotional expression. *BioMed Central Neuroscience,* **4**, 25.

Barris, R.W. & Schuman, H.R. (1953.) Bilateral anterior cingulate gyrus lesions. Syndrome of the anterior cingulate gyri. *Neurology,* **3**, 44–52.

Bauer, R.H. & Fuster, J.M. (1976). Delayed-matching and delayed-response deficit from cooling dorsolateral prefrontal cortex in monkeys. *Journal of Comparative Physiology and Psychology,* **90**, 299–302.

Bauman, M.D., Lavenex, P., Mason, W.A., Capitanio, J.P. & Amaral, D.G. (2004). The development of mother-infant interactions after neonatal amygdala lesions in rhesus monkeys. *Journal of Neuroscience,* **24**, 711–21.

Baxter, M.G., Parker, A., Lindner, C.C., Izquierdo, A.D. & Murray, E.A. (2000). Control of response selection by reinforcer value requires interaction of amygdala and orbital prefrontal cortex. *Journal of Neuroscience,* **20**, 4311–19.

Bechara, A., Damasio, H., Damasio, A.R. & Lee, G.P. (1999). Different contributions of the human amygdala and ventromedial prefrontal cortex to decision-making. *Journal of Neuroscience,* **19**, 5473–81.

Bechara, A., Tranel, D., Damasio, H. & Damasio, A.R. (1996). Failure to respond autonomically to anticipated future outcomes following damage to prefrontal cortex. *Cerebral Cortex,* **6**, 215–25.

Bisley, J.W. & Goldberg, M.E. (2003). The role of the parietal cortex in the neural processing of saccadic eye movements. *Advances in Neurology,* **93**, 141–57.

Boussaoud, D., Ungerleider, L.G. & Desimone, R. (1990). Pathways for motion analysis: Cortical connections of the medial superior temporal and fundus of the superior temporal visual areas in the macaque. *The Journal of Comparative Neurology,* **296**, 462–95.

Broca, P. (1878). Anatomie compareé des enconvolutions cérébrales: Le grand lobe limbique et la scissure limbique dans la serie des mammifères. *Revue Anthropologique,* **1**, 385–498.

Brodmann, K. (1905). Beitrage zur histologischen lokalisation der Grosshirnrinde. III. Mitteilung: Die Rindenfelder der niederen Affen. *Journal of Psychology and Neurology,* **4**, 177–266.

Brodmann, K. (1909). *Vergleichende Lokalizationslehre der Grosshirnrinde in ihren Prinizipien dargestelt auf Grund des Zellenbaues.* Leipzig: Barth.

Buge, A., Escourolle, R., Rancurel, G. & Poisson, M. (1975). Akinetic mutism and bicingular softening. 3 anatomo-clinical cases. *Revue Neurologique (Paris),* **131**, 121–31.

Carmichael, S. T., Clugnet, M.-C. & Price, J. L. (1994). Central olfactory connections in the macaque monkey. *The Journal of Comparative Neurology,* **346**, 403–34.

Carmichael, S. T. & Price, J. L. (1995a). Limbic connections of the orbital and medial prefrontal cortex in macaque monkeys. *The Journal of Comparative Neurology,* **363**, 615–41.

Carmichael, S. T. & Price, J. L. (1995b). Sensory and premotor connections of the orbital and medial prefrontal cortex of macaque monkeys. *The Journal of Comparative Neurology,* **363**, 642–64.

Carmichael, S. T. & Price, J. L. (1996). Connectional networks within the orbital and medial prefrontal cortex of macaque monkeys. *The Journal of Comparative Neurology,* **371**, 179–207.

Castro-Alamancos, M. A. & Connors, B. W. (1997). Thalamocortical synapses. *Progress in Neurobiology,* **51**, 581–606.

Cavada, C., Company, T., Tejedor, J., Cruz-Rizzolo, R. J. & Reinoso-Suarez, F. (2000). The anatomical connections of the macaque monkey orbitofrontal cortex. A review. *Cerebral Cortex,* **10**, 220–42.

Chao, L. L. & Knight, R. T. (1997a). Age-related prefrontal alterations during auditory memory. *Neurobiology of Aging,* **18**, 87–95.

Chao, L. L. & Knight, R. T. (1997b). Prefrontal deficits in attention and inhibitory control with aging. *Cerebral Cortex,* **7**, 63–9.

Chao, L. L. & Knight, R. T. (1998). Contribution of human prefrontal cortex to delay performance. *Journal of Cognitive Neuroscience,* **10**, 167–77.

Chavis, D. A. & Pandya, D. N. (1976). Further observations on corticofrontal connections in the rhesus monkey. *Brain Research,* **117**, 369–86.

Chiba, T., Kayahara, T. & Nakano, K. (2001). Efferent projections of infralimbic and pre-limbic areas of the medial prefrontal cortex in the Japanese monkey, *Macaca fuscata. Brain Research,* **888**, 83–101.

Cicerone, K. D. & Tanenbau, L. N. (1997). Disturbance of social cognition after traumatic orbitofrontal brain injury. *Archives of Clinical Neuropsychology,* **12**, 173–88.

Colby, C. L. & Goldberg, M. E. (1999). Space and attention in parietal cortex. *Annual Review of Neuroscience,* **22**, 319–49.

Conde, F., Lund, J. S., Jacobowitz, D. M., Baimbridge, K. G. & Lewis, D. A. (1994). Local circuit neurons immunoreactive for calretinin, calbindin D-28k or parvalbumin in monkey prefrontal cortex: distribution and morphology. *The Journal of Comparative Neurology,* **341**, 95–116.

Crowell, R. M. & Morawetz, R. B. (1977). The anterior communicating artery has significant branches. *Stroke,* **8**, 272–3.

D'Esposito, M., Alexander, M.P., Fischer, R., McGlinchey-Berroth, R. & O'Connor, M. (1996). Recovery of memory and executive function following anterior communicating artery aneurysm rupture. *Journal of the International Neuropsychological Society*, **2**, 565–70.

Damasio, A.R. (1994). *Descarte's Error: Emotion, Reason, and the Human Brain*. New York: G.P. Putnam's Sons.

Damasio, H., Grabowski, T., Frank, R., Galaburda, A.M. & Damasio, A.R. (1994). The return of Phineas Gage: clues about the brain from the skull of a famous patient. *Science*, **264**, 1102–5.

Davis, M. (1992). The role of the amygdala in fear and anxiety. *Annual Revue of Neuroscience*, **15**, 353–75.

De Lima, A.D., Voigt, T. & Morrison, J.H. (1990). Morphology of the cells within the inferior temporal gyrus that project to the prefrontal cortex in the macaque monkey. *The Journal of Comparative Neurology*, **296**, 159–72.

De Olmos, J. (1990). Amygdaloid nuclear gray complex. In *The Human Nervous System*, ed. G. Paxinos. San Diego: Academic Press, Inc., pp. 583–710.

DeFelipe, J., Hendry, S.H., Hashikawa, T., Molinari, M. & Jones, E.G. (1990). A microcolumnar structure of monkey cerebral cortex revealed by immunocytochemical studies of double bouquet cell axons. *Neuroscience*, **37**, 655–73.

DeFelipe, J., Hendry, S.H. & Jones, E.G. (1989a). Synapses of double bouquet cells in monkey cerebral cortex visualized by calbindin immunoreactivity. *Brain Research*, **503**, 49–54.

DeFelipe, J., Hendry, S.H. & Jones, E.G. (1989b). Visualization of chandelier cell axons by parvalbumin immunoreactivity in monkey cerebral cortex. *Proceedings of the National Academy of Science, U.S.A.*, **86**, 2093–7.

Dermon, C.R. & Barbas, H. (1994). Contralateral thalamic projections predominantly reach transitional cortices in the rhesus monkey. *The Journal of Comparative Neurology*, **344**, 508–31.

Distler, C., Boussaoud, D., Desimone, R. & Ungerleider, L.G. (1993). Cortical connections of inferior temporal area TEO in macaque monkeys. *The Journal of Comparative Neurology*, **334**, 125–50.

Dombrowski, S.M. & Barbas, H. (1998). Distinction of prefrontal architectonic areas using stereologic procedures. *Neuroscience Abstracts*, **24**, 1163.

Dombrowski, S.M., Hilgetag, C.C. & Barbas, H. (2001). Quantitative architecture distinguishes prefrontal cortical systems in the rhesus monkey. *Cerebral Cortex*, **11**, 975–88.

Douglas, R.J., Martin, K.A. & Whitteridge, D. (1991). An intracellular analysis of the visual responses of neurones in cat visual cortex. *Journal of Physiology (London)*, **440**, 659–96.

Dum, R.P. & Strick, P.L. (1991). The origin of corticospinal projections from the premotor areas in the frontal lobe. *Journal of Neuroscience*, **11**, 667–89.

Felleman, D.J. & Van Essen, D.C. (1991). Distributed hierarchical processing in the primate cerebral cortex. *Cerebral Cortex*, **1**, 1–47.

Freedman, L.J., Insel, T.R. & Smith, Y. (2000). Subcortical projections of area 25 (subgenual cortex) of the macaque monkey. *The Journal of Comparative Neurology*, **421**, 172–88.

Funahashi, S., Bruce, C. J. & Goldman-Rakic, P. S. (1990). Visuospatial coding in primate prefrontal neurons revealed by oculomotor paradigms. *Journal of Neurophysiology*, **63**, 814–31.

Funahashi, S., Bruce, C. J. & Goldman-Rakic, P. S. (1991) Neuronal activity related to saccadic eye movements in the monkey's dorsolateral prefrontal cortex. *Journal of Neurophysiology*, **65**, 1464–83.

Fuster, J. M. (1989). *The Prefrontal Cortex*. New York: Raven Press.

Fuster, J. M. (1993). Frontal lobes. *Current Opinions in Neurobiology*, **3**, 160–5.

Gabbott, P. L. & Bacon, S. J. (1996). Local circuit neurons in the medial prefrontal cortex (areas 24a, b,c, 25 and 32) in the monkey: II. Quantitative areal and laminar distributions. *The Journal of Comparative Neurology*, **364**, 609–36.

Gabbott, P. L., Jays, P. R. & Bacon, S. J. (1997). Calretinin neurons in human medial prefrontal cortex (areas 24a, b,c, 32', and 25). *The Journal of Comparative Neurology*, **381**, 389–410.

Galea, M. P. & Darian-Smith, I. (1994). Multiple corticospinal neuron populations in the macaque monkey are specified by their unique cortical origins, spinal terminations, and connections. *Cerebral Cortex*, **4**, 166–94.

Gehring, W. J. & Knight, R. T. (2002). Lateral prefrontal damage affects processing selection but not attention switching. *Brain Research. Cognitive Brain Research*, **13**, 267–79.

Ghashghaei, H. T. & Barbas, H. (2001). Neural interaction between the basal forebrain and functionally distinct prefrontal cortices in the rhesus monkey. *Neuroscience*, **103**, 593–614.

Ghashghaei, H. T. & Barbas, H. (2002). Pathways for emotions: Interactions of prefrontal and anterior temporal pathways in the amygdala of the rhesus monkey. *Neuroscience*, **115**, 1261–79.

Gilbert, C. D. & Kelly, J. P. (1975). The projections of cells in different layers of the cat's visual cortex. *The Journal of Comparative Neurology*, **163**, 81–105.

Goldman-Rakic, P. S. (1987). Motor control function of the prefrontal cortex. *Ciba Foundation Symposium*, **132**, 187–200.

Goldman-Rakic, P. S. (1988). Topography of cognition: Parallel distributed networks in primate association cortex. *Annual Review of Neuroscience*, **11**, 137–56.

Goldman-Rakic, P. S., Isseroff, A., Schwartz, M. L. & Bugbee, N. M. (1983). The neurobiology of cognitive development. In *Handbook of Child Psychology: Biology and Infancy Development*, ed. P. Mussen. New York: Wiley, pp. 281–344.

Goldman-Rakic, P. S., Lidow, M. S. & Gallager, D. W. (1990). Overlap of domaminergic, adrenergic, and serotoninergic receptors and complementarity of their subtypes in primate prefrontal cortex. *Journal of Neuroscience*, **10**, 2125–38.

Goldman-Rakic, P. S. & Porrino, L. J. (1985). The primate mediodorsal (MD) nucleus and its projection to the frontal lobe. *The Journal of Comparative Neurology*, **242**, 535–60.

Gower, E. C. (1989). Efferent projections from limbic cortex of the temporal pole to the magnocellular medial dorsal nucleus in the rhesus monkey. *The Journal of Comparative Neurology*, **280**, 343–58.

Grant, S. & Hilgetag, C.-C. (2004). Structural model explains laminar origins of projections in cat visual cortex. *Neuroscience Abstracts*, **30**, 300.9.

Graybiel, A. M. (2000). The basal ganglia. *Current Biolology*, **10**, R509–R511.

Graybiel, A. M., Aosaki, T., Flaherty, A. W. & Kimura, M. (1994). The basal ganglia and adaptive motor control. *Science*, **265**, 1826–31.

Haber, S. & McFarland, N. R. (2001). The place of the thalamus in frontal cortical-basal ganglia circuits. *The Neuroscientist*, **7**, 315–24.

Hasegawa, R. P., Blitz, A. M. & Goldberg, M. E. (2004). Neurons in monkey prefrontal cortex whose activity tracks the progress of a three-step self-ordered task. *Journal of Neurophysiology*, **92**, 1524–35.

Heckers, S. (1997). Neuropathology of schizophrenia: cortex, thalamus, basal ganglia, and neurotransmitter-specific projection systems. *Schizophrenia Bulletin*, **23**, 403–21.

Heckers, S. & Konradi, C. (2002). Hippocampal neurons in schizophrenia. *Journal of Neural Transmission*, **109**, 891–905.

Heffner, H. E. & Heffner, R. S. (1986). Effect of unilateral and bilateral auditory cortex lesions on the discrimination of vocalizations by Japanese macaques. *Journal of Neurophysiology*, **56**, 683–701.

Heizmann, C. W. (1992). Calcium-binding proteins: Basic concepts and clinical implications. *General Physiology and Biophysics*, **11**, 411–25.

Hendry, S. H. C., Jones, E. G., Emson, P. C., *et al.* (1989). Two classes of cortical GABA neurons defined by differential calcium binding protein immunoreactivities. *Experimental Brain Research*, **76**, 467–72.

Herzog, A. G. & Van Hoesen, G. W. (1976). Temporal neocortical afferent connections to the amygdala in the rhesus monkey. *Brain Research*, **115**, 57–69.

Hikosaka, O., Nakahara, H., Rand, M. K., *et al.* (1999). Parallel neural networks for learning sequential procedures. *Trends in Neurosciences*, **22**, 464–71.

Hikosaka, K. & Watanabe, M. (2000). Delay activity of orbital and lateral prefrontal neurons of the monkey varying with different rewards. *Cerebral Cortex*, **10**, 263–71.

Hilgetag, C. C., O'Neill, M. A. & Young, M. P. (1996). Indeterminate organization of the visual system. *Science* **271**, 776–7.

Hof, P. R., Glezer, I. I., Conde, F., *et al.* (1999). Cellular distribution of the calcium-binding proteins parvalbumin, calbindin, and calretinin in the neocortex of mammals: phylogenetic and developmental patterns. *Journal of Chemical Neuroanatomy*, **16**, 77–116.

Hof, P. R., Nimchinsky, E. A. & Morrison, J. H. (1995). Neurochemical phenotype of corticocortical connections in the macaque monkey: Quantitative analysis of a subset of neurofilament protein-immunoreactive projection neurons in frontal, parietal, temporal, and cingulate cortices, *The Journal of Comparative Neurology*, **362**, 109–33.

Hollerman, J. R., Tremblay, L. & Schultz, W. (2000). Involvement of basal ganglia and orbitofrontal cortex in goal-directed behavior. In *Progress in Brain Research*, ed. H. B. M. Uylings, C. G. van Eden, J. P. C. De Bruin, M. G. P. Feenstra and C. M. A. Pennartz. Paris: Elsevier Science, pp. 193–215.

Huerta, M. F., Krubitzer, L. A. & Kaas, J. H. (1987). Frontal eye field as defined by intracortical microstimulation in squirrel monkeys, owl monkeys, and Macaque monkeys II. Cortical connections. *The Journal of Comparative Neurology*, **265**, 332–61.

Hutchins, K. D., Martino, A. M. & Strick, P. L. (1988). Corticospinal projections from the medial wall of the hemisphere. *Experimental Brain Research*, **71**, 667–72.

Ilinsky, I. A., Jouandet, M. L. & Goldman-Rakic, P. S. (1985). Organization of the nigrothalamocortical system in the rhesus monkey. *The Journal of Comparative Neurology,* **236**, 315–30.

Insausti, R. & Munoz, M. (2001). Cortical projections of the non-entorhinal hippocampal formation in the cynomolgus monkey (Macaca fascicularis). *European Journal of Neuroscience,* **14**, 435–51.

Jacobsen, C. F. (1936). Studies of cerebral function in primates: I. The functions of the frontal association area in monkeys. *Computational Psychology Monographs,* **13**, 3–60.

Jacobson, S., Butters, N. & Tovsky, N. J. (1978). Afferent and efferent subcortical projections of behaviorally defined sectors of prefrontal granular cortex. *Brain Research,* **159**, 279–96.

Jacobson, S. & Trojanowski, J. Q. (1975). Amygdaloid projections to prefrontal granular cortex in rhesus monkey demonstrated with horseradish peroxidase. *Brain Research,* **100**, 132–9.

Jacobson, S. & Trojanowski, J. Q. (1977). Prefrontal granular cortex of the rhesus monkey I. Intrahemispheric cortical afferents. *Brain Research,* **132**, 209–33.

Jones, E. G. (1985). *The Thalamus.* New York: Plenum Press.

Jones, E. G. (2002). Thalamic organization and function after Cajal. *Progress in Brain Research,* **136**, 333–57.

Jones, E. G. & Powell, T. P. S. (1970). An anatomical study of converging sensory pathways within the cerebral cortex. *Brain,* **93**, 793–820.

Jones, E. G. & Wise, S. P. (1977). Size, laminar and columnar distribution of efferent cells in the sensory-motor cortex of monkeys. *The Journal of Comparative Neurology,* **175**, 391–438.

Jongen-Relo, A. L. & Amaral, D. G. (1998). Evidence for a GABAergic projection from the central nucleus of the amygdala to the brainstem of the macaque monkey: a combined retrograde tracing and in situ hybridization study. *European Journal of Neuroscience,* **10**, 2924–33.

Jürgens, U. & Müller-Preuss, P. (1977). Convergent projections of different limbic vocalization areas in the squirrel monkey. *Experimental Brain Research,* **29**, 75–83.

Kawaguchi, Y. & Kubota, Y. (1997). GABAergic cell subtypes and their synaptic connections in rat frontal cortex. *Cerebral Cortex,* **7**, 476–86.

Kennard, M. A. (1945). Focal autonomic representation in the cortex and its relation to sham rage. *Journal of Neuropathology and Experimental Neurology,* **4**, 295–304.

Kievit, J. & Kuypers, H. G. J. M. (1977). Organization of the thalamo-cortical connexions to the frontal lobe in the rhesus monkey. *Experimental Brain Research,* **29**, 299–322.

Kling, A. & Steklis, H. D. (1976). A neural substrate for affiliative behavior in nonhuman primates. *Brain, Behavior and Evolution,* **13**, 216–38.

Knight, R. T., Staines, W. R., Swick, D. & Chao, L. L. (1999). Prefrontal cortex regulates inhibition and excitation in distributed neural networks. *Acta Psychologica (Amsterdam),* **101**, 159–78.

Koechlin, E., Basso, G., Pietrini, P., Panzer, S. & Grafman, J. (1999). The role of the anterior prefrontal cortex in human cognition. *Nature,* **399**, 148–51.

Kondo, H., Saleem, K. S. & Price, J. L. (2003). Differential connections of the temporal pole with the orbital and medial prefrontal networks in macaque monkeys. *The Journal of Comparative Neurology,* **465**, 499–523.

Kosaki, H., Hashikawa, T., He, J. & Jones, E. G. (1997). Tonotopic organization of auditory cortical fields delineated by parvalbumin immunoreactivity in macaque monkeys. *The Journal of Comparative Neurology*, **386**, 304–16.

Kunzle, H. (1978). An autoradiographic analysis of the efferent connections from premotor and adjacent prefrontal regions (Areas 6 and 9) in *Macaca fascicularis*. *Brain, Behavior and Evolution*, **15**, 185–234.

LeDoux, J. (1996). *The Emotional Brain*. New York: Simon & Schuster.

Lund, J. S., Lund, R. D., Hendrickson, A. E., Hunt, A. B. & Fuchs, A. F. (1976). The origin of efferent pathways from the primary visual cortex, area 17, of the macaque monkey as shown by retrograde transport of horseradish peroxidase. *The Journal of Comparative Neurology*, **164**, 287–304.

Lynch, J. C. & Graybiel, A. M. (1983). Comparison of afferents traced to the superior colliculus from the frontal eye fields and from two sub-regions of area 7 of the rhesus monkey. *Neuroscience Abstracts*, **9**, 750.

Mah, L., Arnold, M. C. & Grafman, J. (2004). Impairment of social perception associated with lesions of the prefrontal cortex. *American Journal of Psychiatry*, **161**, 1247–55.

Maioli, M. G., Squatrito, S., Galletti, C., Battaglini, P. P. & Sanseverino, E. R. (1983). Cortico-cortical connections from the visual region of the superior temporal sulcus to frontal eye field in the macaque. *Brain Research*, **265**, 294–9.

Malkova, L., Gaffan, D. & Murray, E. A. (1997). Excitotoxic lesions of the amygdala fail to produce impairment in visual learning for auditory secondary reinforcement but interfere with reinforcer devaluation effects in rhesus monkeys. *Journal of Neuroscience*, **17**, 6011–20.

Markowitsch, H. J. (1982). Thalamic mediodorsal nucleus and memory: A critical evaluation of studies in animals and man. *Neuroscience and Biobehavioral Reviews*, **6**, 351–80.

Mayberg, H. S. (2003). Modulating dysfunctional limbic-cortical circuits in depression: towards development of brain-based algorithms for diagnosis and optimised treatment. *British Medical Bulletin*, **65**, 193–207.

McFarland, N. R. & Haber, S. N. (2002). Thalamic relay nuclei of the basal ganglia form both reciprocal and nonreciprocal cortical connections, linking multiple frontal cortical areas. *Journal of Neuroscience*, **22**, 8117–32.

McGuire, P. K., Silbersweig, D. A., Wright, I., *et al.* (1995). Abnormal monitoring of inner speech: a physiological basis for auditory hallucinations. *Lancet*, **346**, 596–600.

McGuire, P. K., Silbersweig, D. A., Wright, I., *et al.* (1996). The neural correlates of inner speech and auditory verbal imagery in schizophrenia: relationship to auditory verbal hallucinations. *British Journal of Psychiatry*, **169**, 148–59.

Mesulam, M. M. (1981). A cortical network for directed attention and unilateral neglect. *Annals of Neurology* **10**, 309–25.

Mesulam, M. M. (1990). Large-scale neurocognitive networks and distributed processing for attention, language, and memory. *Annals of Neurology*, **28**, 597–613.

Mesulam, M. M. (1999). Spatial attention and neglect: parietal, frontal and cingulate contributions to the mental representation and attentional targeting of salient extrapersonal events. *Philosophical Transactions of the Royal Society of London. Series B, Biological Sciences*, **354**, 1325–46.

Middleton, F. A. & Strick, P. L. (1994). Anatomical evidence for cerebellar and basal ganglia involvement in higher cognitive function. *Science*, **266**, 458–61.

Middleton, F. A. & Strick, P. L. (2000). Basal ganglia and cerebellar loops: motor and cognitive circuits. *Brain Research, Brain Research Reviews*, **31**, 236–50.

Middleton, F. A. & Strick, P. L. (2002). Basal-ganglia 'projections' to the prefrontal cortex of the primate. *Cerebral Cortex*, **12**, 926–35.

Miller, E. K. & Cohen, J. D. (2001). An integrative theory of prefrontal cortex function. *Annual Review of Neuroscience*, **24**, 167–202.

Mitchell, I. J., Cooper, A. J. & Griffiths, M. R. (1999). The selective vulnerability of striatopallidal neurons. *Progress in Neurobiology*, **59**, 691–719.

Moga, M. M. & Gray, T. S. (1985). Peptidergic efferents from the intercalated nuclei of the amygdala to the parabrachial nucleus in the rat. *Neuroscience Letters*, **61**, 13–18.

Morecraft, R. J., Geula, C. & Mesulam, M.-M. (1992). Cytoarchitecture and neural afferents of orbitofrontal cortex in the brain of the monkey. *The Journal of Comparative Neurology*, **323**, 341–58.

Müller-Preuss, J. D., Newman, J. D. & Jürgens, U. (1980). Anatomical and physiological evidence for a relationship between the cingular vocalization area and the auditory cortex in the squirrel monkey. *Brain Research*, **202**, 307–15.

Müller-Preuss, P. & Ploog, D. (1981). Inhibition of auditory cortical neurons during phonation. *Brain Research*, **215**, 61–76.

Narr, K. L., Thompson, P. M., Szeszko, P., *et al.* (2004). Regional specificity of hippocampal volume reductions in first-episode schizophrenia. *Neuroimage*, **21**, 1563–75.

Nauta, W. J. H. (1961). Fibre degeneration following lesions of the amygdaloid complex in the monkey. *Journal of Anatomy*, **95**, 515–31.

Nauta, W. J. H. (1979). Expanding borders of the limbic system concept. In *Functional Neurosurgery*, ed. T. Rasmussen and R. Marino. New York: Raven Press, pp. 7–23.

Nelson, M. D., Saykin, A. J., Flashman, L. A. & Riordan, H. J. (1998). Hippocampal volume reduction in schizophrenia as assessed by magnetic resonance imaging: a meta-analytic study. *Archives of General Psychiatry*, **55**, 433–40.

Nielsen, J. M. & Jacobs, L. L. (1951). Bilateral lesions of the anterior cingulate gyri. *Bulletin of the Los Angeles Neurological Society*, **16**, 231–4.

Nishijo, H., Ono, T. & Nishino, H. (1988). Single neuron responses in amygdala of alert monkey during complex sensory stimulation with affective significance. *Journal of Neuroscience*, **8**, 3570–83.

Nitecka, L. & Ben Ari, Y. (1987). Distribution of GABA-like immunoreactivity in the rat amygdaloid complex. *The Journal of Comparative Neurology*, **266**, 45–55.

Ojima, H. (1994). Terminal morphology and distribution of corticothalamic fibers originating from layers 5 and 6 of cat primary auditory cortex. *Cerebral Cortex*, **4**, 646–63.

Öngur, D., An, X. & Price, J. L. (1998). Prefrontal cortical projections to the hypothalamus in macaque monkeys. *The Journal of Comparative Neurology*, **401**, 480–505.

Pandya, D. N., Seltzer, B. & Barbas, H. (1988). Input-output organization of the primate cerebral cortex. In *Comparative Primate Biology*, Vol. 4, ed. H. D. Steklis and J. Erwin. New York: Alan R. Liss, pp. 39–80.

Pandya, D. N., Van Hoesen, G. W. & Domesick, V. B. (1973). A cingulo-amygdaloid projection in the rhesus monkey. *Brain Research*, **61**, 369–73.

Papez, J. W. (1937). A proposed mechanism of emotion. *AMA Archives of Neurology and Psychiatry*, **38**, 725–43.

Pare, D. & Smith, Y. (1993a). Distribution of GABA immunoreactivity in the amygdaloid complex of the cat. *Neuroscience*, **57**, 1061–76.

Pare, D. & Smith, Y. (1993b). The intercalated cell masses project to the central and medial nuclei of the amygdala in cats. *Neuroscience*, **57**, 1077–90.

Pare, D. & Smith, Y. (1994). GABAergic projection from the intercalated cell masses of the amygdala to the basal forebrain in cats. *The Journal of Comparative Neurology*, **344**, 33–49.

Penfield, W. & Jasper, H. (1954). *Epilepsy and the Functional Anatomy of the Human Brain.* Boston: Little, Brown and Company.

Peters, A., Palay, S. L. & Webster, H. D. (1991). *The Fine Structure of the Nervous System. Neurons and their Supporting Cells.* New York: Oxford University Press.

Peters, A. & Sethares, C. (1997). The organization of double bouquet cells in monkey striate cortex. *Journal of Neurocytology*, **26**, 779–97.

Petrides, M. (1995). Impairments on nonspatial self-ordered and externally ordered working memory tasks after lesions of the mid-dorsal part of the lateral frontal cortex in the monkey. *Journal of Neuroscience*, **15**, 359–75.

Petrides, M. (1996). Lateral frontal cortical contribution to memory. *Seminars in the Neurosciences*, **8**, 57–63.

Petrides, M. & Pandya, D. N. (1988). Association fiber pathways to the frontal cortex from the superior temporal region in the rhesus monkey. *The Journal of Comparative Neurology*, **273**, 52–66.

Petrovich, G. D., Canteras, N. S. & Swanson, L. W. (2001). Combinatorial amygdalar inputs to hippocampal domains and hypothalamic behavior systems. *Brain Research. Brain Research Reviews*, **38**, 247–89.

Petrovich, G. D., Setlow, B., Holland, P. C. & Gallagher, M. (2002). Amygdalo-hypothalamic circuit allows learned cues to override satiety and promote eating. *Journal of Neuroscience*, **22**, 8748–53.

Pitkanen, A. & Amaral, D. G. (1994). The distribution of GABAergic cells, fibers, and terminals in the monkey amygdaloid complex: an immunohistochemical and in situ hybridization study. *Journal of Neuroscience*, **14**, 2200–24.

Poremba, A., Malloy, M., Saunders, R. C., *et al.* (2004). Species-specific calls evoke asymmetric activity in the monkey's temporal poles. *Nature*, **427**, 448–51.

Porrino, L. J., Crane, A. M. & Goldman-Rakic, P. S. (1981). Direct and indirect pathways from the amygdala to the frontal lobe in rhesus monkeys. *The Journal of Comparative Neurology*, **198**, 121–36.

Preuss, T. M. & Goldman-Rakic, P. S. (1987). Crossed corticothalamic and thalamocortical connections of macaque prefrontal cortex. *The Journal of Comparative Neurology*, **257**, 269–81.

Preuss, T. M. & Goldman-Rakic, P. S. (1989). Connections of the ventral granular frontal cortex of macaques with perisylvian premotor and somatosensory areas: Anatomical evidence for somatic representation in primate frontal association cortex. *The Journal of Comparative Neurology*, **282**, 293–316.

Rakic, P. (1988). Specification of cerebral cortical areas. *Science*, **241**, 170–6.

Rakic, P. (2002). Neurogenesis in adult primate neocortex: an evaluation of the evidence. *Nature Reviews. Neuroscience*, **3**, 65–71.

Rauschecker, J. P. (1998). Parallel processing in the auditory cortex of primates. *Audiology and Neuro-otology*, **3**, 86–103.

Rauschecker, J. P., Tian, B. & Hauser, M. (1995). Processing of complex sounds in the macaque nonprimary auditory cortex. *Science*, **268**, 111–14.

Ray, J. P. & Price, J. L. (1993). The organization of projections from the mediodorsal nucleus of the thalamus to orbital and medial prefrontal cortex in macaque monkeys. *The Journal of Comparative Neurology*, **337**, 1–31.

Rempel-Clower, N. L. & Barbas, H. (1998). Topographic organization of connections between the hypothalamus and prefrontal cortex in the rhesus monkey. *The Journal of Comparative Neurology*, **398**, 393–419.

Rempel-Clower, N. L. & Barbas, H. (2000). The laminar pattern of connections between prefrontal and anterior temporal cortices in the rhesus monkey is related to cortical structure and function. *Cerebral Cortex*, **10**, 851–65.

Robson, J. A. & Hall, W. C. (1975). Connections of layer VI in striate cortex of the grey squirrel (Sciurus carolinensis). *Brain Research*, **93**, 133–9.

Rockland, K. S. (1996). Two types of corticopulvinar terminations: round (type 2) and elongate (type1). *The Journal of Comparative Neurology*, **368**, 57–87.

Romanski, L. M. & LeDoux, J. E. (1992). Equipotentiality of thalamo-amygdala and thalamo-cortico-amygdala circuits in auditory fear conditioning. *Journal of Neuroscience*, **12**, 4501–9.

Rouiller, E. M. & Welker, E. (1991). Morphology of corticothalamic terminals arising from the auditory cortex of the rat: a Phaseolus vulgaris-leucoagglutinin (PHA-L) tracing study. *Hearing Research*, **56**, 179–90.

Rouiller, E. M. & Welker, E. (2000). A comparative analysis of the morphology of corticothalamic projections in mammals. *Brain Research Bulletin*, **53**, 727–41.

Saha, S., Batten, T. F. & Henderson, Z. (2000). A GABAergic projection from the central nucleus of the amygdala to the nucleus of the solitary tract: a combined anterograde tracing and electron microscopic immunohistochemical study. *Neuroscience*, **99**, 613–26.

Sandell, J. H. & Schiller, P. H. (1982). Effect of cooling area 18 on striate cortex cells in the squirrel monkey. *Journal of Neurophysiology*, **48**, 38–48.

Sato, M. & Hikosaka, O. (2002). Role of primate substantia nigra pars reticulata in reward-oriented saccadic eye movement. *Journal of Neuroscience*, **22**, 2363–73.

Schall, J. D., Morel, A., King, D. J. & Bullier, J. (1995). Topography of visual cortex connections with frontal eye field in macaque: Convergence and segregation of processing streams. *Journal of Neuroscience*, **15**, 4464–87.

Schiller, P. H. & Tehovnik, E. J. (2001). Look and see: how the brain moves your eyes about. *Progress in Brain Research*, **134**, 127–42.

Schoenbaum, G., Chiba, A. A. & Gallagher, M. (1999). Neural encoding in orbitofrontal cortex and basolateral amygdala during olfactory discrimination learning. *Journal of Neuroscience*, **19**, 1876−84.

Schultz, W., Tremblay, L. & Hollerman, J. R. (2000.) Reward processing in primate orbitofrontal cortex and basal ganglia. *Cerebral Cortex*, **10**, 272−84.

Shao, Z. & Burkhalter, A. (1999). Role of GABAB receptor-mediated inhibition in reciprocal interareal pathways of rat visual cortex. *Journal of Neurophysiology*, **81**, 1014−24.

Shipp, S. (2005). The importance of being agranular: a comparative account of visual and motor cortex. *Philosophical Transactions of the Royal Society of London. Series B, Biological Sciences*, **360**, 797−814.

Simpson, J. R., Snyder, A. Z., Gusnard, D. A. & Raichle, M. E. (2001). Emotion-induced changes in human medial prefrontal cortex: I. During cognitive task performance. *Proceedings of the National Academy of Science USA*, **98**, 683−7.

Squire, L. R. (1992). Memory and the hippocampus: A synthesis from findings with rats, monkeys, and humans. *Psychological Review*, **99**, 195−231.

Squire, L. R. & Zola-Morgan, S. (1988). Memory: Brain systems and behavior. *Trends in Neurosciences*, **11**, 170−5.

Stefanacci, L. & Amaral, D. G. (2002). Some observations on cortical inputs to the macaque monkey amygdala: an anterograde tracing study. *The Journal of Comparative Neurology*, **451**, 301−23.

Steriade, M., Jones, E. G. & McCormick, D. A. (1997). *Thalamus—Organisation and Function.* Oxford: Elsevier Science.

Szeszko, P. R., Goldberg, E., Gunduz-Bruce, H., *et al.* (2003). Smaller anterior hippocampal formation volume in antipsychotic-naive patients with first-episode schizophrenia. *American Journal of Psychiatry*, **160**, 2190−7.

Takagi, S. F. (1986). Studies on the olfactory nervous system of the old world monkey. *Progress in Neurobiology*, **27**, 195−250.

Talland, G. A., Sweet, W. H. & Ballantine, T. (1967). Amnesic syndrome with anterior communicating artery aneurysm. *Journal of Nervous and Mental Disease*, **145**, 179−92.

Toni, I., Rowe, J., Stephan, K. E. & Passingham, R. E. (2002). Changes of cortico-striatal effective connectivity during visuomotor learning. *Cerebral Cortex*, **12**, 1040−7.

Turner, B. H., Mishkin, M. & Knapp, M. (1980). Organization of the amygdalopetal projections from modality- specific cortical association areas in the monkey. *The Journal of Comparative Neurology*, **191**, 515−43.

Van Hoesen, G. W. (1981). The differential distribution, diversity and sprouting of cortical projections to the amygdala of the rhesus monkey. In *The Amygdaloid Complex*, ed. Y. Ben-Ari. Amsterdam: Elsevier/North Holland Biomedical Press, pp. 77−90.

Vogt, B. A. & Barbas, H. (1988). Structure and connections of the cingulate vocalization region in the rhesus monkey. In *The Physiological Control of Mammalian Vocalization*, ed. J. D. Newman. New York: Plenum Publ. Corp., pp. 203−25.

Vogt, B. A. & Pandya, D. N. (1987). Cingulate cortex of the rhesus monkey: II. Cortical afferents. *The Journal of Comparative Neurology*, **262**, 271−89.

Voytko, M. L. (1985). Cooling orbital frontal cortex disrupts matching-to-sample and visual discrimination learning in monkeys. *Physiological Psychology*, **13**, 219–29.

Wallis, J. D. & Miller, E. K. (2003). Neuronal activity in primate dorsolateral and orbital prefrontal cortex during performance of a reward preference task. *European Journal of Neuroscience*, **18**, 2069–81.

Webster, M. J., Bachevalier, J. & Ungerleider, L. G. (1994). Connections of inferior temporal areas TEO and TE with parietal and frontal cortex in macaque monkeys. *Cerebral Cortex*, **4**, 470–83.

Weiss, A. P., DeWitt, I., Goff, D., Ditman, T. & Heckers, S. (2005). Anterior and posterior hippocampal volumes in schizophrenia. *Schizophrenia Research*, **73**, 103–12.

Whalen, P. J., Rauch, S. L., Etcoff, N. L., *et al.* (1998). Masked presentations of emotional facial expressions modulate amygdala activity without explicit knowledge. *Journal of Neuroscience*, **18**, 411–18.

Wood, J. N. (2003). Social cognition and the prefrontal cortex. *Behavioral and Cognitive Neuroscience Reviews*, **2**, 97–114.

Xiao, D. & Barbas, H. (2002). Pathways for emotions and memory II: afferent input to the anterior thalamic nuclei from prefrontal, temporal, hypothalamic areas and the basal ganglia in the rhesus monkey. *Thalamus and Related Systems*, **2**, 33–48.

Xiao, D. & Barbas, H. (2004). Circuits through prefrontal cortex, basal ganglia, and ventral anterior nucleus map pathways beyond motor control. *Thalamus and Related Systems*, **2**, 325–43.

Yakovlev, P. I. (1948). Motility, behavior and the brain: Stereodynamic organization and neurocoordinates of behavior. *Journal of Nervous and Mental Disease*, **107**, 313–35.

Yeterian, E. H. & Pandya, D. N. (1988). Corticothalamic connections of paralimbic regions in the rhesus monkey. *The Journal of Comparative Neurology*, **269**, 130–46.

Young, M. P. (1992). Objective analysis of the topological organization of the primate cortical visual system. *Nature*, **358**, 152–5.

Zald, D. H. & Kim, S. W. (1996). Anatomy and function of the orbital frontal cortex, I: anatomy, neurocircuitry; and obsessive-compulsive disorder. *The Journal of Neuropsychiatry and Clinical Neurosciences*, **8**, 125–38.

Zola-Morgan, S. & Squire, L. R. (1993). Neuroanatomy of memory. *Annual Review of Neuroscience*, **16**, 547–63.

Human prefrontal cortex: processes and representations

Jordan Grafman

1 Introduction

The purpose of this chapter is to familiarize you with a variety of contemporary approaches that place the function(s) of the prefrontal cortex in a cognitive context. Obviously, without a context, interpreting findings from single research studies can be difficult. In addition, without a context, it can be difficult to know whether a specific line of research is clearly verifying or rejecting a proposed prefrontal cortex (PFC) function. Finally, as with posterior cerebral cortex functions, it is much easier to see how a particular cognitive component functions within a system if you have an overall context to place that component in. The broad cognitive context that needs to be articulated is one that explains the cognitive commonality between, and the neural mechanisms shared by, higher cognitive functions. Through evolution, humans have acquired "higher" cognitive skills such as language, abstract reasoning, planning, and complex social behavior. Evidence from lesion and neuroimaging research indicates that the PFC mediates the key components composing these higher cognitive skills. A number of theories have been proposed for how the PFC might achieve this. Although many of these theories focus on the types of "processes" that the PFC carries out, an alternative point of view emphasizes the nature of long-term representations stored in the PFC. This chapter reviews both of these approaches although I place more weight on the representational approach, partly because it has been dominated by the process approach to date and partly because it is the view I espouse. Although it is clear that the PFC is important for higher cognitive skills, particularly in humans, how it supports these functions is unknown. Although the human PFC is not necessarily larger than that of other primate species (Semendeferi *et al.*, 2002), its neural architecture is likely to be more sophisticated or organized differently to accommodate higher cognitive functions that are superior to those of related species (Rilling & Insel, 1999; Semendeferi *et al.*, 2001).

As noted above, researchers have proposed a number of theories of PFC function, many of which center around the representations or processes that are mediated by PFC. A representation can be defined as a long-term memory that is localized in a neural network, that when activated, enables a person access to this stored memory. Processes, on the other hand, are computational procedures or algorithms that are localized in neural networks but are independent of the nature, content, or modality of the stimulus being processed. From a representational viewpoint, processes can be redefined as a set of representations that remain activated over a period of time (and thus give the false impression of a process). For the purpose of this chapter, I will adapt the five minimum criteria that Wood and Grafman (2003) believed a theory should meet if it is to provide a useful framework for the understanding of PFC function(s).

First, it must be explicit about the information stored in the PFC. Does it store information akin to a memory function (representational approach)? Does it store algorithms or computational procedures only for manipulating information stored elsewhere in the brain (processing approach)? Does it do a combination of these things (hybrid approach)? Second, it must be consistent with our knowledge of stimulus representation in the brain. If it is not, then the authors must have explained the inconsistency and provided evidence as to why this is valid. Third, it must be reasonable from an evolutionary perspective (as defined below). Fourth, it must make predictions that enable verification and invalidation of the model. Fifth, it must be supported by the available physiological data (neuroimaging, electrophysiology, animal and human lesion research).

To place these frameworks in context in this chapter, I first briefly describe the biology and structure of the PFC (see Barbas, this volume for a detailed look at the neuroanatomy of the frontal lobes), and introduce the competing representation and processing viewpoints. After briefly describing the primary theories of PFC function, I evaluate the extent to which they meet these criteria. Although this is not a comprehensive review, it should provide you with a reasonable overview of the range of theory-frameworks that are competing to explain PFC functions.

2 Biology, structure, and evolution of the PFC

The PFC is usually grossly divided into ventromedial and dorsolateral regions, each of which is associated with (and connected to) selective posterior and subcortical brain regions. The ventromedial PFC has reciprocal connections with brain regions associated with emotional processing (amygdala), memory (hippocampus) and higher order sensory processing (temporal visual association areas), as well as with dorsolateral PFC. The dorsolateral PFC has reciprocal connections with brain regions associated with motor control (basal ganglia, premotor cortex, supplementary motor area), performance monitoring (cingulate) and higher order sensory processing (association areas, parietal cortex). Thus the ventromedial PFC is well suited to support functions involving the integration of information about emotion, memory and environmental stimuli, and the dorsolateral PFC is well suited to support the regulation of behavior and control of responses to environmental stimuli.

Neurons in the PFC are genetically endowed to fire over extended periods of time (Levy & Goldman-Rakic, 2000) and across events (Fuster & Alexander, 1971; Bodner et al., 1996). This may be due to intrinsic neuronal mechanisms, recurrent or reentry pathway mechanisms, or a combination of these mechanisms. This suggests that the PFC has the neural machinery to maintain stimulus representations across time (Fuster et al., 2000), enabling a subject to engage in behavior to achieve long-term goals. It has also been noted that pyramidal cells in the macaque PFC are more spinous, and thus can handle more excitatory inputs than other cortical pyramidal cells (Elston, 2000). Here is a structural explanation for the PFC's ability to integrate input from many sources and implement more abstract behaviors. The monkey's PFC contains cells that respond to both internally generated and observed behavior — these have been termed mirror neurons (Gallese et al., 1996). Similar regions have been activated in humans when observing and performing actions (Gallese et al., 1996; Grafton et al., 1996). These data are suggestive of a role for the PFC in the *representation* of action in long-term memory. Furthermore, it has been shown that abnormal development of the ventromedial PFC might lead to certain forms of impaired social behavior (Williams et al., 2001) and ventromedial PFC damage later in life can cause impaired social behavior in a similar fashion, arguing for domain specificity within representational knowledge in the PFC.

It is thought that the anterior PFC evolved from motor regions and that the dorsolatereal PFC developed much later than ventromedial PFC (Fuster, 1997; Banyas, 1999). Motor regions *store* motor programs and it seems reasonable, therefore, that if the functions of the "newer" PFC regions would be related to those of older PFC regions then they too should represent information. This also suggests a role for anterior PFC in representing cognitive (as opposed to motoric) action (Fuster, 1997). Given the usually systematic nature of evolution, I believe that a dramatic shift from cortical tissue storing representations to a content-free computational function would be unlikely. Therefore I am persuaded that the PFC stores memory representations; over the course of evolution these became capable of representing more complex behaviors or behaviors that occurred over a longer period of time. While it may be possible for a processing perspective to be accounted for within the evolution of the PFC, such a perspective has not, to my knowledge, been sufficiently articulated and is, in my opinion, inconsistent with the prevalent views of the evolutionary development of the PFC and other cortical regions.

My abbreviated overview and interpretation of the exceptionally rich and contentious neuroscientific and evolutionary research on the PFC would be acceptable to the proponents of both processing and representational approaches. However, I believe that the connectivity of the PFC regions, physiological properties of its neurons, and evolutionary principles are strongly suggestive of its role in the integration of sensory and memory information and in the *representation* and control of actions/behavior. Any testable theory of PFC function should be consistent with these roles.

3　Representation versus processing

It has been suggested that "it is difficult to interpret prefrontal deficits without reference to some form of memory" and "the evolution of a capacity to guide behavior by representation of stimuli rather than by the stimuli themselves introduces the possibility that concepts and plans can govern behavior" (Goldman-Rakic, 1987). Yet, traditionally, PFC function in humans has been studied using a processing approach. The processing approach is often reduced to describing a process (e.g. "conflict resolution") without specifying whether this process is sensitive to repetition, content, or other characteristics that are associated with various forms of stimuli such as objects or words. This approach is a fundamental shift away from how cognitive neuroscientists have previously tried to understand the role of the cerebral cortex in cognition and suggests that the PFC, in contrast to posterior cortex, has little neural commitment to long-term storage of knowledge.

A representational approach, by contrast, seeks to establish the basis by which unique forms of information are stored in the PFC. This approach is much closer to how we seek to understand the functions of posterior cortex (Fuster, 1997) – similar ideas of representation have dominated the scientific understanding of face, word, and object recognition and are accepted descriptions of how features of information are stored and interrelated. In this sense, a representational point of view insists that the PFC would store certain elements of knowledge. When activated, these representations would correspond to a unique brain state that is signified by the strength and pattern of neural activity. In the PFC, a representation would be a "permanent" unit of memory that can be modified by repeated exposure to similar knowledge elements; it would be a member of a local psychological and neural network composed of multiple similar representations. Accordingly, this view would be forced to reinterpret "processes" as a set of representations that, when activated, remain activated *over a period of time* – a possibility that is supported by data regarding sustained firing by PFC neurons – and thus would appear to indicate a process. Yet, this sustained firing would enable the PFC to code, store, and retrieve the more abstract features of behaviors whose goal or end-stage would occur well after a time that exceeds the limits of consciousness in "the present" (Nichelli *et al.*, 1995; Rueckert & Grafman, 1996). Presumably, this unique capability of the PFC would result in unique representations being stored there in long-term memory that are nontransferable to other cortical regions.

An advantage of the representational approach to studying the functions of the human PFC is that it forces investigators to define in detail the nature of the memories stored in the PFC, which leads to a description of the underlying cognitive architecture that is ideally suited to hypothesis testing. Although processes can be studied by emphasizing performance-based analyses, this level of analysis is much harder to constrain theoretically. The well-known models of the functions of the PFC I review below emphasize representations or processes or are hybrids. Are they sufficient to address the five criteria outlined above as being necessary for a comprehensive theory of PFC function?

4   Adaptive coding model

The adaptive coding model (Duncan, 2001) proposes that working memory, attention, and cognitive control are supported by a common underlying process. This is due to the highly adaptable nature of PFC neurons in coding task-relevant information to provide a temporary, task-specific, context-dependent operating space. The operating space is a temporary state, as the *same neurons will code different aspects of a situation if the task or context changes and provides a mechanism for selective attention.* By selecting the inputs that are most task-relevant, the PFC focuses processing in posterior cortical regions on task-relevant representations. Duncan proposes that the flexibility of PFC neurons in coding particular types of information *might vary,* with not all neurons capable of representing all task features to the same extent. Rather, he proposes that overlapping regions of PFC are selective to different task demands. Although Duncan uses the term "representation" in reference to the PFC in his model, these representations are *temporary* and the purpose of PFC is to provide a flexible means to guide activation of representations *stored elsewhere* in the brain. This is inconsistent with our earlier definition of representations as stored memories.

This viewpoint is a processing approach but is consistent with sustained firing of PFC neurons and with a role for the PFC in selecting and integrating sensory information. It is unclear how this model fits in with neurophysiological and evolutionary ideas of action representation and memory integration within the PFC. It is also unclear how task-relevancy of information is determined (e.g. is it simply based on reward and punishment experience?) and how processing in the PFC is coordinated with that in posterior cortex and subcortical regions (although an attentional mechanism could be specified for this purpose I suppose).

Duncan's model proposes that PFC neurons should be involved in almost all tasks with little functional specialization between PFC regions — a claim that is based primarily on electrophysiological studies showing task-specific activity in a large proportion of PFC neurons across a variety of different tasks (Freedman et al., 2001) and stimulus domains (Rao et al., 1997; Rainer et al., 1998; Freedman et al., 2001). He has also analyzed neuroimaging data from 20 studies to demonstrate the involvement of specific PFC regions in a diverse collection of tasks — perception, response selection, language, memory retrieval, and problem solving (Duncan, 2001). However, a different and more comprehensive survey of 275 neuroimaging studies of PFC function (Cabeza & Nyberg, 2000) has demonstrated consistent differences in PFC localization between different broadly defined functions, such as attention, episodic memory, working memory, language, and semantic memory. Furthermore, some electrophysiological studies have demonstrated response selectivity to particular tasks (Asaad et al., 2000; Ramus & Eichenbaum, 2000; Chang et al., 2002) or stimulus types (Ramus & Eichenbaum, 2000; Kawasaki et al., 2001). Therefore, support for the adaptive coding model is mixed.

5 Attentional control model

Norman and Shallice's model of attentional control proposes the existence of two major mechanisms that monitor behavior (Norman & Shallice, 1986; Shallice & Burgess, 1998). The contention scheduler results in automatic priming of stored knowledge and the supervisory attentional system (SAS) controls the setting of priorities for action. The SAS allows conscious awareness and reflection rather than simple reflexive responses to stimuli. The SAS is localized in the PFC; however, the localization of the contention scheduler is somewhat unspecified (it has been hypothesized that basal ganglia structures could mediate contention scheduling). The SAS can override the contention scheduler when necessary; for example, the ring of a telephone will cause priming of "answer the phone" behavior by the contention scheduler, but it might be appropriate for the SAS to override this if the telephone belongs to someone else. While there is some limited discussion of representation-like components, such as action schemas and memory operation packets, the attentional control model focuses on mechanistic procedures rather than information storage and therefore can be considered to be a processing theory. It is consistent with the functions of behavioral control indicated by the biology and structure of the PFC. However, it is unclear how the model relates to the integration of sensory and memory information and to the neurophysiological properties of PFC neurons, and how it fits with knowledge about the PFC's evolution.

Damage to the SAS should result in distractibility due to the retained reflexive-like behaviors controlled by the contention scheduler in the face of impaired conscious behavioral control. Although there is much evidence that damage to the PFC has these effects (Fuster, 1997; Masterman & Cummings, 1997; Dimitrov *et al.*, 1999), the model proposes that the SAS is strongly biased towards novel situations for which no behavioral template (schema) is available. This would predict that routine behavior should not be disrupted by PFC damage. Neuropsychological research has demonstrated that knowledge about routine behavior is impaired following PFC lesions (Sirigu *et al.*, 1996; Allain *et al.*, 1999) and neuroimaging research has demonstrated PFC involvement in event knowledge (Partiot *et al.*, 1996; Crozier *et al.*, 1999; Wood *et al.*, 2005). In addition, novel tasks activate anterior PFC, but overlearned tasks activate medial and slightly more posterior PFC regions (Koechlin *et al.*, 2000). These data are inconsistent with this theory's predictions.

The SAS has further been divided into subprocesses that are localized in dissociable PFC regions. These include strategy generation, episodic memory retrieval, error monitoring, problem solving, and intention generation. However, the model does not specify which regions are implicated in these processes. There is empirical evidence of different PFC regions being implicated in different processes; for example, error monitoring (anterior cingulate) (MacDonald *et al.*, 2000; Braver *et al.*, 2001; Menon *et al.*, 2001), episodic memory retrieval (dorsolateral PFC) (Wagner *et al.*, 1998; Buckner *et al.*, 1999; Rugg & Wilding, 2000), and problem solving (anterior PFC) (Baker *et al.*, 1996; Strange *et al.*, 2001; Braver & Bongiolatti, 2002). These data are consistent with the broad claims of the model. Without detailed a priori hypotheses regarding the nature of how these processes are represented in the PFC, however, experimental data will be unable to verify the Norman and Shallice model.

More recently Burgess *et al.* (2006) has suggested that the anterior part of the PFC serves as a gateway into the Norman and Shallice processing regions for newly acquired experiences.

6 Connectionist model

Burnod and colleagues proposed a connectionist model of cerebral cortex function in which the PFC is crucial for acquisition and expression of complex behavior (Burnod, 1991; Guigon et al., 1994). The model considers four levels of the cortical system (cell, module, tissue, global) that integrate learning experiences to produce a coherent functional system (Burnod, 1991). The levels have different functions: the cellular level processes information and modifies neuronal behavior; the modular level enables computation and learning within a cortical column; the tissue level activates different inputs in parallel and integrates successive learning experiences; and the global level integrates functions from different cortical regions to produce behavior. Different levels of the cortical system would be accessible to different extents by available methodologies; for example, the global and tissue levels might be well suited to neuroimaging and neuropsychological approaches, whereas the cellular and modular levels might be better suited to investigation using electrophysiology.

In this connectionist model, the PFC integrates sensory inputs and motor information; it stores information about past events; it modulates behavior on the basis of past experience, current motivation and available reinforcement; and it is important for structured learning and temporal processing. This viewpoint is *representational* and is consistent with the structure, connectivity, neurophysiology, and evolution of the PFC. However, although the model specifies a hierarchy in PFC organization, it does not elaborate on the nature of this hierarchy. Burnod proposes that units in the PFC correspond to specific sensory or motor events of a specific behavior and are selective for event sequence. Neuropsychological, electrophysiological and fMRI data showing the PFC's involvement in action and event knowledge are consistent with this perspective (Godbout & Doyon, 1995; Gallese et al., 1996; Partiot et al., 1996; Sirigu et al., 1996; Crozier et al., 1999; Murray et al., 2000; Zalla et al., 2000, 2001; Koechlin et al., 2002).

The model provides an overview of cortical function and a useful framework in which to consider the contributions of different functional levels of the cortex. However, the model is very broad and does not lend itself well to specific hypothesis testing or content analysis.

7 Structured event complex framework

The structured event complex (SEC) framework developed by my colleagues and I proposes that the PFC stores unique forms of knowledge (Grafman, 2002). We defined an SEC as a goal-oriented set of events that is structured in sequence and represents thematic knowledge, morals, abstractions, concepts, social rules, event features, event boundaries and grammars. The stored characteristics of these representations (e.g. frequency) form the bases for the strength of representation in memory and the relationships between SEC representations. A SEC is not a single stored memory but instead is viewed as the minimal set of linked subcomponents that can be "memory engine" for performing a functional activity. Thus, the subcomponents of SECs are represented independently (and stored in different PFC regions) but are encoded and retrieved as an episode. The SEC framework is a representational viewpoint that makes specific predictions regarding the properties and localization of SECs in the PFC (Wood & Grafman, 2003). Maintenance of SEC activation depends on the completion of the behavioral goal − this is consistent with sustained firing of PFC neurons, but can be interfered with by supervening goals. The SEC framework is consistent with the structure, connectivity, neurophysiology, and evolution of the PFC.

Specific predictions enable the verification or invalidation of this framework. For example, the theory predicts that different categories of SECs are stored in different regions of the PFC. The localization of different aspects or categories of SECs (e.g. social or emotional) is based on the connectivity between specific PFC and posterior cortical (temporal-parietal) or subcortical (basal ganglia, hippocampus, amygdala) regions. Consistent with this, impairment of social behavior is most evident after ventromedial PFC damage (Grafman et al., 1996; Dimitrov et al., 1999), whereas impairment of reflective, mechanistic behavior is evident following dorsolateral PFC damage (Burgess et al., 2000, Goel & Grafman, 2000). Furthermore, neuroimaging data support the existence of dissociable networks for emotional versus nonemotional (Partiot et al., 1995) and social versus nonsocial (Wood et al., 2003) SECs, and emotion-specificity of neurons in the human ventral PFC (Kawasaki et al., 2001) has been shown in an electrophysiological study. The framework also predicts that online processing of an SEC would enable a person to predict subsequent events, but damage to the PFC that limited retrieval of part or all of a SEC would lead to disruption of day-to-day behavior as individuals would have difficulty detecting behavioral and social errors or anticipating the onset of future episodes. This is supported by available evidence (Stone et al., 1998; Dimitrov et al., 1999; Gehring & Knight, 2000).

8   Guided activation theory

Miller and Cohen's influential guided activation theory proposes that the PFC stores representations of task-specific rules, attentional templates, and goals

(Freedman *et al.*, 2001). Essentially, the PFC "directs" activation to bias the activation of goal-related representations that are stored in posterior cortex. This "guided activation" of posterior representations is important in learning new rules and behaviors. Repeated activation of the same pathway creates stronger associations between them and, consequently, the role of the PFC in guiding posterior representations lessens — *the role of the PFC may be virtually nil with frequently used rules or behaviors*. Would they say the same thing about the role of the temporal-parietal cortex for frequently seen words or objects? Miller and Cohen liken the PFC's role to that of a switch operator determining which railway tracks a train will use — by the same analogy, if a train always uses the same track, then the switch operator is no longer necessary. Miller and Cohen propose that their theory is representational and is consistent with both the PFC's function of behavioral control and its connectivity with other brain regions. It is partially consistent with the evolutionary perspective, but is biased towards novel behavior. Furthermore, it is not explicit about how these novel representations are transferred to the posterior regions that store representations of well-learned behaviors.

Miller and Cohen make specific predictions on the basis of their theory. The role of the PFC is modulatory and, therefore, it should be activated *only* in conjunction with posterior cortex. In addition, PFC involvement should increase as controlled processing demands increase — this is consistent with studies of cognitive control (Frith *et al.*, 1991; MacDonald *et al.*, 2000). The prediction of the PFC's involvement only in novel behaviors is inconsistent with evidence of neural responses in the PFC to known actions (Gallese *et al.*, 1996; Grafton *et al.*, 1996). Miller and Cohen claim that the PFC is important in the integration of information across stimulus domains. The guided activation theory also predicts that learning influences representation, organization, and hence localization. This is supported by evidence of dissociable regions implicated in the representation of different stimulus attributes (Wilson *et al.*, 1993; O Scalaidhe *et al.*, 1997; Rao *et al.*, 1997). However, this evidence appears inconsistent with Miller and Cohen's assertion that localization of representations in the PFC is organized in terms of broad categories with no "modular discretely localized" forms. Rather, categories are determined by the relative strengths of competing responses with strongly asymmetric responses localized in orbitofrontal regions and symmetric/balanced responses in dorsolateral PFC. There is neuropsychological (Rolls, 1996; Anderson *et al.*, 1999; Barrash *et al.*, 2000; Bechara *et al.*, 2000), electrophysiological (Ramus & Eichenbaum, 2000; Kawasaki *et al.*, 2001), and neuroimaging (Northoff *et al.*, 2000; Berthoz *et al.*, 2002; Moll *et al.*, 2002) evidence that orbitofrontal cortex, for example, is prominently implicated in social and emotional responses and behavior. Rather than segregating the PFC on the basis of category distinctiveness, Miller and Cohen suggest that functional differences between orbitofrontal and dorsolateral PFC are, instead, due to different balances of response strength (Roberts & Wallis, 2000; Freedman *et al.*, 2001).

9 Somatic marker hypothesis

This type of framework is a more narrow one as it tries to tackle one major aspect of frontal lobe functions — the role of emotion in decision-making. Damasio and colleagues have argued that somatic markers are important in guiding behavior (Damasio, 1995, 1998). Somatic markers are stored memories of somatic states that are associated with particular behavioral experiences or outcomes — this is consistent with a representational approach. Somatic markers are stored in ventromedial PFC and enable decisions and behaviors to be selected on the basis of prior experience, even in the absence of awareness of that past experience. The ventromedial PFC is critical in the linkage of somatic markers with behavioral experience. The somatic marker hypothesis is primarily a theory of decision-making and its neurological extent within the PFC is limited to ventromedial regions. The ventromedial PFC is described as a "convergence zone" in which information from amygdala, hippocampus, and sensory regions interacts to influence behavior — this is consistent with a processing approach. As the somatic marker hypothesis has both processing and representational components, it is a hybrid of these approaches. The integration of information is consistent with the structure and connectivity of the PFC, although it is unclear how this viewpoint fits with the evolutionary development of the PFC as outlined earlier.

The somatic marker hypothesis predicts that damage to ventromedial PFC results in an impaired ability to utilize somatic markers and consequently in poor decision-making. In addition, it predicts that emotionally charged stimuli should be associated with ventromedial PFC activation and somatic responses (as indexed by changes in electrodermal activity or heart rate). There is evidence consistent with these predictions from electrophysiology (Bechara *et al.*, 1997; Dimitrov *et al.*, 1999; Kawasaki *et al.*, 2001), neuroimaging (Davidson & Irwin, 2000; Northoff *et al.*, 2000), and patients with ventromedial PFC damage (Bechara *et al.*, 1996; Anderson *et al.*, 1999; Bechara *et al.*, 2000). The somatic marker hypothesis is not intended to be a theory of PFC function in general and it would benefit from expansion to consider the functions of other PFC regions in processing social stimuli and how that processing interacts with or modulates the ventromedial PFC.

10 Temporal organization model

Fuster has proposed that the PFC temporally organizes behavior with that process constrained by short-term memory, motor attention, and the inhibitory control of interference (Fuster, 1997). In his framework, he describes mechanisms for monitoring, memory, and attentional selection that prioritize goals and ensure that behavioral sequences are performed in the correct order. Temporal integration is mediated by the activity of PFC neurons and also by interactions between the PFC and posterior cortex; the specific posterior cortical areas involved in these interactions are determined by the modalities of the sensory and motor information. Given the emphasis on attention, short-term memory, and inhibitory control, the model appears to take a processing viewpoint. However, Fuster also describes PFC function in terms of "motor memory" (schemas) with a hierarchy of motor representations within the PFC. Attention and working memory are properties of the representations (embedded within neural networks), rather than explicit "processes" in terms of computational procedures. Fuster's model is a hybrid of the representational and processing approaches and is consistent with the evolution and neurophysiology of the PFC. Motor memories stored in the PFC become more complex or abstract as the region becomes more anterior. He proposes that the functions of the ventromedial PFC parallel those of the dorsolateral PFC, but with the addition of emotional information, given the connectivity between ventromedial PFC and limbic regions (e.g. amygdala).

Fuster believes that automatic actions are stored in the basal ganglia and premotor cortex, with PFC representation reserved for actions/behaviors that are not habitual or well learned. Consistent with this viewpoint, the premotor cortex and basal ganglia are known to be important in movement preparation (Kurata, 1994; Harrington et al., 2000; Toni et al., 2001); however, the PFC has been implicated in both novel and well learned tasks (Koechlin et al., 2000; Averbeck et al., 2002). Decision-making is the result of integration of memorial, experiential, affective, and motivational inputs that select the response after resolution of competition between the available information. Thus, Fuster suggests that decision-making should be associated with networks involving anterior PFC (complex behavior), medial temporal (memory) and limbic (affect and motivation) regions. Neuroimaging studies have implicated prefrontal–parietal (Paulus et al., 2001; Rubinsztein et al., 2001), prefrontal–cingulate (Elliott & Dolan, 1998; Rubinsztein et al., 2001), and orbitofrontal–limbic

(Bechara *et al.*, 2000) networks in decision-making. Clearly, the evidence is mixed with respect to any precise neuroanatomy of decision-making, which may be partly due to the heterogeneity of the decision-making tasks used. Finally, Fuster suggests that inhibitory control of interference, irrespective of its source, is performed by orbitomedial PFC neurons. Although there is evidence consistent with a role for orbital PFC in inhibition (Cummings, 1995; Wallis *et al.*, 2001; Jentsch *et al.*, 2002), there is also evidence consistent with networks including the dorsolateral PFC and anterior cingulate being important in inhibition too (Konishi *et al.*, 1998; Garavan *et al.*, 1999; Konishi *et al.*, 1999; Casey *et al.*, 2000; Leung *et al.*, 2000; MacDonald *et al.*, 2000).

11 Working memory model

Goldman-Rakic suggested that the PFC serves as a working memory structure that keeps stimulus representations active for short periods of time (Goldman-Rakic, 1987, 1998). Her model is primarily based on neuropsychological and electrophysiological research with nonhuman primates, but she proposed that it applies also to humans. In Goldman-Rakic's view, the PFC is part of an integrated network of regions (temporal, parietal, premotor, and limbic regions) involved in the representation of stimuli in the absence of those stimuli; this enables behavior to be guided by internal representations rather than relying on the presence of external stimuli. Goldman-Rakic further proposed that the other brain regions (e.g. brain stem) modulate the PFC. Her model focuses primarily on dorsolateral PFC function, with orbitofrontal cortex implicated in behavioral regulation by maintenance of internal representations of external stimuli. However, the model does not detail what this regulation entails, other than to state that accessibility of central representations of reward and punishment is important. The working memory model is a hybrid of the processing and representational approaches and is consistent with the structure, connectivity, and neurophysiology of the PFC. It is unclear how the model fits in with the evolutionary perspective outlined earlier.

The model states that disruption of behavioral regulation by internal representations of the stimuli will lead to distractibility and perseveration. These problems have been consistently reported in patients with damage to the PFC (Godefroy & Rousseaux, 1996; Koski & Petrides, 2002) and in primates in PFC lesions (Crofts *et al.*, 2001). Goldman-Rakic noted that a variety of tasks should demonstrate impairments in individuals with immature (young children) or damaged PFC – including problems in selective attention (Stuss *et al.*, 1999; Klenberg *et al.*, 2001), response conflict (Helmstaedter *et al.*, 1998; Bunge *et al.*, 2002), processing of temporal order (Sirigu *et al.*, 1996; Allain *et al.*, 1999), planning (Goel & Grafman, 1995; Goel *et al.*, 1997; Colvin *et al.*, 2001), decomposition of a task into goals and subgoals (Goel & Grafman, 1995; Braver & Bongiolatti, 2002), and generation of new or novel responses (Burgess & Shallice, 1996). These tasks all require symbolic representations of stimuli to be maintained "online" in the absence of the stimuli themselves. The evidence is generally supportive of this position. However, there is also some evidence that selective attention may be intact following focal PFC damage (Lee *et al.*, 1999).

Goldman-Rakic proposed that different domains of knowledge representation might be localized to dissociable regions of the PFC. Although the model states that spatial representations *might* be localized to area 46, it does not specify how these representations differ from spatial representations stored in, for example, parietal cortex, where other types of knowledge are stored, nor how these domains are integrated. Inconsistent neuropsychological evidence, taken together with its topographical limitation to dorsolateral PFC, makes the working memory model an incomplete model of PFC function (see Wang, this volume, for an updated view on working memory by a prominent working memory proponent).

12   Summary and conclusions

The aim of this chapter was to briefly describe the state and range of processing and representational models of PFC function. I began by articulating five criteria that could be used to judge a theory's ability to provide a rational account of PFC function. In terms of specific approaches, the models meet this criteria to varying degrees. Those with some claim of representation are consistent with the neurophysiology, connectivity and structure of the PFC, thus providing support for the utility of the representational approach to understanding PFC function. Most models provide specific predictions that enable the testing of their position; however, the specificity of the predictions is also highly variable between models. While all the models are supported to some extent by the available cognitive neuroscience data, it is not the case that each model addresses all of the available data. For example, the somatic marker hypothesis addresses some potential functions of the ventromedial PFC, but is not intended to address any data regarding dorsolateral PFC function and thus is not inconsistent with these data. Finally, there is variability in the degree to which the models meet the evolutionary criterion. With respect to specific theories, without modification, no single theory of PFC function appears to explain all of the available data.

The processing approach dominates frameworks of the human prefrontal cortex. The notion of the prefrontal cortex as a processor is a metaphor that is in keeping with the notion that the PFC mediates executive functioning. It is a location that "controls" and "manipulates" knowledge stored elsewhere that is in a temporarily active state. This is an appealing approach at first glance but there are some outstanding questions that should be raised before adapting one or more of the frameworks. Is it true that posterior cortex is able to store all aspects of knowledge? How can a third of the cerebral cortex be limited to a few key processes? Why would it be necessary to devote such a large amount of cortical space to just a few processes? What are the biological and structural changes that occurred in the PFC that enabled it to subserve processes rather than posterior-cortex-like representations? In my view, there is compelling evidence from the psychology and artificial intelligence domains that certain forms of representation exist that are simply rarely considered in the processing frameworks including thematic knowledge, plan components, social cognition, and similar high-level knowledge. It is my view that such knowledge types would be stored in the PFC based on certain representational principles. This is a parsimonious view since it would continue the increasingly complex chain of representation that began in sensory cortices to the highest level of knowledge representation that is nearly divorced from the sensory qualities of the stimuli. In terms of general approaches, the representational approach seems to be most consistent with the neurophysiology, structure, and connectivity of the PFC — either with or without processing components. In addition, a representational approach is consistent with a modern cognitive neuroscience view of how the brain stores aspects of certain kinds of stimuli (e.g. words or objects) in posterior cortex. The representational approach forces the investigator to describe the features of the high-level representation (e.g. age when representation was first acquired, how often it is activated, its associative strength to other representations) and, by default, enables specific hypothesis testing — this enables identification of the properties influencing knowledge storage and retrieval in the normal brain. In addition, a representational approach makes simple predictions about the effects of brain damage upon the retrievability of representational knowledge (e.g. see Wood & Grafman, 2003 and Figure 3.1). So, there are questions that can be posed to the investigator who makes a representational claim about the PFC. For example, did they use normative data or otherwise have access to parametric characteristics about the stimuli they used (e.g. social strategies) so that their results allow them to claim that such stimuli are at least partially represented in PFC? I believe that the pure processing approaches are inconsistent with the neurophysiology, structure, connectivity, and evolution of the PFC, and that adapting a representational approach to understanding PFC function will prove fruitful. The representational approach does not eliminate the use of the term "process"

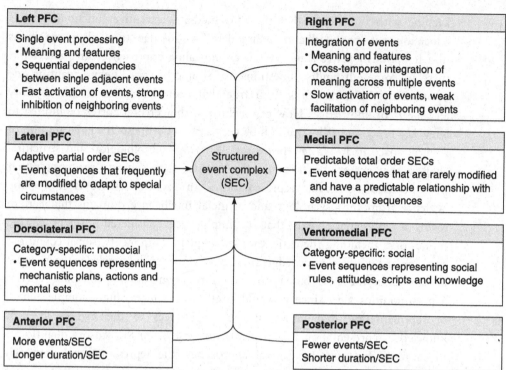

Left PFC	Right PFC
Single event processing • Meaning and features • Sequential dependencies between single adjacent events • Fast activation of events, strong inhibition of neighboring events	Integration of events • Meaning and features • Cross-temporal integration of meaning across multiple events • Slow activation of events, weak facilitation of neighboring events

Lateral PFC	Medial PFC
Adaptive partial order SECs • Event sequences that frequently are modified to adapt to special circumstances	Predictable total order SECs • Event sequences that are rarely modified and have a predictable relationship with sensorimotor sequences

Structured event complex (SEC)

Dorsolateral PFC	Ventromedial PFC
Category-specific: nonsocial • Event sequences representing mechanistic plans, actions and mental sets	Category-specific: social • Event sequences representing social rules, attitudes, scripts and knowledge

Anterior PFC	Posterior PFC
More events/SEC Longer duration/SEC	Fewer events/SEC Shorter duration/SEC

Figure 3.1   The representational forms of the SEC and their proposed localization within the prefrontal cortex. All subcomponents can contribute to the formation of an SEC, with the different subcomponents being differentially weighted in activation depending on the nature of the represented SEC and moment-by-moment behavioral demands. For example, the left anterior ventromedial prefrontal cortex (PFC) would be expected to represent a long multievent sequence of social information with specialized processing of the meaning and features of the single events within the sequence, including the computation of their sequential dependencies and primary meaning. (For a colour version of this figure, please see the colour plate section.)

to describe activation states in the PFC. In the representational approach, "processes" in cognition are a set of representations that, when activated, remain activated over a period of time (rather than the short time span required for the representations in posterior cortex to be activated to enable action or recognition). For example, in this view, working memory is simply a euphemism for the activation of a set of representations over a limited time period (see Ruchkin *et al.* [2003] for a debate on this issue). The time period itself reflects either the actual time required for the representational action to be completed or the time it takes for a compressed version of the representational action to be completed (e.g. recite a verbal description of a plan executed in real time). This is not a trivial debate since the use of the term working memory implies another component or form of memory distinct from episodic or semantic memory. In the strong representational view, there are simply two kinds of memory: representations stored in long-term memory and episodic memories formed by the temporal binding of distinct long-term memories. Given this definition, we predict that local computational procedures (which depend upon a neuronal predisposition to sustain activations within the network or reentrant pathways that allow for same sustained firing) for PFC representations are required to determine and enhance the relationship of one representation to others in the local (and distant) networks and to refine the form of the representational memory itself over time (this would be expected to occur for representations in posterior and PF cortex).

In any case, there is food for thought when considering theories of PFC function. Whether you follow the process, representational, or hybrid approach has implications for the evolution of the human brain and the role of the prefrontal cortex in that evolution. Each approach also has implications for how knowledge is stored and used by humans. Given that a strong (and ultimately revolutionary) explanation about how and why the human PFC would support only temporary processes without a knowledge base has not been offered by any of the process modelers, we think that the most parsimonious approach to understanding its role in human behavior is to explore and examine the nature of higher forms of knowledge stored as representations in the PFC.

REFERENCES

Allain, P., Le Galle, D., Etcharry-Brouyx, F., Aubin, G. & Emile, J. (1999). Mental representation of knowledge following frontal-lobe lesion: Dissociations on tasks using scripts. *Journal of Clinical and Experimental Neuropsychology*, **21**, 643–65.

Andersson, S. W., Bechara, A., Damasio, H., Tranel, D. & Damasio, A. R. (1999). Impairment of social and moral behavior related to early damage in human prefrontal cortex. *Nature*, **2**, 1032–7.

Asaad, W. F., Rainer, G. & Miller, E. K. (2000). Task-specific neural activity in the primate prefrontal cortex. *Journal of Neurophysiology*, **84**, 451–9.

Averbeck, B. B., Chafee, M. V., Crowe, D. A. & Georgopoulos, A. P. (2002). Parallel processing of serial movements in prefrontal cortex. *Proceedings of the National Academy of Science*, **99**, 13172–7.

Baker, S. C., Rogers, R. D., Owen, A. M., *et al.* (1996). Neural systems engaged by planning: A PET study of the Tower of London Task. *Neuropsychologia*, **34**, 515–26.

Banyas, C. A. (1999). Evolution and phylogenetic history of the frontal lobes. In *The Human Frontal Lobes: Functions and Disorders*, ed. B. L. Miller and J. L. Cummings. pp. 83–106. New York: Guilford Press.

Barrash, J., Tranel, D. & Anderson, S. W. (2000). Acquired personality disturbances associated with bilateral damage to the ventromedial prefrontal region. *Developmental Neuropsychology*, **18**, 355–81.

Bechara, A., Damasio, H. & Damasio, A. R. (2000). Emotion, decision making and the orbitofrontal cortex. *Cerebral Cortex*, **10**, 295–307.

Bechara, A., Damasio, H., Tranel, D. & Damasio, A. R. (1997). Deciding advantageously before knowing the advantageous strategy. *Science*, **275**, 1293–5.

Bechara, A., Tranel, D., Damasio, H. & Damasio, A. R. (1996). Failure to respond autonomically to anticipated future outcomes following damage to prefrontal cortex. *Cerebral Cortex*, **6**, 215–25.

Berthoz, S., Armony, J. L., Blair, R. J. & Dolan, R. J. (2002). An fMRI study of intentional and unintentional (embarrassing) violations of social norms. *Brain*, **125**, 1696–708.

Bodner, M., Kroger, J. & Fuster, J. M. (1996). Auditory memory cells in dorsolateral prefrontal cortex. *NeuroReport*, **7**, 1905–8.

Braver, T. S., Barch, D. M., Gray, J. R., Molfese, D. L. & Snyder, A. (2001). Anterior cingulate cortex and response conflict: Effects of frequency, inhibition and errors. *Cerebral Cortex*, **11**, 825–36.

Braver, T. S. & Bongiolatti, S. R. (2002). The role of frontopolar cortex in subgoal processing during working memory. *NeuroImage*, **15**, 523–36.

Buckner, R. L., Kelley, W. M. & Petersen, S. E. (1999). Frontal cortex contributes to human memory formation. *Nature Neuroscience*, **2**, 311–14.

Bunge, S. A., Dudukovic, N. M., Thomason, M. E., Vaidya, C. J. & Gabrieli, J. D. E. (2002). Immature frontal lobe contributions to cognitive control in children: Evidence from fMRI. *Neuron*, **33**, 301–11.

Burgess, P. W., Gilbert, S. J., Okuda, J. & Simons, J. S. (2006). Rostral prefrontal brain regions (area 10): A gateway between inner thought and the external world? In *Disorders of Volition*, ed. N. Sebanz and W. Prinz. pp. 373–395. Cambridge, MA: MIT Press.

Burgess, P. W. & Shallice, T. (1996). Response suppression, initiation and strategy use following frontal lobe lesions. *Neuropsychologia*, **34**, 263–73.

Burgess, P. W., Veitch, E., De Lacy Costello, A. & Shallice, T. (2000). The cognitive and neuroanatomical correlates of multitasking. *Neuropsychologia*, **38**, 848–63.

Burnod, Y. (1991). Organizational levels of the cerebral cortex: An integrated model. *Acta Biotheoretica*, **39**, 351–61.

Cabeza, R. & Nyberg, L. (2000). Imaging cognition II: An empirical review of 275 PET and fMRI studies. *Journal of Cognitive Neuroscience*, **12**, 1–47.

Casey, B. J., Thomas, K. M., Welsh, T. F., et al. (2000). Dissociation of response conflict, attentional selection, and expectancy with functional magnetic resonance imaging. *Proceedings of the National Academy of Science*, **97**, 8728–33.

Chang, J. Y., Chen, L., Lou, F., Shi, L. H. & Woodward, D. J. (2002). Neuronal responses in the frontal cortico-basal ganglia system during delayed matching-to-sample task: Ensemble recording in freely moving rats. *Experimental Brain Research*, **142**, 67–80.

Colvin, M. K., Dunbar, K. & Grafman, J. (2001). The effects of frontal lobe lesions on goal achievement in the water jug task. *Journal of Cognitive Neuroscience*, **13**, 1129–47.

Crofts, H. S., Dalley, J. W., Collins, P., *et al.* (2001). Differential effects of 6-OHDA lesions of the frontal cortex and caudate nucleus on the ability to acquire an attentional set. *Cerebral Cortex*, **11**, 1015–26.

Crozier, S., Sirigu, A., Lehericy, S., *et al.* (1999). Distinct prefrontal activations in processing sequence at the sentence and script level: An fMRI study. *Neuropsychologia*, **37**, 1469–76.

Cummings, J. L. (1995). Anatomic and behavioral aspects of frontal-subcortical circuits. In *Structure and Functions of the Human Prefrontal Cortex*, ed. J. Grafman, K. J. Holyoak and F. Boller. pp. 1–13. New York, NY: Academy of Sciences.

Damasio, A. R. (1995). On some functions of the human prefrontal cortex. In *Structure and Functions of the Human Prefrontal Cortex*, ed. J. Grafman, K. J. Holyoak and F. Boller. pp. 241–251. New York, NY: Academy of Sciences.

Damasio, A. R. (1998). The somatic marker hypothesis and the possible functions of the prefrontal cortex. In *The Prefrontal Cortex: Executive and Cognitive Functions*, ed. A. C. Roberts, T. W. Robbins and L. Weiskrantz. pp. 1413–1420. Oxford: Oxford University Press.

Davidson, R. J. & Irwin, W. (2000). Functional MRI in the study of emotion. In *Functional MRI*, ed. C. T. W. Moonen and P. A. Bandettini. pp. 487–499. New York: Springer-Verlag.

Dimitrov, M., Phipps, M., Zahn, T. & Grafman, J. (1999). A thoroughly modern Gage. *Neurocase*, **5**, 345–54.

Duncan, J. (2001). An adaptive coding model of neural function in prefrontal cortex. *Nature Reviews Neuroscience*, **2**, 820–9.

Elliot, R. & Dolan, R. J. (1998). Activation of different anterior cingulate foci in association with hypothesis testing and response selection. *NeuroImage*, **8**, 17–29.

Elston, G. N. (2000). Pyramidal cells of the frontal lobe: all the more spinous to think with. *Journal of Neuroscience*, **20**, RC95 (1–4).

Freedman, D. J., Riesenhuber, M., Poggio, T. & Miller, E. K. (2001). Categorical representation of visual stimuli in the primate prefrontal cortex. *Science*, **291**, 312–16.

Frith, C. D., Friston, K., Liddle, P. F. & Frackowaik, R. S. J. (1991). Willed action and the prefrontal cortex in man: A study with PET. *Proceedings of the Royal Society London, B*, **244**, 241–6.

Fuster, J. M. (1997). *The Prefrontal Cortex: Anatomy, Physiology, and Neuropsychology of the Frontal Lobe*. New York: Raven Press.

Fuster, J. M. & Alexander, G. E. (1971). Neuron activity related to short-term memory. *Science*, **173**, 652–4.

Fuster, J. M., Bodner, M. & Kroger, J. K. (2000). Cross-modal and cross-temporal association in neurons of frontal cortex. *Nature*, **405**, 347–51.

Gallese, V., Fadiga, L., Fogassi, L. & Rizzolatti, G. (1996). Action recognition in the premotor cortex. *Brain*, **119**, 593–609.

Garavan, H., Ross, T. J. & Stein, E. A. (1999). Right hemispheric dominance of inhibitory control: An event-related fMRI study. *Proceedings of the National Academy of Science USA*, **96**, 8301–6.

Gehring, W. J. & Knight, R. T. (2000). Prefrontal-cingulate interactions in action monitoring. *Nature Neuroscience*, **3**, 516–20.

Godbout, L. & Doyon, J. (1995). Mental representation of knowledge following frontal-lobe or postrolandic lesions. *Neuropsychologia*, **33**, 1671–96.

Godefroy, O. & Rousseaux, M. (1996). Divided and focused attention in patients with lesion of the prefrontal cortex. *Brain and Cognition*, **30**, 155–74.

Goel, V. & Grafman, J. (1995). Are the frontal lobes implicated in "planning" functions? Interpreting data from the Tower of Hanoi. *Neuropsychologia*, **33**, 623–42.

Goel, V. & Grafman, J. (2000). Role of the right prefrontal cortex in ill-structured planning. *Cognitive Neuropsychology*, **17**, 415–36.

Goel, V., Grafman, J., Tajik, J., Gana, S. & Danto, D. (1997). A study of the performance of patients with frontal lobe lesions in a financial planning task. *Brain*, **120**, 1805–22.

Goldman-Rakic, P. S. (1987). Circuitry of primate prefrontal cortex and regulation of behavior by representational memory. In *Handbook of Physiology: A Critical Comprehensive Presentation of Physiological Knowledge and Concepts*, ed. S. R. Geiger. pp. 374–417. Bethesda, MD: American Physiological Society.

Goldman-Rakic, P. S. (1998). The prefrontal landscape: Implications of functional architecture for understanding human mentation and the central executive. In *The Prefrontal Cortex: Executive and Cognitive Functions*, ed. A. C. Roberts, T. W. Robbins and L. Weiskrantz. pp. 87–102. Oxford: Oxford University Press.

Grafman, J. (2002). The human prefrontal cortex has evolved to represent components of structured event complexes. In *Handbook of Neuropsychology*. 2nd edn, ed. J. Grafman. Amsterdam: Elsevier.

Grafman, J., Schwab, K., Warden, D., *et al.* (1996). Frontal lobe injuries, violence, and aggression: A report of the Vietnam Head Injury Study. *Neurology*, **46**, 1231–8.

Grafton, S. T., Arbib, M. A., Fadiga, L. & Rizzolatti, G. (1996). Localization of grasp representations in humans by PET: II. Observation compared with imagination. *Experimental Brain Research*, **112**, 103–11.

Guigon, E., Grandguillaum, P., Otto, I., Boutkhil, L. & Burnod, Y. (1994). Neural network models of cortical functions based on the computational properties of the cerebral cortex. *Journal of Physiology*, **88**, 291–308.

Harrington, D. L., Rao, S. M., Haaland, K. Y., *et al.* (2000). Specialized neural systems underlying representations of sequential movements. *Journal of Cognitive Neuroscience*, **12**, 56–77.

Helmstaedter, C., Gleibner, U., Zentner, J. & Elger, C. E. (1998). Neuropsychological consequences of epilepsy surgery in frontal lobe epilepsy. *Neuropsychologia*, **36**, 681–9.

Jentsch, J. D., Olausson, P., De la Garza, R. & Taylor, J. R. (2002). Impairments of reversal learning and response perseveration after repeated intermittent cocaine administrations to monkeys. *Neuropsychopharmacology*, **26**, 183–90.

Kawasaki, H., Adolphs, R., Kaufman, O., *et al.* (2001). Single-neuron responses to emotional visual stimuli recorded in the human ventral prefrontal cortex. *Nature Neuroscience*, **4**, 15–16.

Klenberg, L., Korkman, M. & Lahti-Nuuttila, P. (2001). Differential development of attention and executive functions in 3- to 12-year-old Finnish children. *Developmental Neuropsychology*, **20**, 407–28.

Koechlin, E., Corrado, G., Pietrini, P. & Grafman, J. (2000). Dissociating the role of the medial and lateral anterior prefrontal cortex in human planning. *Proceedings of the National Academy of Science USA*, **97**, 7651–6.

Koechlin, E., Danek, A., Burnod, Y. & Grafman, J. (2002). Medial prefrontal and subcortical mechanisms underlying the acquisition of motor and cognitive action sequences. *Neuron*, **35**, 371–81.

Konishi, S., Nakajima, K., Uchida, I., *et al.* (1998). Transient activation of inferior prefrontal cortex during cognitive set shifting. *Nature Neuroscience*, **1**, 80–4.

Konishi, S., Nakajima, K., Uchida, I., *et al.* (1999). Common inhibitory mechanisms in the human inferior prefrontal cortex revealed by event-related functional MRI. *Brain*, **22**, 981–91.

Koski, L. & Petrides, M. (2002). Distractibility after unilateral resections from the frontal and anterior cingulate cortex in humans. *Neuropsychologia*, **40**, 1059–72.

Kurata, K. (1994). Information processing for motor control in primate premotor cortex. *Behavioural Brain Research*, **61**, 135–42.

Lee, S. S., Wild, K., Hollnagel, C. & Grafman, J. (1999). Selective visual attention in patients with frontal lobe lesions or Parkinson's disease. *Neuropsychologia*, **37**, 595–604.

Leung, H. C., Skudlarski, P., Gatenby, J. C., Peterson, B. S. & Gore, J. C. (2000). An event-related functional MRI study of the Stroop color word interference task. *Cerebral Cortex*, **10**, 552–60.

Levy, R. & Goldman-Rakic, P. S. (2000). Segregation of working memory functions within the dorsolateral prefrontal cortex. *Experimental Brain Research*, **133**, 23–32.

Macdonald, A. W., Cohen, J. D., Stenger, V. A. & Carter, C. S. (2000). Dissociating the role of the dorsolateral prefrontal and anterior cingulate cortex in cognitive control. *Science*, **288**, 1835–8.

Masterman, D. L. & Cummings, J. L. (1997). Frontal-subcortical circuits: The anatomic basis of executive, social and motivated behaviors. *Journal of Psychopharmacology*, **11**, 107–14.

Menon, V., Adleman, N. E., White, C. D., Glover, G. H. & Reiss, A. L. (2001). Error-related brain activation during a go/nogo response inhibition task. *Human Brain Mapping*, **12**, 131–43.

Moll, J., De Oliveira-Souza, R., Bramati, I. E. & Grafman, J. (2002). Functional networks in emotional moral and nonmoral social judgments. *NeuroImage*, **16**, 696–703.

Murray, E. A., Bussey, T. J. & Wise, S. P. (2000). Role of prefrontal cortex in a network for arbitrary visuomotor mapping. *Experimental Brain Research*, **133**, 114–29.

Nichelli, P., Grafman, J., Pietrini, P., *et al.* (1995). Where the brain appreciates the moral of a story. *NeuroReport*, **6**, 2309–13.

Norman, D. A. & Shallice, T. (1986). Attention to action. In *Consciousness and Self-Regulation*, ed. R. J. Davidson, G. E. Schwartz and D. Shapiro. pp. 1–18. New York: Plenum Press.

Northoff, G., Richter, A., Gessner, M., *et al.* (2000). Functional dissociation between medial and lateral prefrontal cortical spatiotemporal activation in negative and positive emotions: A combined fMRI/MEG study. *Cerebral Cortex*, **10**, 93–107.

O'Scalaidhe, S. P., Wilson, F. A. & Goldman-Rakic, P. S. (1997). Areal segmentation of face-processing neurons in prefrontal cortex. *Science*, **278**, 1135–8.

Partiot, A., Grafman, J., Sadato, N., Flitman, S. & Wild, K. (1996). Brain activation during script event processing. *NeuroReport*, **7**, 761–6.

Partiot, A., Grafman, J., Sadato, N., Wachs, J. & Hallett, M. (1995). Brain activation during the generation of non-emotional and emotional plans. *NeuroReport*, **6**, 1397–400.

Paulus, M. P., Hozack, N., Zauscher, B., *et al.* (2001). Prefrontal, parietal, and temporal cortex networks underlie decision-making in the presence of uncertainty. *NeuroImage*, **13**, 91–100.

Rainer, G., Asaad, W. F. & Miller, E. K. (1998). Selective representation of relevant information by neurons in the primate prefrontal cortex. *Nature*, **393**, 277–579.

Ramus, S. J. & Eichenbaum, H. (2000). Neural correlates of olfactory recognition memory in the rat orbitofrontal cortex. *Journal of Neuroscience*, **20**, 8199–208.

Rao, S. C., Rainer, G. & Miller, E. K. (1997). Integration of what and where in the primate prefrontal cortex. *Science*, **276**, 821–4.

Rilling, J. K. & Insel, T. R. (1999). The primate neocortex in comparative perpective using magnetic resonance imaging. *Journal of Human Evolution*, **37**, 191–223.

Roberts, A. C. & Wallis, J. D. (2000). Inhibitory control and affective processing in the prefrontal cortex: Neuropsychological studies in the common marmoset. *Cerebral Cortex*, **10**, 252–62.

Rolls, E. T. (1996). The orbitofrontal cortex. *Philosophical Transactions of the Royal Society of London B*, **351**, 1433–44.

Rubinsztein, J. S., Fletcher, P. C., Rogers, R. D., *et al.* (2001). Decision-making in mania: A PET study. *Brain*, **124**, 2550–63.

Ruchkin, D., Grafman, J., Cameron, K. & Berndt, R. (2003). Working memory retention systems: A state of activated long-term memory. *Behavioral and Brain Sciences*, **26**, 709–77.

Rueckert, L. & Grafman, J. (1996). Sustained attention deficits in patients with right frontal lesions. *Neuropsychologia*, **34**, 953–63.

Rugg, M. D. & Wilding, E. L. (2000). Retrieval processing and episodic memory. *Trends in Cognitive Sciences*, **4**, 108–15.

Semendeferi, K., Armstrong, E., Schleicher, A., Zilles, K. & Van Hoesen, G. W. (2001). Prefrontal cortex in humans and apes: a comparative study of area 10. *American Journal of Physical Anthropology*, **114**, 224–41.

Semendeferi, K., Lu, A., Schenker, N. & Damasio, H. (2002). Humans and great apes share a large frontal cortex. *Nature Neuroscience*, **5**, 272–6.

Shallice, T. & Burgess, P. (1998). The domain of supervisory processes and the temporal organization of behaviour. In *The Prefrontal Cortex: Executive and Cognitive Functions*, ed. A. C. Roberts, T. W. Robbins and L. Weiskrantz. Oxford: Oxford University Press.

Sirigu, A., Zalla, T., Pillon, B., *et al.* (1996). Encoding of sequence and boundaries of scripts following prefrontal lesions. *Cortex*, **32**, 297–310.

Stone, V. E., Baron-Cohen, S. & Knight, R. T. (1998). Frontal contributions to theory of mind. *Journal of Cognitive Neuroscience*, **10**, 640–56.

Strange, B. A., Henson, R. N. A., Friston, K. J. & Dolan, R. J. (2001). Anterior prefrontal cortex mediates rule learning in humans. *Cerebral Cortex*, **11**, 1040–6.

Stuss, D. T., Toth, J. P., Franchi, D., *et al.* (1999). Dissociation of attentional processes in patients with focal frontal and posterior lesions. *Neuropsychologia*, **37**, 1005–27.

Toni, I., Thoennissen, D. & Zilles, K. (2001). Movement preparation and motor intention. *NeuroImage*, **14**, S110–117.

Wagner, A. D., Desmond, J. E., Glover, G. H. & Gabrieli, J. D. (1998). Prefrontal cortex and recognition memory: Functional-MRI evidence for context-dependent retriveval processes. *Brain*, **121**, 1985–2002.

Wallis, J. D., Dias, R., Robbins, T. W. & Roberts, A. C. (2001). Dissociable contributions of the orbitofrontal and lateral prefrontal cortex of the marmoset to performance on a detour reaching task. *European Journal of Neuroscience*, **13**, 1797–808.

Williams, J. H. G., Whiten, A., Suddendorf, T. & Perrett, D. I. (2001). Imitation, mirror neurons and autism. *Neuroscience and Biobehavioral Reviews*, **25**, 287–95.

Wilson, F. A. W., O'Scalaidhe, S. P. & Goldman-Rakic, P. S. (1993). Dissociation of object and spatial processing domains in primate prefrontal cortex. *Science*, **260**, 1955–8.

Wood, J. N. & Grafman, J. (2003). Human prefrontal cortex: processing and representational perspectives. *Nature Reviews Neuroscience*, **4**, 139–47.

Wood, J. N., Knutson, K. M., & Grafman, J. (2005). Cerebral Cortex. *Psychological Structure and Neural Correlates of Event Knowledge*, **15**(8), 1155–61.

Wood, J. N., Romero, S. G., Makale, M. & Grafman, J. (2003). Category-specific representations of social and nonsocial knowledge in the human prefrontal cortex. *Journal of Cognitive Neuroscience*, **15**, 236–48.

Zalla, T., Plassiarti, C., Pillon, B., Grafman, J. & Sirigu, A. (2001). Action planning in a virtual context after prefrontal cortex damage. *Neuropsychologia*, **39**, 759–70.

Zalla, T., Sirigu, A., Pillon, B., *et al.* (2000). How patients with Parkinson's disease retrieve and manage cognitive event knowledge. *Cortex*, **36**, 163–79.

A microcircuit model of prefrontal functions: Ying and Yang of reverberatory neurodynamics in cognition

Xiao-Jing Wang

1 Introduction

In contrast to neural systems responsible for sensory processing or motor behavior, the prefrontal cortex is a quintessentially "cognitive" structure. A bewildering gamut of complex higher brain processes depend on prefrontal cortex. It is thus a particularly challenging quest to elucidate the neurobiology of prefrontal functions at the mechanistic level. Patricia S. Goldman-Rakic voiced this difficulty in 1987:

Unlike largely sensory and motor skills, the mnemonic, associative, and command functions of the mammalian brain have eluded precise neurological explanation. The proposition that cognitive function(s) can be localized to specialized neuronal circuits is not easy to defend because the neural interactions that underlie even the most simple concept or solution of an abstract problem have not been convincingly demonstrated. Also it does not seem possible to conceptualize in neural terms what it means to generate an idea, to grasp the essentials of a situation, to be oriented in space and time, or to plan for long-range goals. Furthermore we are still learning how to formulate the structure-function problem in a way that can lead to fruitful experimentation, theory building, or modeling in terms of neural systems or synaptic mechanisms.

Since these words were written, some of the impediments have begun to yield ground, partly thanks to the development of novel techniques linking cognitive functions with underlying neural processes. The advent of functional magnetic resonance imagining (fMRI) has opened up a window with which brain activity can be probed and dissected during behavior. Therefore, internal representations and processes that are not necessarily reflected by overt motor responses can now be directly observed and quantitatively analyzed. Stimulated by a confluence of experimental psychology, computer science, clinic neurology, and brain imaging, theory building in cognitive science has evolved from predominantly "conceptual models" (in words and box diagrams) to more quantitative "connectionist" neural network models (Dehaene & Changeux, 1995; Cohen et al., 1996; O'Reilly et al., 1999; O'Reilly & Munakata, 2000). Meanwhile, neurobiologists have developed laboratory paradigms that combine psychophysics and neuronal recordings with behaving animals, especially nonhuman primates. While an alert monkey performs a cognitive task (such as working memory, perceptual discrimination, selection of motor response), psychophysical data are collected to quantitatively measure the animal's performance. At the same time and under the same conditions, spike firing activities of individual neurons are recorded from identified brain areas and linked to the animal's behavior (for reviews, see Parker & Newsome, 1998; Romo & Salinas, 2000; Schall, 2001; Pasternak & Greenlee, 2005). Therefore, in many cases, a quantifiable relationship can be established between specific aspects of behavior and spike firing activity of single cells at the spatial resolution of microns and the temporal resolution of milliseconds.

Yet, correlations are not explanations. To build a neurobiological foundation of cognition, we need to understand network behavior underlying higher brain functions in terms of the biophysics of neurons and synapses, microcircuit anatomy, and collective neural dynamics. Past decades have seen tremendous progress in our understanding of the "hardware" of cortex and its plasticity. The vast amount of information gained from these advances has helped our efforts in a mechanistic understanding of sensory processing such as orientation selectivity in primary visual cortex, and long-term plasticity such as development of barrels in somatosensory cortex. By contrast, relatively little has been firmly established regarding cellular mechanisms of higher cognitive functions. This situation is changing in recent years, when neuroscientists of various subfields begin to join force in studying prefrontal cortex (Wang & Goldman-Rakic, 2003). The question must be raised: can cognitive functions, such as working memory and decision-making, be described and explained in terms of what we know about the brain: be it the rich repertoire of electroresponsiveness of single neurons (Llinas, 1988), intricate active properties of neuroral dendrites (Magee et al., 1998), dynamics of synaptic connections between individual neurons (Markram et al. 1998; Abbott & Regehr, 2004), and microcircuit wiring connectivity (Somogyi et al., 1998; Douglas & Martin, 2004)? In this chapter, I will explore this question from a computational perspective. At the interface between cognitive science and neurobiology, realistic modeling offers a valuable approach for at least two reasons. First, existing experimental methods are limited in linking neural processes observed in behaving animals with the underlying cellular mechanisms; models can serve to bridge these different levels. Second, cognitive functions involve cortical circuits that are strongly recurrent.

Predicting behaviors of such nonlinear systems with positive and negative feedback loops is not easy or even possible by intuition alone, a mathematical framework based on dynamical systems theory and computational methods is needed.

I will discuss models of prefrontal cortex that are constructed based on the known cortical anatomy and electrophysiology. To be concrete, I have chosen to focus on a cardinal prefrontal function which is nevertheless simple enough for detailed mechanistic analysis at the microcircuit level. I will thus devote the bulk of this chapter to delayed response behavior that engages working memory. As we shall see later, the same models designed for working memory are also suitable for decision-making processes. Finally, I will argue that theory of microcircuit neural dynamics provides a framework for understanding how alternations at the molecular level (e.g. deficits in glutamate, GABA, dopamine transmission) give rise to impaired network behaviors associated with mental diseases such as schizophrenia.

2   Mnemonic persistent neural activity

In delayed response tasks (Hunter, 1913), the sensory stimulus and motor response are separated by a brief delay period, during which time the sensory information must be actively held in mind by the subject. The behavior goes beyond simple stimulus-response reflexes and engages active short-term memory or "working memory." In the 1930s, C. F. Jacobsen (Jacobsen 1936) demonstrated that lesion of prefrontal cortex in monkeys induced specific deficits in delayed response tests. It is worth noting that such deficits did not occur with temporal lobe lesions, a result that was confirmed by later monkey lesion studies (Bachevalier *et al.*, 2002) and in consonance with evidence from the human clinical literature (H. M. had essentially intact active short-term memory) (Milner, 1972). Subsequent work by K. H. Pribram, H. E. Rosvold, M. Mishkin and others substantiated Jacobsen's finding and established delayed response tasks as a paradigm of choice for studying prefrontal cortex (see Curtis & D'Esposito [2004] for a recent critical review). The delayed response task is simple compared to other cognitive tasks, and thus offers a paradigm amenable to rigorous experimentation for studying prefrontal function in the laboratory.

When single neuron recordings from awake monkeys became possible Fuster and Alexander (1971) discovered that, during delayed response tasks, cells in prefrontal cortex displayed elevated spike discharges throughout the delay period while the animal was required to maintain sensory information internally in the absence of sensory stimulation. Persistent neural activity was immediately recognized as candidate neural correlate of working memory. Over the last

35 years, there has been a large body of work documenting mnemonic persistent activity in prefrontal cortex (Funahashi *et al.*, 1989; Miller *et al.*, 1996; Rainer *et al.*, 1998; Romo *et al.*, 1999), posterior parietal cortex (Gnadt & Andersen, 1988; Chafee & Goldman-Rakic, 1998), inferotemporal cortex (Fuster & Jervey, 1982; Miyashita, 1988), and basal ganglia (Hikosaka & Wurtz, 1983).

An especially elegant paradigm is the spatial delayed oculomotor task (Figure 4.1A). Using this task Funahashi *et al.* (1989) found that many neurons in the dorsolateral prefrontal cortex, including and surrounding the principal sulcus, and in the frontal eye field, exhibited mnemonic persistent activity during the delay period (Figure 4.1B). Remarkably, the delay activity of a recorded neuron was selective for preferred spatial cues (the cell's "memory field"), and this selectivity could be quantified by a bell-shaped tuning curve (Figure 4.1C). The discovery of "memory fields" demonstrated an internal representation of visuospatial information in the prefrontal cortex. This representation is observable and can be quantitatively described in terms of a Gaussian tuning of persistent delay activity at the single-cell level. However Gaussian tuning is commonplace among cortical neurons. Perhaps the best known example is orientation selectivity in primary visual cortex, the mechanisms of which have been extensively studied in cortical physiology (Sompolinsky & Shapley, 1997; Ferster & Miller, 2000). Thus, the question of prefrontal microcircuitry underlying working memory could be formulated in cellular and synaptic terms (Goldman-Rakic, 1995; Wang, 2001): what are the excitatory-inhibitory synaptic mechanisms for the formation of memory fields? What are the microcircuitry properties of the prefrontal cortex, such as local horizontal connections, that give rise to persistent activity?

The persistence time (up to 10 s) of sustained firing activity during working memory is orders of magnitude longer than the biophysical time constants (tens of milliseconds) of fast electrical signals in neurons and synapses. For this reason, persistent activity is believed to be generated by feedback dynamics, or reverberation, in a neural circuit (Lorente de Nó, 1933; Hebb, 1949; Amit, 1995). The characteristic horizontal connections found in the superficial layers II—III of the dorsolateral PFC may provide the anatomical substrate for such a recurrent circuit (Levitt *et al.*, 1993; Kritzer & Goldman-Rakic, 1995). This idea is made precise in theoretical work where persistent activity is described as "dynamical attractors" (Wilson & Cowan, 1973; Amari, 1977; Amit, 1995; Wang, 2001). The mathematical term "attractor" simply means any self-sustained and stable state of a dynamical system, such as a neural network. For example, according to this picture, in a working memory system, the spontaneous state and stimulus-selective memory states are assumed to represent multiple attractors, such that a memory state can be switched on and off by transient inputs.

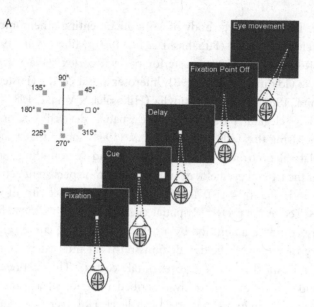

A

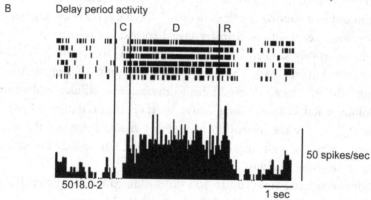

B   Delay period activity

50 spikes/sec

5018.0-2

1 sec

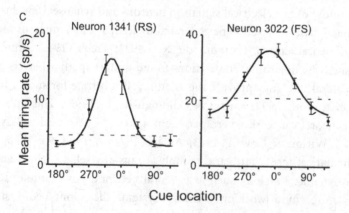

C

Neuron 1341 (RS)

Neuron 3022 (FS)

Mean firing rate (sp/s)

Cue location

This formulation is plausible, inasmuch as stimulus-selective persistent firing patterns are dynamically stable and approximately tonic in time (e.g. across a delay). However, it remains unproven that attractor networks can be realized in the brain. To determine the realistic synaptic properties and circuit dynamics that are required for a robust network-induced persistent activity, biologically-constrained models of persistent activity were needed, which became possible only recently thanks to the advances in quantitative neurophysiology (Wang, 2001; Major & Tank, 2004). Broadly speaking, feedback mechanisms underlying reverberation can either arise from recurrent network dynamics (Amit & Brunel, 1997; Lisman *et al.*, 1998; Wang, 1999; Durstewitz *et al.*, 2000b; Compte *et al.*, 2000; Seung *et al.*, 2000; Brunel & Wang, 2001; Miller *et al.*, 2003), or from intrinsic membrane/intracellular dynamics of single cells (Camperi & Wang, 1998; Egorov *et al.*, 2002; Koulakov *et al.*, 2002; Goldman *et al.*, 2003; Loewenstein & Sompolinsky, 2003). This chapter will mostly deal with circuit mechanisms but, as we shall see, network functions strongly depend on the biophysical properties of single cells, even though the latter alone are not sufficient to account for mnemonic persistent activity.

3   A biophysically based model of working memory

A network model for the Funahashi experiment of spatial working memory is illustrated in Figure 4.2A. The key feature is the preeminence of recurrent connections ("loops") between neurons, so that a cell receives not only external stimulation (via afferents from upstream neurons) but also inputs from other cells within the same microcircuit (via "horizontal" connections). A commonly assumed network architecture is the so-called "Mexican-hat": localized recurrent excitation between pyramidal cells with similar preference to spatial cues, and broader inhibition mediated by interneurons. Models of synapses and single cells

Figure 4.1   (A) Oculomotor delayed response task. Trials begin with the appearance of a fixation point at the center of the screen, which the monkey is required to foveate throughout the trial. A spatial cue is subsequently presented, typically at one of eight locations (inset at left). After a delay period of a few seconds, the disappearance of the fixation light spot signals the end of the delay. At that moment the monkey must make an accurate saccadic eye movement to the location where the cue was shown before the delay period, in order to collect a liquid reward. (B) Activity of a single prefrontal neuron, exemplifying persistent discharges during working memory. (C) Tuning curves of mnemonic delay period activity in a regular spiking putative pyramidal cell (left) and a fast-spiking putative interneuron (right). ([A–C] are adopted from Constantinidis & Wang [2004]; Funahashi *et al.* [1989], and Constantinidis & Goldman-Rakic [2002] respectively, with permission.)

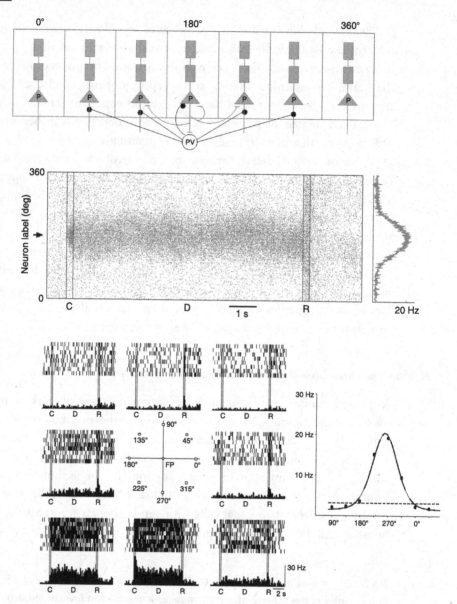

Figure 4.2   Working memory maintained by a spatially tuned network activity pattern (a "bump attractor"). Top: model architecture. Excitatory pyramidal cells are labeled by their preferred locational cues (0° to 360°). Pyramidal cells of similar preferred cues are connected through local E-to-E connections. Interneurons receive inputs from excitatory cells and send feedback inhibition by broad projections. Middle: a network simulation of delayed oculomotor response experiment. C: cue period; D: delay period; R: response period. Pyramidal neurons are labeled along the y-axis according to their preferred cues. The x-axis represents time. A dot in the rastergram indicates a spike of a neuron whose preferred location is at y, at time x. Note the enhanced and localized neural activity that is triggered by

are calibrated quantitatively by cortical electrophysiological studies. This is important: as we will discuss below, even though network function is determined by the collective dynamics of many thousands of neurons, the emergent population behavior depends critically on the properties of single cells and synapses.

Figure 4.2B shows a model simulation of the delayed oculomotor task (Compte *et al.*, 2000; Renart *et al.*, 2003) (for movie presentation of this model, go to http://wanglab.ccs.brandeis.edu). Initially, the network is in a resting state in which all cells fire spontaneously at low rates. A transient input (in this case at 180°) drives a subpopulation of cells to fire at high rates. As a result they send recruited excitation to each other via horizontal connections. This internal excitation is large enough to sustain elevated activity, so that the firing pattern persists after the stimulus is withdrawn. Synaptic inhibition ensures that the activity does not spread to the rest of the network, and persistent activity has a bell shape ("bump attractor"). At the end of a mnemonic delay period the cue information can be retrieved by reading out the peak location of the persistent activity pattern; and the network is reset back to the resting state. In different trials, a cue can be presented at different locations. For example, across eight cue presentations the firing activity of a single cell (Figure 4.2C) can be compared with the single-unit recording data from monkey's prefrontal cortex (Funahashi *et al.*, 1989). At the network level, each cue triggers a persistent firing pattern of the same bell-shape but peaked at a different location. A spatial working memory network thus requires a continuous family of "bump attractors," each encoding a potential location (Ben-Yishai *et al.*, 1995; Camperi & Wang, 1998; Compte *et al.*, 2000; Renart *et al.*, 2003; Song & Wang, 2005). The instantiation of such a continuous attractor can be rendered robust by regulatory homeostatic mechanisms in a biophysically realistic cortical network in spite of cellular heterogeneities (Renart *et al.*, 2003).

Thus, this biologically constrained model captures salient experimental observations from behaving monkeys. What lessons have we learned from such a model?

Figure 4.2 (contd.) a transient cue stimulus and persists during the delay period. The population firing profile, averaged over the delay period, is shown on the right. Bottom left: firing activities of a single cell when the cue was shown in one of the eight locations indicated in the center diagram. This neuron exhibits an elevated persistent activity in the delay only for one direction (270°), and is suppressed relative to intertrial spontaneous activity in the upper visual field. Bottom right: the delay period tuning curve shows the average discharge rate during the delay period (circles), together with a Gaussian fit of the data. The horizontal line indicates average intertrial spontaneous activity. Data provided by A. Compte. (For a color version of this figure, please see the color plate section.)

4   Excitation-inhibition balance

A conspicuous feature of our network model is multistability: a resting state coexists with a number of stimulus-selective memory states, so that transient inputs lead to switching between self-sustained network firing patterns, or "attractors" (Figure 4.3). When the attractor network scenario for working memory was tested with biophysically realistic models, it was recognized that such a system with strong recurrent loops is prone to instability. For instance, the resting state should be stable to small perturbations due to noisy spontaneous neural firing, in spite of strong excitatory recurrency. This is realized by a tight balance between excitation and inhibition (E-I balance), like Ying and Yang in ancient Chinese philosophy. In fact, in the resting state, feedback inhibition is slightly larger than excitation, hence the overall recurrent input to a neuron is inhibitory (Figure 4.4A) and spontaneous spike firing is driven by random background external inputs. Interestingly, in a memory state in which stronger reverberatory excitation is recruited to sustain an elevated firing rate, synaptic inhibition increases proportionally with excitation (Figure 4.4B—C); this dynamically maintained E-I balance contributes to controlling the firing rates and preventing runaway excitation. Other experimental and theoretical work suggests that a fixed E-I balance, regardless of changing neuronal firing rates, may be

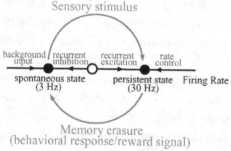

Figure 4.3   Schematic illustration of the biophysics underlying an attractor dynamics. An attractor is a neural firing state that is stable to perturbations: when a small input perturbs the network to a lower or higher activity level, there is a "restoring force" to bring the network back to the attractor state. In this case, the spontaneous state is stabilized from below by background inputs, and from above by feedback synaptic inhibition. A sufficiently powerful sensory stimulus can drive a cell assembly to "escape" from the spontaneous state, and after the stimulus is withdrawn the system settles in one of the active memory states at an elevated firing rate. The persistent activity state is stabilized from below by excitatory reverberation, and from above by various negative feedback "rate control" mechanisms. Finally, a behavioral response or reward signal can turn the network off and erase the memory. (Adopted from Wang [2001] with permission.) (For a color version of this figure, please see the color plate section.)

(A) Spontaneous Activity

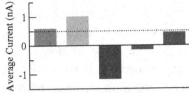

(B) Delay activity – preferred stimulus

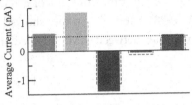

(C) Delay activity – nonpreferred stimulus

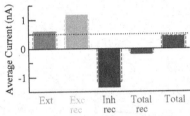

Ext   Exc   Inh   Total   Total
        rec   rec   rec

Figure 4.4   Balanced excitation and inhibition in the spatial working memory model (same as in Figure 4.2). Various components of synaptic current in a single cell during spontaneous activity (top), during delay activity following presentation of a preferred stimulus (middle), and during delay activity following presentation of a nonpreferred stimulus (bottom). The dotted line indicates the value of excitatory synaptic currents needed to reach the (deterministic) firing threshold. In the two lower panels, the dotted boxes indicate the value of the corresponding component during spontaneous activity, to show the differences between delay and spontaneous activity. Background external inputs are superthreshold. Recurrent circuit is dominated by inhibition (brown) over excitation (orange) in the spontaneous state, so that the net recurrent synaptic current is hyperpolarizing (blue). During delay activity both recurrent excitation and inhibition are larger and dynamically balance each other, in such a way that the overall synaptic excitation becomes slightly larger following a preferred stimulus (leading to persistent activity at an elevated rate) than after a nonpreferred stimulus. (For a color version of this figure, please see the color plate section.)

a general characteristic of cortical network dynamics (Shadlen & Newsome, 1994; Shu *et al.*, 2003; Compte *et al.*, 2003b; Liu, 2004).

    The balancing act of recurrent excitation and inhibition may contribute to an explanation for the highly irregular spike discharges in prefrontal cells

(Compte *et al.*, 2003a). On the other hand, we found that the E-I balance often manifests itself in the form of coherent network oscillations, typically in the gamma (40 Hz) frequency range (Wang, 1999; Compte *et al.*, 2000; Tegnér *et al.*, 2002) (Figure 4.5). This is because fast excitation followed by slower inhibition is a common recipe for rhythmogenesis in neural networks (Wilson & Cowan, 1972; Wang, 2003). Synaptic inhibition mediated by GABA_A receptors is typically about 3–5 times slower than fast synaptic excitation mediated by AMPA receptors, the latter having a decay time constant of a few milliseconds (Hestrin *et al.*, 1990b; Xiang *et al.*, 1998). Modeling studies showed that coherent oscillations resulting from an interplay between AMPAR-mediated excitation

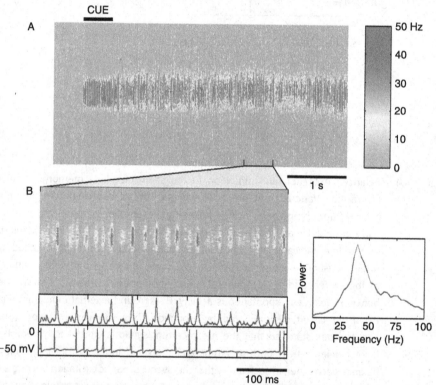

Figure 4.5   Gamma oscillations during working memory. (A) Spatiotemporal firing pattern of a spatial working memory model same as in Figure 4.2 (with slightly different parameters) except that firing rates are color-coded. (B) 500-ms blowup of (A) to show synchronous oscillations in the spatiotemporal activity pattern (top), the local field potential (middle) and membrane potential of a single neuron (bottom). On the right is shown the power spectrum of the local field, demonstrating a large peak at about 40 Hz. (Adopted from Compte *et al.* [2000] with permission.) (For a color version of this figure, please see the color plate section.)

and GABA$_A$R-mediated inhibition have a preferred frequency range around 40 Hz (Brunel & Wang, 2003). This theoretical finding suggests that synchronous 40-Hz oscillations may be observed in mnemonic persistent activity, a notion that has found some experimental support (Pesaran *et al.*, 2002). In this view, fast γ rhythms may be a characteristic sign of the engagement of strongly reverberatory cortical circuits in cognition and memory.

5   The importance of being slow: role of NMDA receptors

A system with fast positive and slow negative feedbacks, both powerful, is prone to dynamical instability. Persistent activity is often disrupted in the middle of a delay period, thereby the memory is lost (Wang, 1999; Compte *et al.*, 2000; Tegnér *et al.*, 2002; Renart *et al.*, 2003). The same destabilization problem is present if negative feedback is instantiated by spike-frequency adaptation (McCormick *et al.*, 1985) or short-term synaptic depression (Markram *et al.*, 1998; Abbott & Regehr, 2004). Such instability does not occur, if the excitation is sufficiently slow, when compared to negative feedback, i.e. when recurrent synapses are primarily mediated by NMDA receptors (time constant 50−100 ms) (Wang, 1999; Compte *et al.*, 2000). Moreover, the slow NMDAR unbinding to glutamate gives rise to saturation of the NMDA synaptic current with repetitive stimulation at high frequencies (Figure 4.6). As a result further increase in neural firing rates does not lead to a larger excitatory drive, and the explosive positive feedback is curtailed. Therefore it helps to control the firing rate in a persistent activity state (Wang, 1999).

A specific suggestion from modeling work, then, is that in a working memory microcircuit, *if persistent activity is primarily sustained by synaptic reverberation,* local excitatory synapses should have a sufficiently high NMDA/AMPA ratio. How high is high enough? The answer depends on the details of network biophysics and connectivity. For instance, the time constant of a synaptic current depends on the subunit composition of its receptors. If GABA$_A$-receptor-mediated inhibition is unusually fast in a working memory circuit, instability due to the time constant mismatch with AMPA-receptor-mediated excitation would be less severe, and the required NMDA/AMPA ratio would be lower (Tegnér *et al.*, 2002). Furthermore, if a slow ion channel in single cells contributes to positive feedback, then less NMDA/AMPA ratio would also be needed, as shown in Figure 4.7 (Tegnér *et al.*, 2002). The general idea is that positive feedback should not be too fast compared to negative feedback, when both are powerful in a working memory circuit. This remains true if persistent activity is generated not by a synaptic mechanism, but by intrinsic membrane dynamics of single neurons.

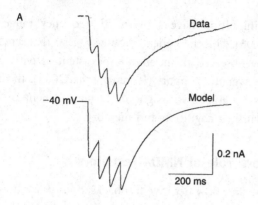

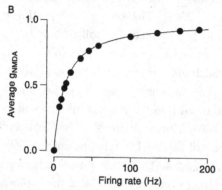

Figure 4.6   Temporal summation of the NMDAR-mediated excitatory postsynaptic currents (EPSCs). (A) NMDAR-mediated EPSCs elicited by four stimuli, when the membrane potential is clamped at −40 mV. Upper panel: data from a pyramidal neuron in CA1 of the rat hippocampus (redrawn from [Hestrin *et al.*, 1990b] with permission). The stimulus is at 25 Hz. Note the significant summation and saturation. These properties are mediated postsynaptically by the NMDARs, since they are absent in the non-NMDR-mediated EPSCs recorded in the same cell at −100 mV. Lower panel: NMDAR-mediated EPSCs produced by a model synapse in response to a stimulus at 20 Hz. (B) The average NMDAR-mediated EPSC as function of stimulus frequency. (Adopted from Wang [1999] with permission.)

6   Stimulus selectivity and resistance against distractors

As I discussed earlier, like Ying and Yang, reverberatory excitation should be balanced by synaptic inhibition to ensure proper function of a working memory circuit. Synaptic inhibition plays a critical role in sculpturing stimulus selectivity of mnemonic persistent firing patterns, in consonance with the observation that GABA$_A$ receptor antagonists resulted in the loss of spatial tuning of prefrontal neurons during a delayed oculomotor task (Rao *et al.*, 2000). Note that it is useful to distinguish between "feedforward" inhibition (from GABAergic cells driven

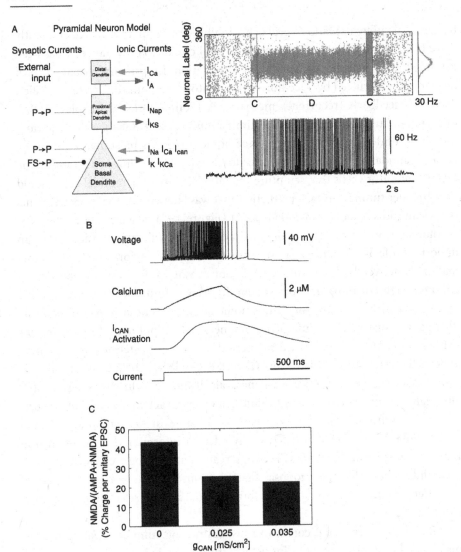

Figure 4.7   A spatial working memory model, with single neurons endowed with three compartments (soma, proximate and distal dendrites) and a number of voltage-gated ion channels. (A) Left: schematic single pyramidal cell model; right: spatiotemporal network activity (top) and membrane potential of a single cell (bottom) in a simulation of the delayed oculomotor experiment. Data provided by J. Tegnér (2002). (B) Electroresponsiveness of an isolated pyramidal cell model with a nonselective cation current I_{Can}. The calcium-dependent activation of I_{Can} is slow, leading to a ramping-up time course of the neural response. A few action potentials are still fired after stimulus extinction, in parallel with a slow deactivation of I_{Can}. Notice that the neuron is not bistable; it returns to stable resting state. (C) Slow ionic currents (here I_{Can}) reduce the minimum level of NMDAR that is required for sustained delay activity. Further increase in g_{Can} renders the neuron intrinsically bistable (not shown). (Adopted from Tegnér et al. [2002] with permission.) (For a color version of this figure, please see the color plate section.)

by external afferents) and "feedback" inhibition (from those predominantly driven by pyramidal cells within the same local circuit). For instance, it has been proposed that bell-shaped tuning of orientation in primary visual cortical neurons is constructed by a feedforward inhibitory mechanism (Ferster & Miller, 2000), or feedback (recurrent) mechanisms (Sompolinsky & Shapley, 1997), or a combination of both. Because stimulation is absent during a delay period, inhibition underlying selectivity of mnemonic activity is presumably driven by local pyramidal cells, hence of the feedback type. According to Compte et al. (2000), inhibitory cells that sculpture spatial selectivity of pyramidal cells should have broader tuning curves, a prediction that was later confirmed by experiments (Constantinidis & Goldman-Rakic, 2002) (Figure 4.1, bottom panel).

Another key aspect of memory maintenance, in which inhibition plays an important role, is resistance against distractors: while behaviorally relevant information is actively held in mind, irrelevant sensory stimuli should be denied entrance to the working memory system. In delayed response experiments using intervening stimuli (distractors), mnemonic activity has been shown to be easily disrupted by distractors in inferotemporal neurons but not in prefrontal neurons (Miller et al., 1996). Similarly, delay period activity in posterior parietal cortex appears to be sensitive to distractors (Powell & Goldberg, 2000; Constantinidis & Procyk, 2004). Therefore the evidence, albeit not conclusive, suggests that although multiple cortical areas exhibit delay period activity, mnemonic neural signals in prefrontal cortex may persist when those in the temporal lobe and parietal lobe are lost, so that behaviorally relevant information is maintained in the brain in spite of distractors. This observation at the single-cell level suggests a candidate basis for the proposal that prefrontal cortex is a pivotal part of the attention network that focuses brain resources on selective information (Mesulam, 2000).

What enables prefrontal cortex to resist distracting stimuli? A gating mechanism may be involved in deciding which stimulus is behaviorally relevant and thus should be held in working memory (Cohen et al., 1996, 2002). On the other hand, it is desirable that a working memory circuit be endowed with mechanisms to filter out, "by default," external inputs that constantly bombard our senses. We found that synaptic inhibition naturally gave rise to this capability (Compte et al., 2000; Brunel & Wang, 2001). This is because, in a memory delay period, active neurons recruit inhibition which project to the rest of the network. Consequently, those cells not encoding the initial cue are less excitable than when they are in the resting state (see Figures 4.2 and 4.7A), hence less responsive to distracting stimuli presented during the delay. For spatial working memory, the impact of a distractor depends on its strength (saliency) and the distance to the memorized cue (Figure 4.8A). More generally, we found that the network's

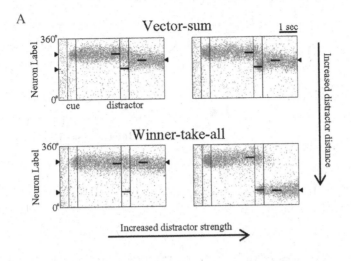

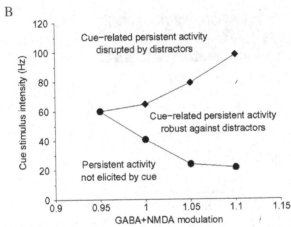

Figure 4.8   Resistance against distractors. (A) In the spatial working memory model, the initial cue (upper arrow on the left) triggers persistent activity centered at 180°. During the delay, a second cue (distractor) is shown briefly (lower arrow on the left). When the distractor is close to the initial stimulus, the network performs a vector sum so that the final remembered cue is half-way between the two (arrow on the right). On the other hand, when the distractor is far away from the initial stimulus, the network operates in a winner-take-all regime, so that the final remembered cue is either the initial stimulus or the distractor, depending on the strength of the stimuli. (B) Behavior of an object working memory model as function of dopamine modulation of NMDAR-mediated recurrent excitation and GABA$_A$R inhibition (x-axis) and amplitude of cue stimulation (y-axis). A very weak stimulus (initial cue) cannot elicit persistent activity (lower left region), whereas a powerful stimulus (distractor) can override recurrent dynamics and disrupt delay activity (upper left region). The desirable behavior (robust persistent activity in spite of distractors) (middle right region) is sensitive to dopamine modulations. (Adopted from Brunel & Wang [2001] with permission.) (For a color version of this figure, please see the color plate section.)

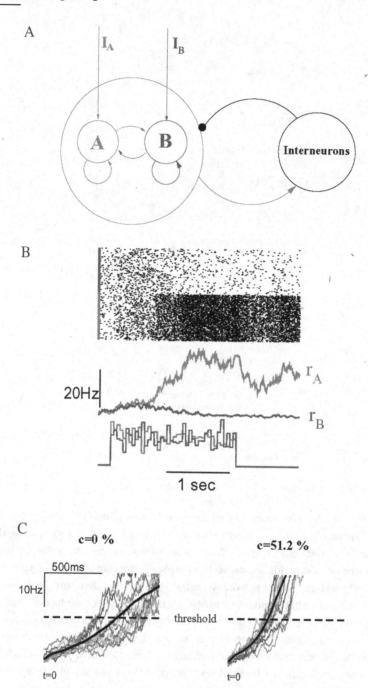

Figure 4.9   (A) A simple model for two-alternative forced-choice tasks. There are two pyramidal cell groups, each of which is selective to one of the two directions (A = left, B = right) of random moving dots in a visual motion discrimination experiment. Within each pyramidal neural group there are strong recurrent excitatory connections which can sustain persistent activity

ability to ignore distractors is sensitive to modulation of recurrent excitation and inhibition (Figure 4.8B). This finding has important implications for dopaminergic signaling in prefrontal cortex (see below).

7 Decision-making

So far, I have focused on delayed response tasks. We have seen that this approach provides a valuable probe into the detailed mechanisms of prefrontal microcircuitry. However, currently there is a heated debate as to whether prefrontal function should be conceptualized by internal representation (memory maintenance) or processes (decision-making, executive control) (Miller & Cohen, 2001; Curtis & D'Esposito, 2003; Wood & Grafman, 2003). Unexpectedly, it turns out that the same models originally developed for working memory can account for decision-making processes as well (Wang, 2002; Machens *et al.*, 2005). An example is shown in Figure 4.9 from model simulations of visual motion discrimination (Newsome *et al.*, 1989; Parker & Newsome, 1998). In this two-alternative forced choice task, monkeys are trained to make a judgment about the direction of motion (say, left or right) in a near-threshold stochastic random dot display, and to report the perceived direction with a saccadic eye movement. Neurons in posterior parietal cortex (Shadlen & Newsome, 2001; Roitman & Shadlen, 2002) and prefrontal cortex (Kim & Shadlen, 1999) were found to exhibit firing activity correlated with the animal's perceptual choice. We used the same model designed for working memory to simulate this decision experiment; with the only difference that for delayed response task only one stimulus is presented, whereas for perceptual discrimination tasks conflicting sensory inputs are fed into competing neural subpopulations in a decision circuit (Figure 4.9A). Our model accounts for not only salient characteristics of the observed decision-correlated neural activity (Figure 4.9B–C), but also

Figure 4.9 (contd.) triggered by a transient preferred stimulus. The two neural groups compete through feedback inhibition from interneurons. The motion coherence is expressed as $c = (\mu_A - \mu_B)/(\mu_A + \mu_B)$, where μ_A and μ_B are the mean values of inputs IA and IB. (B) A network simulation with zero coherence. Top to bottom: network spiking raster, population firing rates r_A and r_B, stochastic inputs I_A and I_B. Note the initial slow ramping (time integration) and eventual divergence of r_A and r_B (categorical choice). (C) In reaction time simulations, when one of the two neural groups reaches a fixed threshold (15 Hz) of population firing activity, the decision is made and the deliberation or decision time is read out. The decision time is longer and more variable at low coherence (left) than at high coherence (right). (Adopted from Wang [2002] with permission.) (For a color version of this figure, please see the color plate section.)

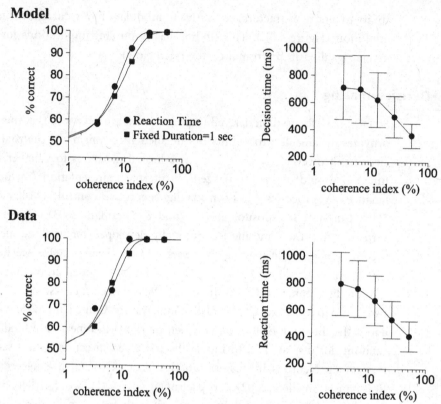

Figure 4.10 Top: left panel: psychometric functions for the reaction time stimulation (circle) and with fixed stimulus duration of 1 s (square); right panel: average decision time as function of the coherence level, ranging from 200 ms at high c to 800 ms at low c. At very low coherence there is a saturation. Note the large standard deviation of decision time, especially at low coherence. (Adopted from Wang [2002] with permission.) Bottom: monkey's behavioral data reproduced with permission from Roitman & Shadle (2002).

quantitatively for the animal's behavioral performance (psychometric function and reaction times) (Figure 4.10).

8 Distinct features of prefrontal microcircuitry

Quantitative differences breed qualitatively different behaviors. That a cortical area exhibits a new type of behavior does not necessarily mean that the circuit must possess unique biological machineries completely different from other areas. Hence, persistent activity may be generated in the prefrontal cortex when the strength of recurrent excitation (mediated by AMPA+NMDA receptors combined) exceeds a critical threshold, whereas this may not be the case for a sensory area such as the primary visual cortex. Based on our modeling results,

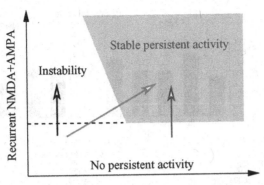

NMDA/AMPA Ratio at Recurrent Synapses

Figure 4.11 Schematic depiction of the dependence of stable persistent activity on both sufficiently strong recurrency (y-axis) and large NMDA/AMPA ratio at local excitatory synapses (x-axis). A circuit that does not exhibit persistent activity may be endowed with this ability by strengthening excitatory connections while preserving a relatively large NMDA/AMPA ratio (blue arrow). However, an enhancement of recurrency at a low NMDA/AMPA ratio can lead to network dynamical instability (black arrow), in which case the NMDA/AMPA ratio needs to be increased simultaneously (red arrow). (For a color version of this figure, please see the color plate section.)

we can extend this idea and propose that, for stable function of a working memory circuit, the NMDA/AMPA ratio at recurrent synapses should also be above a certain threshold, as illustrated in Figure 4.11. It is important to emphasize that what matters for persistent activity is not the unitary amplitude of EPSCs at resting potential, but the ratio of the average NMDA and AMPA synaptic currents during repetitive neural discharges. This ratio depends on multiple factors such as presynaptic short-term plasticity, postsynaptic summation and saturation and voltage-dependence of the NMDA channel conductance. Further, a relatively high NMDA/AMPA ratio at local synapses can be compatible with a low total NMDA/AMPA ratio in a neuron, for instance if feedforward inputs from outside of the network are predominantly mediated by AMPA receptors. Last but not least, this ratio can be enhanced by neuromodulators, such as dopamine (Chen *et al.*, 2004; Huang *et al.*, 2004; Seamans & Yang, 2004).

Immunochemical analysis revealed a significantly larger amount of mRNA expression of NMDA receptor subunits in prefrontal neurons, compared to primary visual cortical neurons (Figure 4.12). It is unknown whether this simply correlates with a larger number of spines (hence synaptic connections) per pyramidal cell in prefrontal cortex (Elston, 2000). In any event, contribution of NMDA receptors to synaptic transmission locally between prefrontal pyramidal cells remains to be established by direct electrophysiological measurements, e.g. using intracellular recording from connected pairs of neighboring

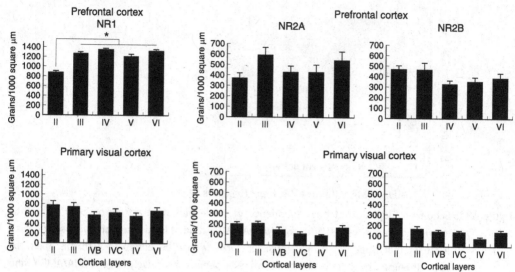

Figure 4.12 mRNA expression of NMDA receptor subunits NR1, NR2A and NR2B in human prefrontal cortex (top) and primary visual cortex (bottom). (Adopted from Scherzer *et al.* [1998] with permission.)

cells in prefrontal slices. On the other hand, iontophoresis can be used to selectively block NMDARs in recorded prefrontal cells of behaving monkeys during working memory (Williams & Goldman-Rakic, 1995; Shima & Tanji, 1998; Wang *et al.*, 2004b). Traditionally, the function of NMDA conductance is almost exclusively emphasized in terms of its role in long-term synaptic potentiation and depression. Thus, an abundance of NMDA receptors could reflect a high degree of plasticity of prefrontal microcircuit, which could subserve learning flexible and adaptive behaviors (Miller & Cohen, 2001; Stuss & Knight, 2002). That may be, but we propose that NMDA receptors also directly mediate slow excitatory synaptic transmission critically important to working memory, and that this may explain why NMDA receptor antagonists produce working memory impairment in healthy human subjects (Krystal *et al.*, 1994). Taken one step further, effects on cognitive behavior by genetic manipulation of NMDARs may also be partly caused by altered short-term memory, in addition to long-term memory.

On the other side of Ying and Yang, prefrontal cortex may also be endowed with specialized inhibitory circuitry. A salient feature of cortical organization is the presence of a wide diversity of GABAergic interneurons, with regards to their morphology, electrophysiology, chemical markers, synaptic connections and short-term plasticity, molecular characteristics (Freund & Buzsaki, 1996; Cauli *et al.*, 1997; DeFelipe, 1997; Kawaguchi & Kubota, 1997; Somogyi *et al.*, 1998; Buzsaki *et al.*, 2004; Markram *et al.*, 2004). How do different interneuron types work together in prefrontal cortex? To investigate this question, we have extended our model of spatial working memory to incorporate three subclasses of interneurons classified according to their synaptic targets (Wang *et al.*, 2004a). In this model (Figure 4.13A), in addition to widespread inhibition mediated by perisoma-targeting and parvalbumin-containing (PV) interneurons, dendrite-targeting (calbindin-containing, CB) interneurons receive inputs from interneuron-targeting (calretinin-containing, CR) interneurons, leading to an activity-dependent local disinhibition of pyramidal cells.

Note that the three interneuron types in our model should be more appropriately interpreted according to their synaptic targets, rather than calcium-binding protein expressions. For example, PV cells display a variety of axonal arbors, among which the large basket cells (Krimer & Goldman-Rakic, 2001; Kisvarday *et al.*, 2003) are likely candidates for our widely-projecting cells. Similarly, CB interneurons show a high degree of heterogeneity, but some of them (such as double bouquet cells) are known to act locally and preferentially target dendritic spines and shafts of pyramidal cells (DeFelipe, 1997; Somogyi *et al.*, 1998). Finally, although many CR interneurons do project to pyramidal cells (DeFelipe, 1997), anatomical studies show that a subset of CR cells avoid pyramidal cells (Gulyás *et al.*, 1996), at least in the same cortical layer (Meskenaite, 1997), and preferentially target CB interneurons (DeFelipe *et al.*, 1999). It is also possible that axonal innervations of a CR cell project onto pyramidal cells in a different cortical layer, while selectively targeting inhibitory neurons in the same layer (Meskenaite, 1997; Gonchar & Burkhalter, 1999). Whether such selective connection pattern holds true as a general principle can only be settled by further anatomical studies. Moreover, electro-physiological evidence is presently lacking about the preferred innervations of a subset of CR interneurons onto GABAergic cells; progress in this direction would be most welcome.

We found that the disinhibition mechanism, mediated by CR inhibition of CB interneurons, contributes significantly to the formation of memory field, as well as the network's ability to filter out distracting stimuli (Wang *et al.*, 2004a). Interestingly, the distributions of PV, CB and CR interneurons appear to be quite different in macaque monkey prefrontal cortex (Conde *et al.*, 1994; Gabbott & Bacon, 1996) compared to primary visual cortex (Brederode *et al.*, 1990; Meskenaite, 1997) (Figure 4.13B). In the prefrontal cortex the proportions are 24% (PV), 24% (CB) and 45% (CR), respectively, according to Conde *et al.* (1994) and Gabbott and Bacon (1996). Other studies reported different estimates (Kondo *et al.*, 1999; Dombrowski *et al.*, 2001; Elston & Gonzalez-Albo, 2003), presumably due to species differences and technical factors (different cell-counting methods and antibodies used for calcium-binding proteins,

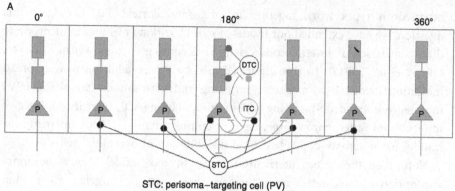

A

0°   180°   360°

STC: perisoma–targeting cell (PV)
DTC: peridendrite–targeting cell (CB)
ITC: interneuron–targeting cell (CR)

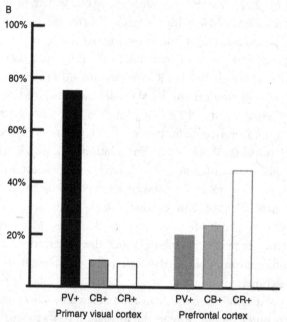

B

Figure 4.13 (A) A spatial working memory model with three subclasses of GABAergic interneurons.
Pyramidal (P) neurons are arranged according to their preferred cues (0 – 360°). There are
localized recurrent excitatory connections, and broad inhibitory projections from perisoma-
targeting (parvalbumin-containing, PV) fast-spiking neurons to P cells. Within a column,
calbindin-containing (CB) interneurons target the dendrites of P neurons, whereas
calretinin-containing (CR) interneurons preferentially project to CB cells. Excitation of a
group of pyramidal cells recruits locally CR neurons, which sends enhanced inhibition to CB
neurons, leading to dendritic disinhibition of the same pyramidal cells. (Adopted from Wang
et al. [2004] with permission.) (B) Proportional distribution of PV, CB and CR expressing
GABAergic cells in primary visual cortex and prefrontal cortex. See text for details. (For a
colour version of this figure, please see the colour plate section.)

overlapping CB expression by GABAergic cells and pyramidal neurons, etc). Future work is needed to resolve these discrepancies, and to test the hypothesized disinhibition mechanism and assess whether it may be especially prominent in working memory circuit.

9 Insights into prefrontal dysfunction in schizophrenia

Our modeling work has given rise to a number of specific candidate explanations for frontal lobe dysfunction associated with schizophrenia and other mental disorders.

We showed that impairment of NMDARs at intrinsic prefrontal synapses is detrimental to persistent activity underlying working memory. If borne out, these results may shed insights into why working memory dysfunction similar to that observed in schizophrenic patients can be induced in healthy subjects by subanesthetic doses of ketamine, a noncompetitive NMDA receptor antagonist (Krystal *et al.*, 1994). Postmortem studies showed significant alterations of the NMDAR mRNA expression (Akbarian *et al.*, 1996), but did not reveal abnormality (Healy *et al.*, 1998) or a slight increase (Dracheva *et al.*, 2005) in the AMPAR level. Available information does not yet permit a more precise explanation as to why and how impairment of the NMDA receptor system causes cognitive deficits associated with schizophrenia. It has been previously suggested that impairment can occur outside of prefrontal cortex, such as in hippocampus (Grunze *et al.*, 1996; Jodo *et al.*, 2005; Rowland *et al.*, 2005) or in the dopamine system (Carlsson *et al.*, 2001). Again, functional implications tend to be discussed in the realm of learning and synaptic modification. By contrast, our modeling work suggests a novel scenario focused on the role of NMDARs in persistent activity. Of course, this scenario is compatible with other proposals, given that impairment of NMDARs may not be restricted to a single pathway, and that NMDARs play a major role in long-term synaptic plasticity. These different facets of NMDAR function are also under influence of dopamine modulation (Chen *et al.*, 2004; Huang *et al.*, 2004).

On the other side of Ying-Yang, there is mounting evidence that the dorsolateral prefrontal cortex of schizophrenic patients shows abnormality of selective interneuron subtypes, especially fast-spiking basket and chandelier cells (Lewis *et al.*, 2005). Our theory suggests that this may be the case for two reasons. Modeling work (Compte *et al.*, 2000; Brunel & Wang, 2001; Wang *et al.*, 2004a), in concordance with physiological experiments (Rao *et al.*, 2000; Constantinidis & Goldman-Rakic, 2002), demonstrates that inhibition mediated by fast spiking and broadly projecting interneurons is critical to the stimulus selectivity, hence information specificity, of mnemonic persistent activity. Moreover, fast spiking

GABAergic cells are critical to the generation of coherent gamma (40 Hz) oscillations (Traub et al., 1996; Wang & Buzsaki, 1996; Wang, 2003; Traub et al., 2004), which may contribute to cognitive processes such as feature integration in perception (Singer & Gray, 1995) or selective attention (Fries et al., 2001). Revealingly, gamma oscillations appear to be decreased in schizophrenic brain compared to control subjects (Lee et al., 2003; Spencer et al., 2004). Thus, deficits in synaptic inhibition could impair the quality of information stored in working memory as well as the brain's ability to bind distributed neural activity.

We found that inhibition is also crucial for robust working memory despite ongoing sensory flow. This result provides another insight into how dopamine may affect prefrontal functions (Durstewitz et al., 2000a; Brunel & Wang, 2001). It is known that dopamine acts on prefrontal cortex partly through modulation of gluatamergic and GABAergic synaptic transmissions (see Arnsten [1998] and Seamans & Yang [2004] for reviews). Our modeling showed that a relatively small increase by dopamine of recurrent connections (while preserving the E-I balance) can lead to significant enhancement of the network's resistance against distractors. Conversely, mild impairment of dopamine signaling in the prefrontal cortex can result in behavioral distractibility associated with mental disorders such as schizophrenia. Moreover, according to the disinhibition mechanism (Figure 4.13), dendritic inhibition is reduced locally in activated pyramidal cells, but increased in those pyramidal cells not engaged in encoding the shown stimulus. This mechanism mediated by CB interneurons could serve to filter out distracting stimuli, and that this mechanism is enhanced with a larger dendritic/somatic inhibition ratio (Wang et al., 2004a). A high dendritic/somatic inhibition ratio in a working memory circuit may be hard-wired, for example with a large proportion of CB cells in prefrontal cortex. Alternatively, it can also be dynamically controlled by neuromodulators such as dopamine.

Interestingly, an in vitro work suggests that dopamine D1 receptor activation precisely increases the ratio of dendritic/somatic inhibition onto pyramidal cells in prefrontal cortex (Gao et al., 2003). Using double intracellular recording in prefrontal cortex slices and morphological reconstruction, it was found that bath application of dopamine has a dual effect on the inhibitory synaptic transmission in a pyramidal cell of the prefrontal cortex. Dopamine was found to reduce the efficacy of inhibitory synapses onto the perisomatic domains of a pyramidal cell, mediated by fast-spiking interneurons; whereas it enhances inhibition at synapses from accommodating or low-threshold spiking inter-neurons that target the dendritic domains of a pyramidal cell (Gao et al., 2003). Our model predicts a specific function for such a dual dopamine action, namely it could boost the ability of a working memory network to filter out behaviorally irrelevant distracting stimuli. Our modeling work (Brunel & Wang, 2001), as well as brain imaging (Sakai *et al.*, 2002), points to a possible physiological basis of the clinical literature documenting distractibility as a common symptom of frontal lobe damage (Goldman-Rakic, 1987; Fuster, 1988; Mesulam, 2000).

10   Concluding remarks

In this chapter I discussed biophysically based neural modeling that, in concert with experiments, offers a powerful tool for investigating the cellular and circuit mechanisms of mnemonic persistent activity in delayed response tasks. This approach has been used to assess whether the attractor model for working memory and decision-making can be instantiated by biologically plausible mechanisms. Our theoretical work suggests that slow excitatory reverberation underlies persistent activity in working memory and time integration in decision-making (Figure 4.14). A candidate cellular substrate is the NMDA receptors at local recurrent synapses; an alternative/complementary scenario involves intrinsic channels and calcium dynamics in single cells. Recurrent excitation must be balanced by feedback inhibition, which is mediated by several types of GABAergic interneurons. We found that inhibitory circuitry plays a key role in stimulus selectivity (similarly as in sensory areas) and the network's resistance against distracting stimuli (a cardinal requirement for robust working memory), as well as winner-take-all competition in decision-making. These modeling predictions can be tested experimentally, such as by in vitro physiology or iontophoresis of transmitter receptor blockers with behaving nonhuman primates.

We have confined ourselves to models in which working memory storage is maintained by roughly tonic (constant) spike discharges in a neural assembly

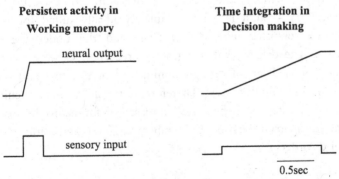

Figure 4.14   Working memory requires neurons to convert a transient input pulse into a self-sustained persistent activity, whereas decision-making involves neuronal ramping activity for accumulation of sensory information. Both types of time integration can be subserved by slow reverberatory dynamics in a recurrent neural network.

across a delay period. However, many cortical cells exhibit delay activity that is not stationary but ramps up or down over time (Fuster, 1988; Chafee & Goldman-Rakic, 1998; Brody *et al.*, 2003). Such ramping activity can conceivably be realized in a two-layer network, in which first-layer neurons show tonic delay activity whereas second-layer neurons slowly integrate inputs from the first-layer neurons in the form of ramping activity (Miller *et al.*, 2003). Moreover, self-sustained network activity can occur as a firing pattern that propagates in a neural network (Sanchez-Vives & McCormick, 2000; Cossart *et al.*, 2003). It remains unclear how the specificity of stored information can be preserved in dynamically moving neural activities (Baeg *et al.*, 2003).

Our emphasis on *internal representations* by no means underestimates the importance of processes such as action selection. Rather, we propose that prefrontal cortex does not simply send out nonspecific "control signals" and that representational information is indispensable to processes. As it turns out, our model is capable of both working memory maintenance and decision-making computations. These results suggest that it may not be a mere coincidence that decision-related neural activity has been found in the same cortical areas that also exhibit persistent activity during working memory (Romo & Salinas, 2000; Schall, 2001). In our model, both working memory and decision-making rely on slow reverberatory dynamics that gives rise to persistent activity and time integration (Figure 4.14), and inhibitory circuitry that leads to selectivity and winner-take-all competition. Thus, we are beginning to unravel the microcircuit properties of a "cognitive" cortical area (such as prefrontal cortex as in contrast to, for example, primary visual cortex) that enable it to serve multiple cognitive functions. At a fundamental level, these studies point to a unified view about why and how "cognitive" cortical area can serve both internal representation (active working memory) and processing (decision, action selection, etc).

Microcircuitry is at a level of complexity ideally suited for bridging the gap between cognitive network functions and the underlying biophysical mechanisms. The delicate balancing act of recurrent excitation and feedback inhibition is at the heart of strongly nonlinear dynamics that underlie cognitive processes in prefrontal cortex. Therefore, ultimately, microcircuit neurodynamics hold the key to a theoretical foundation for neuropharmacology and molecular psychiatry (Harrison & Weinberger, 2005), and a full understanding of mental disorders.

Acknowledgments

I am grateful to Albert Compte, Nicolas Brunel, Alfonso Renart and Jesper Tegnér for their contributions, and to Pengcheng Song for his help in preparing

Figures 4.4 and 4.8A. This work was partly supported by NIH (MH62349, DA016455) and the Swartz Foundation.

REFERENCES

Abbott, L. F. & Regehr, W. G. (2004). Synaptic computation. *Nature*, **431**, 796–803.

Akbarian, S., Sucher, N. J., Bradley, D., *et al.* (1996). Selective alterations in gene expression for NMDA receptor subunits in prefrontal cortex of schizophrenics. *Journal of Neuroscience*, **16**, 19–30.

Amari, S. (1977). Dynamics of pattern formation in lateral-inhibition type neural fields. *Biological Cybernetics*, **27**, 77–87.

Amit, D. J. (1995). The Hebbian paradigm reintegrated: local reverberations as internal representations. *Behavioral and Brain Sciences*, **18**, 617–26.

Amit, D. J. & Brunel, N. (1997). Model of global spontaneous activity and local structured activity during delay periods in the cerebral cortex. *Cerebral Cortex*, **7**, 237–52.

Arnsten, A. F. T. (1998). Catecholamine modulation of prefrontal cortical cognitive function. *Trends in Cognitive Sciences*, **2**, 436–47.

Bachevalier, J., Nemanic, S. & Alvarado, M. C. (2002). The medial temporal lobe structures and object recognition memory in nonhuman primates. In *Neuropsychology of Memory*, 3rd edn, eds. Squire, L. R. and Schacter, D. L. New York: Guilford Press, pp. 326–338.

Baeg, E. H., Kim, Y. B., Huh, K., *et al.* (2003). Dynamics of population code for working memory in the prefrontal cortex. *Neuron*, **40**, 177–88.

Ben-Yishai, R. R., Bar-Or, L. & Sompolinsky, H. (1995). Theory of orientation tuning in visual cortex. *Proceedings of the National Academy of Science USA*, **92**, 3844–8.

Brederode, J. F., Mulligan, V. K. A. & Hendrickson, A. E. (1990). Calcium-binding proteins as markers for subpopulations of GABAergic neurons in monkey striate cortex. *The Journal of Comparative Neurology*, **298**, 1–22.

Brody, C. D., Hernandez, A., Zainos, A. & Romo, R. (2003). Timing and neural encoding of somatosensory parametric working memory in macaque prefrontal cortex. *Cerebral Cortex*, **13**, 1196–207.

Brunel, N. & Wang, X.-J. (2001). Effects of neuromodulation in a cortical network model of object working memory dominated by recurrent inhibition. *Journal of Computational Neuroscience*, **11**, 63–85.

Brunel, N. & Wang, X.-J. (2003). What determines the frequency of fast network oscillations with irregular neural discharges? I. Synaptic dynamics and excitation-inhibition balance. *Journal of Neurophysiology*, **90**, 415–30.

Buzsaki, G., Geisler, C., Henze, D. A. & Wang, X.-J. (2004). Interneuron Diversity series: Circuit complexity and axon wiring economy of cortical interneurons. *Trends in the Neurosciences*, **27**, 186–93.

Camperi, M. & Wang, X.-J. (1998). A model of visuospatial short-term memory in prefrontal cortex: recurrent network and cellular bistability. *Journal of Computational Neuroscience*, **5**, 383–405.

Carlsson, A., Waters, N., Holm-Waters, S., et al. (2001). Interactions between monoamines, glutamate, and GABA in schizophrenia: new evidence. *Annual Review of Pharmacology and Toxicology*, **41**, 237–60.

Cauli, B., Audinat, E., Lambolez, B., et al. (1997). Molecular and physiological diversity of cortical nonpyramidal cells. *Journal of Neuroscience*, **17**, 3894–906.

Chafee, M. V. & Goldman-Rakic, P. S. (1998). Neuronal activity in macaque prefrontal area 8a and posterior parietal area 7ip related to memory guided saccades. *Journal of Neurophysiology*, **79**, 2919–40.

Chen, G., Greengard, P. & Yan, Z. (2004). Potentiation of NMDA receptor currents by dopamine D1 receptors in prefrontal cortex. *Proceedings of the National Academy of Science USA*, **101**, 2596–600.

Cohen, J. D., Braver, T. S. & Brown, J. W. (2002). Computational perspectives on dopamine function in prefrontal cortex. *Current Opinion in Neurobiology*, **12**, 223–9.

Cohen, J. D., Braver, T. S. & O'Reilly, R. C. (1996). A computational approach to prefrontal cortex, cognitive control and schizophrenia: recent developments and current challenges. *Philosophical Transactions of the Royal Society of London, B Biological Sciences*, **351**, 1515–27.

Compte, A., Brunel, N., Goldman-Rakic, P. S. & Wang, X.-J. (2000). Synaptic mechanisms and network dynamics underlying spatial working memory in a cortical network model. *Cerebral Cortex*, **10**, 910–23.

Compte, A., Constantinidis, C., Tegner, J., et al. (2003a). Temporally irregular mnemonic persistent activity in prefrontal neurons of monkeys during a delayed response task. *Journal of Neurophysiology*, **90**, 3441–54.

Compte, A., Sanchez-Vives, M. V., McCormick, D. A. & Wang, X.-J. (2003b). Cellular and network mechanisms of slow oscillatory activity (<1 Hz) and wave propagations in a cortical network model. *Journal of Neurophysiology*, **89**, 2707–25.

Conde, F., Lund, J. S., Jacobowitz, D. M., Baimbridge, K. G. & Lewis, D. A. (1994). Local circuit neurons immunoreactive for calretinin, calbindin D-28k or parvalbumin in monkey prefrontal cortex: distribution and morphology. *The Journal of Comparative Neurology*, **341**, 95–116.

Constantinidis, C. & Goldman-Rakic, P. S. (2002). Correlated discharges among putative pyramidal neurons and interneurons in the primate prefrontal cortex. *Journal of Neurophysiology*, **88**, 3487–97.

Constantinidis, C. & Procyk, E. (2004). The primate working memory networks. *Cognitive, Affective & Behavioral Neuroscience*, **4**, 444–65.

Constantinidis, C. & Wang, X.-J. (2004). A neural circuit basis for spatial working memory. *Neuroscientist*, **10**, 553–65.

Cossart, R., Aronov, D. & Yuste, R. (2003). Attractor dynamics of network UP states in the neocortex. *Nature*, **423**, 283–8.

Curtis, C. E. & D'Esposito, M. (2003). Persistent activity in the prefrontal cortex during working memory. *Trends in Cognitive Sciences*, **7**, 415–23.

Curtis, C. E. & D'Esposito, M. (2004). The effects of prefrontal lesions on working memory performance and theory. *Cognitive, Affective & Behavioral Neuroscience*, **4**, 528–39.

DeFelipe, J. (1997). Types of neurons, synaptic connections and chemical characteristics of cells immunoreactive for calbindin-D28K, parvalbumin' and calretinin in the neocortex. *Journal of Chemical Neuroanatomy*, **14**, 1–19.

DeFelipe, J., Gonzalez-Albo, M. C., Del Rio, M. R. & Elston, G. N. (1999). Distribution and patterns of connectivity of interneurons containing calbindin, calretinin, and parvalbumin in visual areas of occipital and temporal lobes of the macaque monkeys. *The Journal of Comparative Neurology*, **412**, 515–26.

Dehaene, S. & Changeux, J. P. (1995). Neuronal models of prefrontal cortical functions. *Annals of the New York Academy of Science*, **769**, 305–19.

Dombrowski, S. M., Hilgetag, C. C. & Barbas, H. (2001). Quantitative architecture distinguishes prefrontal cortical systems in the rhesus monkey. *Cerebral Cortex*, **11**, 975–88.

Douglas, R. J. & Martin, K. A. C. (2004). Neuronal circuits of the neocortex. *Annual Review of Neuroscience*, **27**, 419–51.

Dracheva, S., McGurk, S. R. & Haroutunian, V. (2005). mRNA expression of AMPA receptors and AMPA receptor binding proteins in the cerebral cortex of elderly schizophrenics. *Journal of Neuroscience Research*, **79**, 868–78.

Durstewitz, D. J., Seamans, K. & Sejnowski, T. J. (2000a). Dopamine-mediated stabilization of delay-period activity in a network model of prefrontal cortex. *Journal of Neurophysiology*, **83**, 1733–50.

Durstewitz, D. J., Seamans, K. & Sejnowski, T. J. (2000b). Neurocomputational models of working memory. *Nature Neuroscience*, **3**, 1184–91.

Egorov, A. V., Hamam, B. N., Fransen, E., Hasselmo, M. E. & Alonso, A. A. (2002). Graded persistent activity in entorhinal cortex neurons. *Nature*, **420**, 173–8.

Elston, G. N. (2000). Pyramidal cells of the frontal lobe: all the more spinous to think with. *Journal of Neuroscience*, **20-RC95**, 1–4.

Elston, G. N. & Gonzalez-Albo, M. C. (2003). Parvalbumin-, calbindin-, and calretinin-immunoreactive neurons in the prefrontal cortex of the owl monkey (aotus trivirgatus): a standardized quantitative comparison with sensory and motor areas. *Brain Behavior and Evolution*, **62**, 19–30.

Ferster, D. & Miller, K. D. (2000). Neural mechanisms of orientation selectivity in the visual cortex. *Annual Review of Neuroscience*, **23**, 441–71.

Freund, T. F. & Buzsaki, G. (1996). Interneurons of the hippocampus. *Hippocampus*, **6**, 347–470.

Fries, P., Reynolds, J. H., Rorie, A. E. & Desimone, R. (2001). Modulation of oscillatory neuronal synchronization by selective visual attention. *Science*, **291**, 1560–3.

Funahashi, S., Bruce, C. J. & Goldman-Rakic, P. S. (1989). Mnemonic coding of visual space in the monkey's dorsolateral prefrontal cortex. *Journal of Neurophysiology*, **61**, 331–49.

Fuster, J. M. (1988). *The Prefrontal Cortex*, 2nd edn. New York: Raven.

Fuster, J. M. & Alexander, G. (1971). Neuron activity related to short-term memory. *Science*, **173**, 652–4.

Fuster, J. M. & Jervey, J. P. (1982). Neuronal firing in the inferotemporal cortex of the monkey in a visual memory task. *Journal of Neuroscience*, **2**, 361–75.

Gabbott, P. L. A. & Bacon, S. J. (1996). Local circuit neurons in the medial prefrontal cortex (areas 24a,b,c, 25 and 32) in the monkey: II. Quantitative areal and laminar distributions. *The Journal of Comparative Neurology*, **364**, 609–36.

Gao, W.-J., Wang, Y. & Goldman-Rakic, P. S. (2003). Dopamine modulation of perisomatic and peridendritic inhibition in prefrontal cortex. *Journal of Neuroscience*, **23**, 1622–30.

Gnadt, J. W. & Andersen, R. A. (1988). Memory related motor planning activity in posterior parietal cortex of macaque. *Experimental Brain Research*, **70**, 216–20.

Goldman, M. S., Levine, J. H., Major, G., Tank, D. W. & Seung, H. S. (2003). Robust persistent neural activity in a model integrator with multiple hysteretic dendrites per neuron. *Cerebral Cortex*, **13**, 1185–95.

Goldman-Rakic, P. S. (1987). Circuitry of primate prefrontal cortex and regulation of behavior by representational memory. In *Handbook of Physiology – The Nervous System V*, eds. Plum, F. and Mountcastle, V. Bethesda, Maryland: American Physiological Society, pp. 373–417.

Goldman-Rakic, P. S. (1995). Cellular basis of working memory. *Neuron*, **14**, 477–85.

Gonchar, Y. & Burkhalter, A. (1999). Connectivity of GABAergic calretinin-immunoreactive neurons in rat primary visual cortex. *Cerebral Cortex*, **9**, 683–96.

Grunze, H. C., Rainnie, D. G., Hasselmo, M. E., *et al.* (1996). NMDA-dependent modulation of CA1 local circuit inhibition. *Journal of Neuroscience*, **16**, 2034–43.

Gulyás, A. I., Hájos, N. & Freund, T. (1996). Interneurons containing calretinin are specialized to control other interneurons in the rate hippocampus. *Journal of Neuroscience*, **16**, 3397–411.

Harrison, P. J. & Weinberger, D. R. (2005). Schizophrenia genes, gene expression, and neuropathology: on the matter of their convergence. *Molecular Psychiatry*, **10**, 40–68.

Healy, D. J., Haroutunian, V., Powchik, P., *et al.* (1998). AMPA receptor binding and subunit mRNA expression in prefrontal cortex and striatum of elderly schizophrenics. *Neuropsychopharmacology*, **19**, 278–86.

Hebb, D. O. (1949). *Organization of Behavior*. New York: Wiley.

Hestrin, S., Perkel, D. J., Sah, P., *et al.* (1990a). Physiological properties of excitatory synaptic transmission in the central nervous system. *Cold Spring Harbor Symposia on Quantitative Biology*, **55**, 87–93.

Hestrin, S., Sah, P. & Nicoll, R. (1990b). Mechanisms generating the time course of dual component excitatory synaptic currents recorded in hippocampal slices. *Neuron*, **5**, 247–53.

Hikosaka, O. & Wurtz, R. H. (1983). Visual and oculomotor functions of monkey substantia nigra pars reticulata. III. Memory-contingent visual and saccade responses. *Journal of Neurophysiology*, **49**, 1268–84.

Huang, Y.-Y., Simpson, E., Kellendonk, C. & Kandel, E. R. (2004). Genetic evidence for the bidirectional modulation of synaptic plasticity in the prefrontal cortex by D1 receptors. *Proceedings of the National Academy of Science USA*, **101**, 3236–41.

Hunter, W. S. (1913). The delayed reactions in animals and children. *Behavoral Monographs*, **2**, 1–86.

Jacobsen, C. F. (1936). Studies of cerebral function in primates: I. the functions of the frontal association areas in monkeys. *Comparative Psychological Monographs*, **13**, 1–68.

Jodo, E., Suzuki, Y., Katayama, T., *et al.* (2005). Activation of medial prefrontal cortex by phencyclidine is mediated via a hippocampo-prefrontal pathway. *Cerebral Cortex*, **15**, 663–9.

Kawaguchi, Y. & Kubota, Y. (1997). GABAergic cell subtypes and their synaptic connections in rat frontal cortex. *Cerebral Cortex*, **7**, 476–86.

Kim, J. N. & Shadlen, M. N. (1999). Neural correlates of a decision in the dorsolateral prefrontal cortex of the macaque. *Nature Neuroscience*, **2**, 176–85.

Kisvarday, Z. F., Ferecska, A. S., Kovaics, K., *et al.* (2003). One axon-multiple functions: Specificity of lateral inhibitory connections by large basket cells. *Journal of Neurocytology*, **31**, 255–64.

Kondo, H., Tanaka, K., Hashikawa, T. & Jones, E. G. (1999). Neurochemical gradients along monkey sensory cortical pathways: calbindin-immunoreactive pyramidal neurons in layers II and III. *European Journal of Neuroscience*, **11**, 4197–203.

Koulakov, A. A., Raghavachari, S., Kepecs, A. & Lisman, J. E. (2002). Model for a robust neural integrator. *Nature Neuroscience*, **5**, 775–82.

Krimer, L. S. & Goldman-Rakic, P. S. (2001). Prefrontal microcircuits: membrane properties and excitatory input of local, medium, and wide arbor interneurons. *Journal of Neuroscience*, **21**, 3788–96.

Kritzer, M. F. & Goldman-Rakic, P. S. (1995). Intrinsic circuit organization of the major layers and sublayers of the dorsolateral prefrontal cortex in the rhesus monkey. *The Journal of Comparative Neurology*, **359**, 131–43.

Krystal, J. H., Karper, L. P., Seibyl, J. P., *et al.* (1994). Subanesthetic effects of the noncompetitive NMDA antagonist, ketamine, in humans. psychotomimetic, perceptual, cognitive, and neuroendocrine responses. *Archives of General Psychiatry*, **51**, 199–214.

Lee, K.-H., Williams, L. M., Breakspear, M. & Gordon, E. (2003). Synchronous gamma activity: a review and contribution to an integrative neuroscience model of schizophrenia. *Brain Research. Brain Research Reviews*, **41**, 57–78.

Levitt, B., Lewis, D. A., Yoshioka, T. & Lund, J. (1993). Topography of pyramidal neuron intrinsic connections in macaque monkey prefrontal cortex (areas 9 and 46). *The Journal of Comparative Neurology*, **338**, 360–76.

Lewis, D. A., Hashimoto, T. & Volk, D. W. (2005). Cortical inhibitory neurons and schizophrenia. *Nature Reviews. Neuroscience*, **6**, 312–24.

Lisman, J. E., Fellous, J. M. & Wang, X.-J. (1998). A role for NMDA-receptor channels in working memory. *Nature Neuroscience*, **1**, 273–5.

Liu, G. (2004). Local structural balance and functional interaction of excitatory and inhibitory synapses in hippocampal dendrites. *Nature Neuroscience*, **7**, 373–9.

Llinas, R. R. (1988). The intrinsic electrophysiological properties of mammalian neurons: insights into central nervous system function. *Science*, **242**, 1654–64.

Loewenstein, Y. & Sompolinsky, H. (2003). Temporal integration by calcium dynamics in a model neuron. *Nature Neuroscience*, **6**, 961–7.

Lorente de Nó, R. (1933). Vestibulo-ocular reflex arc. *Archives of Neurology and Psychiatry*, **30**, 245–91.

McCormick, D., Connors, B., Lighthall, J. & Prince, D. (1985). Comparative electrophysiology of pyramidal and sparsely spiny stellate neurons in the neocortex. *Journal of Neurophysiology*, **54**, 782–806.

Machens, C. K., Romo, R. & Brody, C. D. (2005). Flexible control of mutual inhibition: a neural model of two-interval discrimination. *Science*, **307**, 1121–4.

Magee, J., Hoffman, D., Colbert, C. & Johnston, D. (1998). Electrical and calcium signaling in dendrites of hippocampal pyramidal neurons. *Annual Review of Physiology*, **60**, 327–46.

Major, G. & Tank, D. (2004). Persistent neural activity: prevalence and mechanisms. *Current Opinion in Neurobiology*, **14**, 675–84.

Markram, H., Gupta, A., Uziel, A., Wang, Y. & Tsodyks, M. (1998). Information processing with frequency-dependent synaptic connections. *Neurobiology of Learning and Memory*, **70**, 101–12.

Markram, H., Toledo-Rodriguez, M., Wang, Y., *et al.* (2004). Interneurons of the neocortical inhibitory system. *Nature Reviews. Neuroscience*, **5**, 793–807.

Meskenaite, V. (1997). Calretinin-immunoreactive local circuit neurons in the area 17 of the cynomolgus monkey, Macaca fascicularis. *The Journal of Comparative Neurology*, **379**, 113–32.

Mesulam, M.-M. (2000). *Principles of Behavioral and Cognitive Neurology*, 2nd edn. New York: Oxford University Press.

Miller, P., Brody, C. D., Romo, R. & Wang, X.-J. (2003). A recurrent network model of somatosensory parametric working memory in the prefrontal cortex. *Cerebral Cortex*, **13**, 1208–18.

Miller, E. K. & Cohen, J. D. (2001). An integrative theory of prefrontal cortex function. *Annual Review of Neuroscience*, **24**, 167–202.

Miller, E. K., Erickson, C. A. & Desimone, R. (1996). Neural mechanisms of visual working memory in prefrontal cortex of the macaque. *Journal of Neuroscience*, **16**, 5154–67.

Milner, B. (1972). Disorders of learning and memory after temporal lobe lesions in man. *Clinical Neurosurgery*, **19**, 421–46.

Miyashita, Y. (1988). Neuronal correlate of visual associative long-term memory in the primate temporal cortex. *Nature*, **335**, 817–20.

Newsome, W. T., Britten, K. H. & Movshon, J. A. (1989). Neuronal correlates of a perceptual decision. *Nature*, **341**, 52–4.

O'Reilly, R. L., Braver, T. S. & Cohen, J. D. (1999). A biologically based computational model of working memory. In *Models of Working Memory: Mechanisms of Active Maintenance and Executive Control*, Miyake, A. and Shah, V. New York: Cambridge University Press, pp. 375–411.

O'Reilly, R. L. & Munakata, Y. (2000). *Computational Explorations in Cognitive Neuroscience: Understanding the Mind by Simulating the Brain*. MA: MIT Press.

Parker, A. J. & Newsome, W. T. (1998). Sense and the single neuron: Probing the physiology of perception. *Annual Review of Neuroscience*, **21**, 227–77.

Pasternak, T. & Greenlee, M. W. (2005). Working memory in primate sensory systems. *Nature Reviews. Neuroscience*, **6**, 97–107.

Pesaran, B., Pezaris, J. S., Sahani, M., Mitra, P. P. & Andersen, R. A. (2002). Temporal structure in neuronal activity during working memory in macaque parietal cortex. *Nature Neuroscience*, **5**, 805−11.

Powell, K. D. & Goldberg, M. E. (2000). Response of neurons in the lateral intraparietal area to a distractor flashed during the delay period of a memory-guided saccade. *Journal of Neurophysiology*, **84**, 301−10.

Rainer, G., Assad, W. F. & Miller, E. K. (1998). Memory fields of neurons in the primate prefrontal cortex. *Proceedings of the National Academy of Science USA*, **95**, 15008−13.

Rao, S. G., Williams, G. V. & Goldman-Rakic, P. S. (2000). Destruction and creation of spatial tuning by disinhibition: GABA(A) blockade of prefrontal cortical neurons engaged by working memory. *Journal of Neuroscience*, **20**, 485−94.

Renart, A., Brunel, N. & Wang, X.-J. (2003a). Mean-field theory of recurrent cortical networks: Working memory circuits with irregularly spiking neurons. In *Computational Neuroscience: A Comprehensive Approach*, ed. J. Feng. Boca Raton: CRC Press.

Renart, A., Song, P. & Wang, X.-J. (2003b). Robust spatial working memory through homeostatic synaptic scaling in heterogeneous cortical networks. *Neuron*, **38**, 473−85.

Roitman, J. D. & Shadlen, M. N. (2002). Response of neurons in the lateral intraparietal area (LIP) during a combined visual discrimination reaction time task. *Journal of Neuroscience*, **22**, 9475−89.

Romo, R., Brody, C. D., Hernandez, A. & Lemus, L. (1999). Neuronal correlates of parametric working memory in the prefrontal cortex. *Nature*, **399**, 470−3.

Romo, R. & Salinas, E. (2000). Touch and go: Decision-making mechanisms in somatosensation. *Annual Review of Neuroscience*, **24**, 107−37.

Rowland, L. M., Astur, R. S., Jung, R. E., *et al.* (2005). Selective cognitive impairments associated with NMDA receptor blockade in humans. *Neuropsychopharmacology*, **30**, 633−9.

Sakai, K., Rowe, J. B. & Passingham, R. E. (2002). Active maintenance in prefrontal area 46 creates distractor-resistant memory. *Nature Neuroscience*, **5**, 479−84.

Sanchez-Vives, M. V. & McCormick, D. A. (2000). Cellular and network mechanisms of rhythmic recurrent activity in neocortex. *Nature Neuroscience*, **3**, 1027−34.

Schall, J. D. (2001). Neural basis of deciding, choosing and acting. *Nature Neuroscience*, **2**, 33−42.

Scherzer, C. R., Landwehrmeyer, G. B., Kerner, J. A., *et al.* (1998). Expression of N-methyl-D-aspartate receptor subunit mRNAs in the human brain: hippocampus and cortex. *The Journal of Comparative Neurology*, **390**, 75−90.

Seamans, J. K. & Yang, C. R. (2004). The principal features and mechanisms of dopamine modulation in the prefrontal cortex. *Progress in Neurobiology*, **74**, 1−58.

Seung, H. S., Lee, D. D., Reis, B. Y. & Tank, D. W. (2000). Stability of the memory of eye position in a recurrent network of conductance-based model neurons. *Neuron*, **26**, 259−71.

Shadlen, M. N. & Newsome, W. T. (1994). Noise, neural codes and cortical organization. *Current Opinion in Neurobiology*, **4**, 569−79.

Shadlen, M. N. & Newsome, W. T. (2001). Neural basis of a perceptual decision in the parietal cortex (area LIP) of the rhesus monkey. *Journal of Neurophysiology*, **86**, 1916–36.

Shima, K. & Tanji, J. (1998). Involvement of NMDA and non-NMDA receptors in the neuronal responses of the primary motor cortex to input from the supplementary motor area and somatosensory cortex: studies of task-performing monkeys. *Japanese Journal of Physiology*, **48**, 275–90.

Shu, Y., Hasenstab, A. & McCormick, D. A. (2003). Turning on and off recurrent balanced cortical activity. *Nature*, **423**, 288–93.

Singer, W. & Gray, C. M. (1995). Visual feature integration and the temporal correlation hypothesis. *Annual Review of Neuroscience*, **18**, 555–86.

Somogyi, P., Tamas, G., Lujan, R. & Buhl, E. H. (1998). Salient features of synaptic organisation in the cerebral cortex. *Brain Research Reviews*, **26**, 113–35.

Sompolinsky, H. & Shapley, R. (1997). New perspectives on the mechanisms for orientation selectivity. *Current Opinion in Neurobiology*, **7**, 514–22.

Song, P. & Wang, X.-J. (2005). Angular path integration by moving "hill of activity": a spiking neuron model without recurrent excitation of the head-direction system. *Journal of Neuroscience*, **25**, 1002–14.

Spencer, K. M., Nestor, P. G., Perlmutter, R., *et al.* (2004). Neural synchrony indexes disordered perception and cognition in schizophrenia. *Proceedings of the National Academy of Science USA*, **101**, 17288–93.

Stuss, D. T. & Knight, R. T. (2002). *Principles of Frontal Lobe Function.* New York: Oxford University Press.

Tegnér, J., Compte, A. & Wang, X.-J. (2002). Dynamical stability of reverberatory neural circuits. *Biological Cybernetics*, **87**, 471–81.

Traub, R. D., Whittington, M. A., Collins, S. B., Buzsáki, G. & Jefferys, J. G. R. (1996). Analysis of gamma rythms in the rat hippocampus *in vitro* and *in vivo*. *Journal of Physiology*, **493**, 471–84.

Traub, R. D., Bibbig, A., LeBeau, F. E. N., Buhl, E. H., &. Whittington, M. A. (2004). Cellular mechanisms of neuronal population oscillations in the hippocampus in vitro. *Annual Review of Neuroscience*, **27**, 247–78.

Wang, X.-J. (1999). Synaptic basis of cortical persistent activity: the importance of NMDA receptors to working memory. *Journal of Neuroscience*, **19**, 9587–603.

Wang, X.-J. (2001). Synaptic reverberation underlying mnemonic persistent activity. *Trends in the Neurosciences*, **24**, 455–63.

Wang, X.-J. (2002). Probabilistic decision making by slow reverberation in cortical circuits. *Neuron*, **36**, 955–68.

Wang, X.-J. (2003). Neural oscillations. In *Encyclopedia of Cognitive Science*, (ed.) Nadil, L. London: MacMillan Reference Ltd., pp. 272–80.

Wang, X.-J. & Buzsaki, G. (1996). Gamma oscillations by synaptic inhibition in a hippocampal interneuronal network. *Journal of Neuroscience*, **16**, 6402–13.

Wang, X.-J. & Goldman-Rakic, P. S. (eds) (2003). Special issue: Persistent neural activity: theory and experiments. *Cerebral Cortex*, **13**, 1123–269.

Wang, X.-J., Tegner, J., Constantinidis, C. & Goldman-Rakic, P. S. (2004a). Division of labor among distinct subtypes of inhibitory neurons in a cortical microcircuit of working memory. *Proceedings of the National Academy of Science USA*, **101**, 1368–73.

Wang, M., Vijayraghavan, S. & Goldman-Rakic, P. S. (2004b). Selective D2 receptor actions on the functional circuitry of working memory. *Science*, **303**, 853–6.

Williams, G. V. & Goldman-Rakic, P. S. (1995). Modulation of memory fields by dopamine D1 receptors in prefrontal cortex. *Nature*, **376**, 572–5.

Wilson, H. R. & Cowan, J. D. (1972). Excitatory and inhibitory interactions in localized populations of model neurons. *Biophysical Journal*, **12**, 1–24.

Wilson, H. R. & Cowan, J. D. (1973). A mathematical theory of the functional dynamics of cortical and thalamic nervous tissue. *Kybernetik*, **13**, 55–80.

Wood, J. N. & Grafman, J. (2003). Human prefrontal cortex: processing and representational perspectives. *Nature Reviews. Neuroscience*, **4**, 139–47.

Xiang, Z., Huguenard, J. R. & Prince, D. A. (1998). GABAA receptor mediated currents in interneurons and pyramidal cells of rat visual cortex. *Journal of Physiology*, **506**, 715–30.

Prefrontal cortex: typical and atypical development

Maureen Dennis

1 Introduction

The ability to bind the past and the future, to become privileged to the contents of other peoples' minds and to share with them the contents of our own minds, and to use both emotion and thought to guide how we make decisions and what we express socially, all make us uniquely human and able to reflect on our past, our present, our future, our own mind, and others' minds, and to experience emotions and modulate them with thought. In some manner, these abilities are associated with the normal function of the prefrontal cortex.

All cortex in front of the central sulcus is frontal cortex. The primary motor cortex (Brodmann area [BA] 4) is the area in front of the central sulcus (Figure 5.1). The premotor cortex and supplementary motor area (BA 6) lie in front of the primary motor cortex. Everything in front of BA 6 is prefrontal cortex: BA 8, 9, 10, 12, 44, 45, 46, 47, and 9/46. The anterior cingulate gyrus and the posteromedial orbitofrontal cortex are important limbic areas within the prefrontal cortex, and the central frontal lobes also contain the orbitofrontal olfactory area. Functionally, the prefrontal cortex consists of multimodal association cortex, with different architectonic areas having distinct connections with cortical, subcortical, and subtentorial structures (Petrides & Pandya, 2002).

The dorsolateral prefrontal cortex (BA 46 and 9) is above and below the superior frontal sulcus, and is bordered posteriorly by Area 6 and anteriorly by the frontal polar cortex (BA 10). The ventromedial area includes the medial surface and parts of the lateral orbitofrontal region (BA 25, lower 24, 32, and medial parts of 11, 12, and 10, with adjacent white matter). The orbitofrontal cortex constitutes the inferior surface, and includes the orbital gyri and the rectus gyrus. The three main surfaces, lateral, medial, and orbitofrontal correspond to broad functional subdivisions.

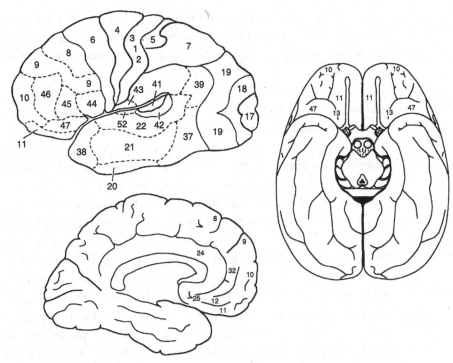

Figure 5.1. Brodmann areas (see text).

2 History of studies of prefrontal cortex function

Interest in the functions of the prefrontal cortex burgeoned after the publication of, arguably, the most famous case in behavioral neurology, that of Phineas Gage (Harlow, 1868; Macmillan, 2000). While at work in Vermont setting explosive charges for the Rutland and Burlington Railroad, Gage's tamping iron reversed direction, and penetrated his left and right prefrontal cortices (Damasio *et al.*, 1994). As a young adult foreman, Gage had been shrewd, energetic, and persistent in executing plans. Postaccident, he showed intact movement, speech, memory, new learning, and reasoning, but became impulsive, restless, impatient, and capricious, alternately rigid and vacillating, forming multiple plans that he could not sustain, and exhibiting impaired social behavior. The Gage case showed that significant prefrontal insult could spare motor function, memory, and intellect, while disrupting cognitive inhibition, planning, and psychosocial function.

From the mid nineteenth century to the present time, the nature of prefrontal cortex function has been actively investigated in relation to a range of questions, most related to the structure and function of the mature brain. The early era of research on prefrontal cortex development was concerned with three questions: the time course of development of the frontal lobe compared to posterior brain regions; the time course of maturation of subcomponents of the prefrontal cortex; and the emergence of frontal lobe functions during development.

Broca compared the timing of frontal lobe and posterior cortex development. Studying a series of 15 fetal brains, he attempted to establish the sequence in which the convolutions and fissures could be seen in the frontal lobes compared to the temporal and parietal lobes (Broca, 1877). Although he was unable to provide an answer to the question, it is of interest that the question itself was considered worthy of investigation as early as 1877.

In a series of studies describing her work in Fulton's laboratory in Yale between 1932 and 1934, Kennard reported correlations between anterior cortex brain lesions and behavioral outcomes in infant rhesus monkeys in relation to motor function, frontal eye field function, and behavior. Her complex findings, which later were erroneously interpreted as showing that early-onset lesions had little effect on motor function, actually formed the first framework for a true developmental neuropsychology. She showed that lesions in BA 8 produce paralysis of conjugate deviation of the eyes, whether the lesions are made in infancy or in adulthood (Kennard, 1938), suggesting that lesions to a functional brain region will produce identical effects in infants and adults; and also that there is a complex evolution of functional deficits after some early lesions, depending on what is functionally mature at the time of evaluation (Kennard, 1940). Kennard was perhaps the first individual to study behavioral changes after early prefrontal lesions. She showed that bilateral prefrontal lesions produce permanent hyperactivity, immediately after the lesion in the adult but later in development after lesions in infancy (Kennard et al., 1941). Kennard also made lesions at different time points in development and compared lesion-induced behavioral regressions to younger, normal stages of motor development (Kennard & Fulton, 1942).

Earlier research into the development of frontal lobe function was limited in a number of ways. A conceptual bias in favor of age-based functional plasticity meant that brain lesion outcome was assumed to correlate negatively with age, even when the data suggested otherwise. For example, the incidence of aphasia was greater following left-sided than right-sided lesions in the literature of the last quarter of the nineteenth century, although interpretation of these and later childhood lesion data continued to be interpreted in terms of lateralized equipotentiality for language (discussed in Dennis & Whitaker, 1977). Poor understanding of the different etiologies that produced brain insult in children and adults meant that studies of expressive aphasia compared children with trauma to adults with strokes (discussed in Dennis, 2003). The time lag between lesion onset and frontal lobe symptoms was much longer in children than in adults, making it difficult to associate early lesions with late-onset behavioral changes. For example, Gage's psychosocial changes were apparent shortly after his frontal lobe trauma, whereas the social and emotional maladjustment following perinatal bilateral frontal damage in the Ackerly and Benton (1948) case emerged gradually, as he reached adulthood. For many years, assessment tools were limited to global measures of IQ, so that the complex neurocognitive disorders of frontal lobe patients could not be formally assessed. Ackerly (1964) provided psychometric information on his 1948 case of perinatal bilateral frontal damage, but it was his clinical descriptions of the psychosocial deficits that caused him to conclude that the prefrontal cortex was the nursery for the faculties that distinguish man as man (pp. 214–15). Although Kennard had described frontal lobe lesion effects in monkeys that emerged slowly in the course of development, it was many years before the biological features of the insult, the age at insult, and the available family, educational, and social reserve became formalized in models of the outcome of brain lesions in children (e.g. Dennis, 1988, 2000). Early studies of frontal development relied on postmortem data, which meant that it was not possible, except retrospectively, to correlate prefrontal brain lesions with contemporaneous changes in function.

The modern era of research into frontal lobe function was brought into being by a number of advances. One was the emergence of developmental psychology as a field with assessment tools to fractionate infant and child behavior. Whereas the earlier era had lacked all but the crudest tools for studying human infants and children, the modern era has been able to study functions such as attention in newborns and infants by the use of habituation techniques. A second advance came with developmental change models and growth curve modeling to measure age effects and to assess the magnitude of developmental change. A third advance was the modern era of structural and functional neuroimaging, which has made it possible, not only to identify frontal lobe pathologies during life, but also to correlate them with concurrent neurocognitive function.

Even today, the assessment of prefrontal function in human children is challenging. Many aspects of self-regulation, inhibition, working memory, and planning emerge only gradually in the course of development. The precursors of prefrontal capacities in infants and preschoolers are not always obvious. In addition, the younger the child, the more limited the number of contexts demanding executive and prefrontal implementation. Some tests of prefrontal function presuppose complex academic competencies such as reading decoding fluency, which younger children have not yet acquired. Almost all prefrontal skills involve a degree of self-awareness or metacognitive monitoring, which are challenging to measure in young children, even after they have begun to emerge.

3   Prefrontal functional model

Recent clinical and experimental research has provided a perspective on the structural and functional development of the frontal lobes, its anatomical and functional relations with other, more remote brain regions, and has proposed developmental functional models (e.g. Dennis, 1991; Stuss & Anderson, 2004). To organize this new material, a working model of prefrontal cortex function is proposed (Figure 5.2) that involves five assumptions:

The overarching function of the prefrontal cortex is to bind together what cannot be sensed (i.e. what cannot be seen, heard, touched, smelled, or tasted) and to bring it into the world of actual or possible action.

The functional organization of the prefrontal cortex involves the establishment of bound representations that are effected by processing resources that allow top-down control (Miller, 2000); the model is therefore a hybrid (Wood & Grafman, 2003) that includes both memory representations and computational processes.

Representations, which are related to the operations of the orbitofrontal and ventromedial prefrontal cortices, have a grammar that concerns organized knowledge structures of the kind described by Grafman as

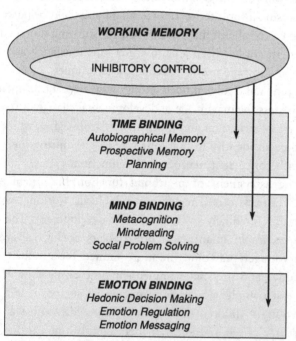

Figure 5.2.   Model of frontal lobe processing resources and frontal lobe representations.

structured event complexes (Grafman, 2002, Chapter 3 in this volume) and a content that concerns time binding (past+future), mind binding (own+other), and emotion binding (affect+thought).

The capacity-limited processing resources (working memory and inhibitory control) effect top-down modulation of attention and memory, and are related to operations of the dorsolateral prefrontal cortex.

Integrated prefrontal function develops gradually, but key elements are present early in life and reconfigure throughout childhood before the adult pattern emerges.

Using Figure 5.2 as a heuristic, this paper explores four developmental issues about the prefrontal cortex:

1. Typical and atypical development of prefrontal cortex microstructure and macrostructure.
2. Typical and atypical development of prefrontal cortex processing resources.
3. Typical and atypical development of prefrontal cortex representations.
4. Models of the developmental relations between prefrontal cortex processing resources and prefrontal cortex representations.

4   Prefrontal cortex development

In humans, fundamental cycles of brain development occur prenatally, although aspects of central nervous system development that are important for organizing and processing sensory input and for higher-level cognition continue throughout childhood and into adult life. Synaptic development occurs in a complex sequence and pattern (Goldman-Rakic et al., 1997). Myelogenesis, the coating of axons in a lipid and protein sheath, also occurs in a specific sequence or cycle over the course of pre-and postnatal development. Glial cells, which continue to proliferate throughout the life span, produce myelin in a pattern of progressive encephalization, starting in the spinal cord prenatally and ending in the higher cortical association areas in mid-life.

A variety of methods have been used to study the structural development of the prefrontal cortex, including electrophysiological recordings (Thatcher, 1997; Segalowitz & Davies, 2004). Fetal brains and the brains of children who died from nonneurological causes have been a source of significant information about frontal development. Postmortem studies have shown that the progression of frontal myelination is a protracted operation that continues well into the third decade of life (Yakovlev & Lecours, 1967). Postmortem work (Rabinowicz, 1986) has shown a decrease in cortical thickness of the frontal pole between the ages of 6 and 22 years, consistent with earlier postmortem work that revealed synaptic density to decline in the frontal cortex between ages 2 and 16 (Huttenlocher, 1979).

An important source of information about prefrontal structural maturation is a set of recent studies of quantified in vivo magnetic resonance imaging (MRI). Empirical data from newer MRI studies have confirmed the older postmortem evidence that the cortical ribbon of the frontal lobes thins during late childhood and adolescence, as a result of regressive activity within the gray matter and/or progressive activity such as myelination within white matter (Yakovlev & Lecours, 1967). There are rapid growth spurts in the frontal lobes relative to the temporal lobes in the first 2 years after birth (Matsuzawa et al., 2001). After age 5, brain volumes are relatively stable (Reiss et al., 1996), although the proportion of gray-to-white matter lessens with increasing age (e.g. Sowell & Jernigan, 1998). Specifically, there is a reduction in gray matter volume between childhood and early adulthood (Gogtay et al., 2004), which contributes to the decreasing ratio of cortical gray-to-white matter shown to occur up to age 20 (Pfefferbaum et al., 1994). Gray matter loss progresses linearly at an early age, whereas more rostral regions of the frontal lobe (superior, inferior frontal gyri) mature successively in an anterior progression, also indicated by progressively later peaks of nonlinear gray matter loss. By adolescence, this decreasing ratio is localized to the frontal and parietal lobes (Sowell et al., 1999, 2002).

4.1   Cross-sectional quantified MRI studies

In a recent cross-sectional study of typically developing children and adolescents, O'Donnell and coworkers (2005) identified in vivo thickness changes in the frontal polar cortex (BA 10), the dorsolateral prefrontal cortex (BA 46 and the lateral aspect of BA 9), and the striate cortex. T1-weighted structural MRI scans from 35 typically developing participants aged 8—20 years were used to construct 3D models of the brain, from which cortical thickness was measured. For the two frontal regions, although not for the striate cortex, cortical thickness decreased with increasing age between 8 and 20 years. The process underlying gray matter loss may involve cerebral white matter changes, synaptic pruning, trophic glial and vascular changes, or cell shrinkage. Paus (2005) has suggested that the asynchronous age-related changes in gray matter volume might equally represent loss ("pruning") or gain (intracortical myelination).

4.2   Longitudinal quantified MRI studies

Recent longitudinal studies have provided a detailed perspective on frontal lobe development. Gogtay et al. (2004) obtained MRI scans on 13 children every 2 years for 8—10 years, which enabled them to visualize the dynamical anatomical sequence of cortical gray matter development over the age range of 4–21 years, using quantitative 4-dimensional maps and time-lapse movies. Higher order association cortices matured only after lower order somatosensory and visual cortices, the functions of which they integrate. Phylogenetically older areas mature earlier than newer ones. Frontal maturation proceeds in a back-to-front direction, beginning in primary motor cortex (precentral gyrus) and spreading anteriorly over the superior and inferior frontal gyri, with the prefrontal cortex developing last. Within the prefrontal cortex, the frontal pole and precentral cortex mature early. In the frontal cortex, the dorsolateral cortex matures last, coinciding with its later myelination.

4.3   Atypical prefrontal development

Prefrontal brain development may be abnormal because of problems in organizational genetic-metabolic processes or because of pathological conditions acquired after a period of normal early development. Chief among the organizational abnormalities is phenylketonuria, a developmental disorder associated with abnormal dopamine metabolism. Among acquired pathologies, some may involve direct structural or functional effects on frontal gray or white matter (e.g. penetrating brain injury, see Marlowe, 1992), traumatic brain injury (TBI), frontal lobe seizure disorders (Culhane-Shelburn et al., 2002), and frontal lobe brain tumors (Dennis et al., 2004), while others may affect frontal function through remote effects (e.g. lesions of the cerebellum). Further, some disorders defined primarily in terms of aberrant behavior (attention deficit hyperactivity disorder, Tourette syndrome) may be associated with prefrontal cortex anomalies, such as volume reductions in gray and white matter or abnormal long association and projection fiber bundles (Kates et al., 2002).

The prefrontal cortex is relatively intact in some forms of significant developmental brain insult. For example, children with spina bifida meningomyelocele have normal frontal volumes (on voxel-based morphometry), despite volume loss and loss of connectivity in the posterior cortex (Fletcher et al., 2005). Of added interest, these children have deficits in the posterior attention functions of attention orienting and inhibition of return, but retain normal top-down attentional control on endogenous orienting tasks (Dennis et al., 2005). In this particular neurodevelopmental disorder, frontal lobe volume and frontal lobe functions are spared relative to posterior brain structure and functions.

4.4   Phenylketonuria

Dopamine has an important organizational effect on the development of the dorsolateral prefrontal cortex (Diamond, 1996). The fact that the distribution of dopamine axons within the dorsolateral prefrontal cortex changes over the same time frame that young monkeys acquire key dorsolateral prefrontal cortex skills has promoted a series of investigations about the functional effects of human developmental dopamine anomalies.

Phenylketonuria is a genetic disorder associated with atypically high levels of phenylalanine. Children with this condition and high phenylalanine levels have impairments, not only in the dorsolateral prefrontal cortex functions of inhibitory control and working memory, but also in visual contrast sensitivity, which is sensitive to retinal dopamine levels (Diamond, 1996).

The catechol gene affects the duration of dopamine activity in the prefrontal cortex, and the methionine polymorphism results in a slower breakdown of prefrontal dopamine. Children homozygous for the methionine polymorphism perform poorly on tasks sensitive to the level of dopamine (Diamond et al., 2004). In brief, the level of prefrontal neurotransmitters predicts children's performance on tests of prefrontal function.

4.5   TBI

TBI, a common form of acquired brain disorder, is often associated with damage to anterior brain regions. Children with TBI have disproportionate reduction in prefrontal and temporal lobe volumes (Wilde et al., 2005). The prefrontal damage following childhood TBI is of three types. The first is contusional injury to the frontal cortex, which, like the temporal lobe, is especially vulnerable to contusional injuries (Levin et al., 1996). The second is diffuse axonal injury, which is seen on late MRI in the form of gliosis, hemosiderin deposits, and volume loss, occurs throughout the corpus callosum and frontal lobe white matter, and becomes more evident in the 3 years following severe childhood TBI (Levin et al., 2000). The third is a reduction in brain connectivity, as shown by changes in the directionality and integrity of white matter tracts after childhood brain trauma (Lee et al., 2003).

Given the proposed role of frontal regions in cognitive control and behavioral self-regulation (Mendelsohn et al., 1992; Miller & Cohen, 2001), it is not surprising that children with closed head injury often show a range of impairments in dorsolateral, orbitofrontal, and ventromedial functions, and, further, that these impairments are correlated with the presence of frontal lobe injury (Scheibel & Levin, 1997). A significant amount of information about the developmental effects of prefrontal lesions has emerged from studies of childhood TBI.

4.6   Cerebellar lesions

The phylogenetically newer areas of the cerebellum (neocerebellum, which includes the posterior lobe of the lateral hemispheres of cerebellar cortex (lobules VI through VIII, lobules VI and VII of the vermis in the medial portion of the cerebellar vermis, and one of the deep nuclei, the dentate) are functionally connected to the dorsolateral prefrontal cortex. The structural organization of the interactions between the cerebellum and the prefrontal cortex involves multiple, topographically closed loops (Middleton & Strick, 2001).

The dentate nuclei comprise output channels directed at different areas of the prefrontal cortex (Middleton & Strick, 2001). Output from ventral portions of the dentate nucleus of the cerebellum project to dorsal prefrontal areas (BA 9 and 46) via the thalamus, although not to more ventral areas of the prefrontal areas (BA 12 and 46v) (Dunn & Strick, 2003). Cerebellar output to prefrontal cortex is topographically organized, such that output projections to prefrontal nonmotor areas are derived from topographically distinct areas within the dentate nucleus. Input to the cerebellum originates in the same region that receives input from the cerebellum via the thalamus, prefrontal areas 9 and 46, which project to the pontine nuclei that provide input to the cerebellum (Schmahmann & Pandya, 1995, 1997).

The cerebellar-frontal connection has become a topic of considerable interest in recent years. Diamond (2000) has highlighted the close coactivation of the neocerebellum and dorsolateral prefrontal cortex in functional neuroimaging, the similarities in the effects of cerebellar and dorsolateral prefrontal damage, and the presence of abnormalities in both cerebellum and prefrontal cortex in some neurodevelopmental disorders. Further stimulating interest in the developmental cerebellar-frontal connection is the increasing evidence that childhood cerebellar lesions show little or no functional age-based plasticity in gross motor function (Dennis et al., 1999) or in nonmotor functions such as short-duration timing, which is impaired after cerebellar damage in both adults (Ivry & Keele, 1989) and children (Dennis et al., 2004). Finally, some effects of cerebellar lesions are phenotypically similar to those that follow prefrontal lesions.

Adult patients with cerebellar lesions exhibit problems in frontal lobe skills: executive function (Grafman et al., 1992; Appollonio et al., 1993), cognitive planning (Kim et al., 1994), shifting attention (Allen et al., 1997), emotional modulation (Reiman et al., 1989), grammatical production (Silveri et al., 1994), and verbal fluency (Fiez et al., 1992). Cerebellar lesions also produce a pattern of cognitive and behavioral changes, termed the *cerebellar cognitive-affective syndrome*, that include executive dysfunction in planning, mental flexibility, working memory, inhibitory control, and personality changes (Schmahmann & Sherman, 1998).

The cerebellar cognitive-affective syndrome has been reported in children (Levisohn et al., 2000; Sadeh & Cohen, 2001). Childhood tumors of the cerebellar vermis are associated with affective dysregulation and complex alterations in social and communicative behavior, some involving autistic-like symptomatology (Riva & Giorgi, 2000). Of interest, deficits in the regulation of affect are sometimes evident in children with cerebellar tumors treated with surgery but with neither radiotherapy nor chemotherapy (Levisohn et al., 2000).

Cognitive-affective changes are more evident after lesions of the posterior lobe and vermis than after anterior lobe lesions, their putative neural substrate being a disruption of the cerebellar modulation of prefrontal, posterior parietal, superior temporal, and limbic regions (Levisohn et al., 2000). The functional relations between the cerebellum and the prefrontal cortex, in particular, the relation between the cerebellar cognitive-affective syndrome and medial cerebellar lesions and the developmental relevance of the neocerebellum-dorsolateral prefrontal cortex connection, are yet to be fully understood.

5 Prefrontal function: Processing resources

5.1 Working memory and inhibitory control

Two processing resources fuel the top-down control and formation of representations in the prefrontal cortex, working memory and inhibitory control. Inhibitory control is the ability to stop or modulate ongoing actions or to hold competing representations; working memory is the process by which information is temporarily activated in memory for rapid manipulation and retrieval.

There are several reasons for considering working memory and inhibitory control as resources: both have a limited capacity, in keeping with the idea that top-down modulation is resource-limited (Gazzeley et al., 2005); both operate over a wide range of domains; many prefrontal cortex neurons are modality nonspecific (Miller, 2000); and cognitive control is broadly distributed in the prefrontal cortex (Derrfuss et al., 2004). The reason to depict inhibitory control as embedded within working memory is that the neural circuitry activated during inhibitory control tasks is a subset of that activated during working memory tasks (Bunge et al., 2001).

In the mature brain, working memory has been linked to operations of the dorsolateral prefrontal cortex (Petrides et al., 1993; D'Esposito et al., 1999; Goldman-Rakic & Leung, 2002; Fletcher & Henson, 2001). The neural basis of age-related changes in working memory performance is related to age-related changes in the dorsolateral but not the ventrolateral prefrontal cortex (Rypma & D'Esposito, 2000).

A variety of studies have identified the functions of working memory and inhibitory control in terms of both typical and atypical development. More recently, functional imaging studies have begun to map the neural circuitry underlying the development of these functions.

5.1.1 Typical development

Inhibitory control may be automatic or effortful (Friedman & Miyake, 2004). Automatic inhibitory control, such as the ability to avoid returning gaze to a previously explored location, develops in infancy or early in childhood (Richards, 2003). Effortful forms of inhibitory control involve the ability to resist interference, and to stop performing automatic or routine behaviors when they become undesirable due to changing circumstances or to altered intentions. Within the broad domain of effortful control, there exists a distinction between inhibitory control that involves consciously stopping an ongoing action, *response inhibition*, and inhibitory control that requires resisting interference, set shifting, the maintenance of competing rules, and conflict monitoring, termed *cognitive inhibition* (Perner *et al.*, 2002).

Effortful forms of inhibitory control have a more protracted developmental course (Houghton & Tipper, 1994; Harnishfeger & Pope, 1996; Williams *et al.*, 1999; Band *et al.*, 2000; Pascual-Leone, 2001). Throughout the preschool years, children become more able to delay responding, to suppress responding in a go-no go paradigm, and to respond correctly in the presence of a conflicting response option (Livesey & Morgan, 1991; Gerstadt *et al.*, 1994; Diamond & Taylor, 1996; Kochanska *et al.*, 1996).

Working memory and inhibitory control develop in tandem (Hulme & Roodenrys, 1995; Cowan, 1997). The relation between working memory and inhibitory control begins to develop during the preschool years, although coordination of these cognitive resources is not manifest until about the fifth year (Dowsett & Livesey, 2000). Inhibitory control keeps irrelevant information out of working memory (Dempster, 1993; Harnishfeger & Bjorklund, 1994; Engle *et al.*, 1995), and, in some views, inhibitory control accounts for working memory growth during childhood (Bjorklund & Harnishfeger, 1990; Dempster, 1993). Later in development, working memory and inhibitory control are in a constant state of recalibration within a limited resource processing system (Oberauer & Suess, 2001).

5.1.2 Atypical development

Childhood closed head injury is associated with deficits in inhibitory control. These deficits include inability to resist perceptual interference, to stop an ongoing action, and to activate and inhibit competing rules.

Children with TBI have difficulty in perceptual interference. At 6 months or more postinjury, children with TBI have difficulty maintaining vigilance in response to distraction, and the degree of interference is inversely correlated with age at injury and time since injury (Dennis *et al.*, 1995).

The ability to withhold responding in response to a signal is impaired in children with TBI tested 2 years postinjury (Levin *et al.*, 1993). Pervasive deficits in stop inhibition occur in children with closed head injury in the acute phase; recovery is greater in younger children and in those with fewer structural brain lesions. Although Konrad and coworkers (2000) reported stop inhibition to be generally impaired following moderate to severe TBI in children, more recent studies have shown that this sequel is restricted to children who have experienced a more severe injury or who have comorbid clinical attention disorders (Purvis & Schachar, 2001; Schachar *et al.*, 2004). Response inhibition, the ability to stop an ongoing action, is impaired in a subgroup of children with closed head injury (Schachar *et al.*, 2004).

Executive inhibition deficits have also been reported. Compared to their noninjured peers, children with closed head injury have difficulty maintaining a counterfactual rule (Manly *et al.*, 1999), or switching between salient and nonsalient responses (Roncadin *et al.*, 2003).

Childhood TBI of moderate or severe degree is associated with working memory deficits, with moderately or severely injured children being most impaired in both cross-sectional (Roncadin *et al.*, 2004) and longitudinal (Levin *et al.*, 2004) studies. Deficits in working memory are consequential for higher language functions, being associated with impairments in sentence comprehension (Dennis & Barnes, 1990; Montgomery, 1995; Hanten *et al.*, 1999), inferencing (Barnes & Dennis, 2001), and discourse (Dennis & Barnes, 1990, 2000; Chapman *et al.*, 1992).

5.1.3 Neuroimaging correlates

In children after TBI, inhibitory processes are correlated with the presence of prefrontal injury. On a response inhibition task, GO/NOGO performance is impaired in children 2 years postinjury, and the performance is related to volume of left prefrontal lesions (Levin *et al.*, 1993).

Using event-related functional magnetic resonance imaging (fMRI) and parametric variation of a GO-NOGO task, Durston *et al.* (2002) examined the effect of interference on the neural processes involved in inhibitory control. Although both adults and 6-to-10-year-old children showed increased errors with more interference, successful response inhibition was associated with stronger prefrontal activation on children than in adults. In adults, activation in the ventral prefrontal regions increased with increasing interference from GO trials; in children, this circuitry was maximally activated regardless of the number of GO trials. Compared to adults, children's response inhibition is less differentiated, and more globally susceptible to interference.

Prefrontal gray matter thinning has functional consequences for memory. A more mature (i.e. thinner) frontal cortex is associated with better verbal memory retrieval, regardless of age, and the relation is specific because the same association does not hold for mesial temporal lobe gray matter volume (Sowell *et al.*, 2001).

Adolescence, a time of important changes in both brain and behavior, is also a time of potential disjunctions between the developing brain, cognition, and behavior, which mature along different timetables (Steinberg, 2005). Concurrent analyses of brain maturation and cognitive development during adolescence have verified a continuous increase in the global and local volume of white matter, and have begun to address the relation between brain maturation and social cognition; for example, there is an increased ability in adolescents relative to younger children to suppress reflective saccades and to respond to socially salient stimuli (Paus, 2005).

6   Prefrontal function: time binding

The ability to link the past and the future, termed *time travel* (Fuster, 2000) or *chronesthesia* (Tulving, 2002), is an important frontal lobe function, possibly a distinctly humanly one (Roberts, 2002). Time travel enables autobiographical memory, prospective memory, and planning.

6.1   Autobiographical memory

Autobiographical memory, which binds awareness of the self as continuous over time and as having a past and a future, is mediated by a distributed neural system that includes the anteromedial prefrontal cortex, which integrates sensory information with self-specific information (Levine, 2004).

6.1.1   Typical development

Autobiographical memory is difficult to assess before age 4, because early time event knowledge is fragmented, cue-dependent, and inconsistent (Fivush & Hamond, 1990). There is little information about the emergence of time binding in relation to frontal lobe development, although it has been suggested that there is a temporal coincidence between the emergence of recollections of self and the timing of some regressive cortical and progressive white matter changes (Levine, 2004).

6.1.2   Atypical development

There has been no systematic study of autobiographical memory in children with prefrontal lobe injury.

6.2 Prospective memory

Prospective memory is the recall of intentions to be activated in the future (in contrast with retrospective memory, the recall of events or information from the past). Depending on the retrieval context, prospective memory can be event based (e.g. delivering a message to a particular person), time based (e.g. remembering to keep an appointment at a specific hour), or activity based (e.g. remembering to take a pill after dinner, whenever dinner occurs) (Kvavilashvili & Ellis, 1996).

6.2.1 Typical development

Prospective memory improves from age 2 to the high school years. Children as young as 2—4 years can perform future intentions such as reminding their mothers to get ice cream (Sommerville et al., 1983). In typically developing school age children, prospective memory performance changes with a number of variables, including external retrieval cues (Kreutzer et al., 1975) intervening or ongoing task complexity (Wichman & Oyasato, 1983), interference (Kvavilashvili et al., 2001), time monitoring (Ceci & Bronfenbrenner, 1985), and encoding manipulations (Passolunghi et al., 1995).

6.2.2 Atypical development

School-age children who have sustained a TBI at least 2 years prior to testing are impaired on event-based and activity-based prospective memory tasks (McCauley & Levin, 2000, 2001). For adolescents with TBI, event-based prospective memory worsens with increased cognitive demands (Shum, 2005). Compared to children with mild TBI, children with severe TBI do not benefit from prospective memory reminders (McCauley & Levin, 2004).

6.3 Planning

Planning involves formulating a series of operations in order to achieve a goal; in practical terms, it requires the ability to project several moves ahead during active problem solving. Efficient planning is a multidirectional process, and the best planning is not linear and inflexible, but rather opportunistic, leaving room for online revision. Planning activates prefrontal cortex areas 9, 46, and 10 (Cabeza & Nyberg, 2000). Adults with prefrontal damage show immature, inefficient planning (Grafman, 1989).

6.3.1 Typical development

As they develop, children show increasing ability to plan. The ability to plan further into the future improves with normal development. The Tower of London task requires configuring beads on vertical rods from one model into another, with the models varying in the number of moves required to effect the reconfiguration. Children by age 4 can solve a 2-move reconfiguration, and older children can solve reconfigurations with a higher number of moves (Levin *et al.*, 1991). The nature of planning also changes throughout development. Young children are rigid in their planning, whereas older children and adults show flexible, more opportunistic planning (Hayes-Roth & Hayes-Roth, 1979).

6.3.2 Atypical development

Planning deficits are evident in children with various forms of frontal lobe damage, including frontal lobe seizures (Culhane-Shelburne *et al.*, 2002) and TBI (Levin *et al.*, 2001). After childhood TBI, performance on the Tower of London task varies with task difficulty (performance is poorer when more planning moves are required), TBI severity (children with severe TBI perform more poorly and break more rules than children with milder forms of TBI), and lesion volume, including orbitofrontal, dorsolateral, and frontal white matter lesions (Levin *et al.*, 1994). Children with severe TBI are impaired on the Porteus Maze Task, a graded series of pencil-and-paper mazes that must be traversed by planning rather than by feedback about blind alleys (Porteus, 1959), and Porteus task performance is correlated with prefrontal lesion volume (Levin *et al.*, 2001). Adolescents with early damage to the prefrontal cortex are inaccurate planners, like younger, typically developing children (Ratterman *et al.*, 2001).

7 Prefrontal function: mind binding

Evidence for the developmental role of the prefrontal cortex in mind binding comes from studies of metacognition and theory of mind. Flexible access to one's own mind (through metacognition) and to the minds of others (through theory of mind) is important for the development of socially appropriate behavior.

7.1 Metacognition

Metacognition is the ability to think about one's own mental processes and state of knowledge. Metacognition involves a number of components, including metacognitive monitoring, the awareness of ongoing cognitive processes, such as the online determination of whether material or instructions are adequate, or whether one is making progress in performing a task; and metacognitive knowledge, information about one's own abilities, state of knowledge, and resources (Mazzoni & Nelson, 1998). Adults with frontal lesions have metacognitive deficits, such as overestimating their ability to learn (Shimamura & Squire, 1986).

7.1.1 Typical development

Metacognitive ability improves with age, with the different components of metacognition developing at different rates (Schneider, 1998). While young children understand that remembering takes effort, it requires some years before this understanding translates into strategic effort (Garrity, 1975), increased study time (Rogoff *et al.*, 1974), and effective allocation of study time between easy and difficult items (Dufresne & Kobasigawa, 1989). Other aspects of metacognition develop over a number of years, such as the ability to integrate both parts of an instruction to determine overall ambiguity (Flavell *et al.*, 1985).

7.1.2 Atypical development

Children with TBI exhibit problems with a variety of forms of metacognition. They have difficulty with metacognitive monitoring, being unable to judge the adequacy of ambiguous directions or to detect anomalies in sentences (Dennis *et al.*, 1996), especially sentences presented under conditions of high memory load (Hanten *et al.*, 1999). Children with severe TBI have difficulty with metacognitive knowledge, being unable to predict the ease with which they will learn specific items or to estimate their memory span accurately (Hanten *et al.*, 2004). Problems in metacognition are especially apparent when TBI occurs early in development and/or includes CT evidence of contusional damage to the frontal lobes (Dennis *et al.*, 1996).

7.2 Theory of mind

Theory of mind involves the ability to think about mental states (thoughts, beliefs, intentions, and desires) and use them to understand and predict what other people need to know and how they will act (Bibby & McDonald, 2005). In adults, frontal lesions impair the ability to infer mental states in others (Stuss *et al.*, 2001).

7.2.1 Typical development

Conceptualizations of theory of mind have varied according to the age of the study population. Several studies of adults (e.g. Happé *et al.*, 2001) have proposed that theory of mind is a distinct module of mind that, like the hypothetical cognitive module (Fodor, 1983), is domain specific, neuro-anatomically distinct, informationally encapsulated, and independent of broader cognitive resources. Studies of children, on the other hand, have focused on the contingent emergence of theory of mind and higher cognitive and executive functions, such as working memory and inhibitory control (e.g. Moses, 2001).

7.2.2   Atypical development

Childhood TBI in the school-age years is associated with deficits in components of theory of mind such as comprehension of mental state words and the production of speech acts. Children with TBI have difficulty making pragmatic inferences about the presuppositions, entailments, and implications of mental state verbs (Dennis & Barnes, 2000), a class of words that includes *know, remember, forget, think, believe,* and *pretend* (Kiparsky & Kiparsky, 1970; Karttunen, 1971; Hall & Nagy, 1986). Children with TBI also have trouble producing speech acts (Dennis & Barnes, 2000), prototypical forms of pragmatic communication that express the mutual intentions of a speaker and a listener. Children with severe TBI, although not those with mild TBI, have difficulty understanding literal statements concerned with first and second-order beliefs and intentions (Dennis *et al.*, 2001).

7.3   Social problem solving

Social problem solving is the ability to think about the social world and to generate and implement solutions to everyday social problems. It is tested by tasks such as the Interpersonal Negotiation Strategies (INS) interview (Yeates *et al.*, 1990), in which children are presented with hypothetical interpersonal dilemmas involving social conflicts and asked to define the problem, generate and select a strategy, consider possible outcomes, and implement a particular outcome.

7.3.1   Typical development

As they mature, children are increasingly able to solve more complex social dilemmas, which contributes to more successful social function (Crick & Dodge, 1994). They progress through several steps during acquisition of problem-solving process, ranging from the retrieval or construction of possible solutions through the evaluation, selection, and enactment of behavioral responses (Mize & Ladd, 1988). Young children have knowledge about prosocial problem solving that is not reflected in their spontaneous behavior (Rudolph & Heller, 1997). With development, social problem solving moves from being automatic to becoming controlled, conscious, and reflective (Crick & Dodge, 1994).

7.3.2   Atypical development

Children with TBI have deficits in social information processing that predict their social and academic function (Warschausky *et al.*, 1997). They do not select a specific solution to social dilemmas or evaluate the outcome of dilemmas, although they are able to define the problem and generate alternative solutions (Janusz *et al.*, 2002). Using online videotape tasks, Turkstra and coworkers (2001) found that adolescents with TBI had poorer social information processing than age peers.

8   Prefrontal function: emotion binding

Emotion binding, the ability to link affect and cognition, is important for at least three reasons. It fosters hedonic encoding and decision-making that combines affect and thought. It allows the expression of emotions to be regulated according to the cognitive understanding of the situation. It allows social-affective messages to be communicated with a softening of the negative affect (e.g. in ironic criticism) or a heightening of the positive affect (e.g. in empathic lies). Studies of emotion binding have concerned hedonic decision-making, emotion regulation, and emotion messaging.

8.1   Hedonic decision-making

People make decisions, not only by evaluating consequences and probabilities, but also on the basis of affect, a concept termed the Somatic Marker Hypothesis (Bechara, 2004). Decision-making depends on neural substrates, including the orbitofrontal prefrontal cortex, that regulate homeostasis, emotion, and affect. Adults with lesions in these prefrontal regions have abnormalities in emotion, feeling, and hedonic encoding and decision-making in the laboratory and in real-life situations (e.g., Tranel, 2002; Bechara, 2004).

8.1.1   Typical development

Although very young children are able to make advantageous decisions (Kerr & Zelazo, 2004), children improve with age in terms of how they make decisions, their decision-making errors, and how they take risks. Younger children are less able than older children to process information relevant to decision-making (Davidson, 1991) and to discount irrelevant information (Demetre et al., 1992). The ability to make advantageous choices improves from school age to adolescence, and again from adolescence to young adulthood (Crone & van der Molen, 2004).

8.1.2   Atypical development

At present, there is limited information about hedonic decision-making in children with prefrontal lesions, in part because of the lack of published studies of children with prefrontal lesions using child-appropriate versions of gambling, betting, and delayed discounting tasks. Adults with prefrontal lesions sustained early in life fail to learn from their mistakes and exhibit poor decision-making (Grattan & Eslinger, 1992; Eslinger et al., 2004).

8.2 Emotion regulation

8.2.1 Typical development

Emotion regulation has been studied in children in relation to the distinction between felt and socially expressed emotions. Facial expressions may express an internal emotional state, *emotional expression*, or communicate a social display, *emotive communication* (Buck, 1994a, 1994b), the latter developing later and requiring the ability to be socially deceptive (Saarni, 1999), and to understand display rules for the social expression of feelings (Ekman & Friesen, 1978).

8.2.2 Atypical development

Children with TBI have trouble with the cognitive regulation of emotions. They understand emotional facial expressions, but do not regulate the social display of emotive facial expressions (Dennis *et al.*, 1998). Emotive identification is particularly impaired in children with early-onset injuries or injuries that involve the frontal lobes (Dennis *et al.*, 1998).

8.3 Emotion messaging

Intentional-affective language is about sending messages about mental states and feelings. Irony and empathy are concerned with affective evaluations that manipulate the mental states and feelings of the hearer. For ironic criticism, the affective valence of the intended meaning is different from the valence of the situation and from the valence of the literal meaning. "Nice that you came early!" uttered with a sarcastic tone to a tardy individual expresses a negative evaluation that matches the situation but that contrasts with the positive evaluation in the semantic content of the words. For an empathic lie, the intended evaluation matches the literal meaning, although not the situation. "You did a great job!" uttered with an empathic tone to an individual who has performed a task poorly expresses a positive evaluation that contrasts with the situation but matches the positive evaluation in the words.

Irony has complex social functions. Through the use of the rhetorical functions of praise and blame, irony conveys social messages that include formulating a judgment while muting its evaluative force (Dews & Winner, 1997), muting criticism (Harris & Pexman, 2003), or establishing social distance through a negative assessment of the actions of the hearer (Haverkate, 1990). Empathy is a means of giving comfort or maintaining social connectedness in complex or difficult situations. One might use an empathic lie, for instance, to make someone feel better about a bad haircut (e.g. "Your hair looks really nice like that!").

8.3.1 Typical development

The ability to use and understand forms of nonliteral language, such as irony and empathy, in which the affective message is opaque with respect to the words, follows a protracted developmental course (reviewed in Dennis *et al.*, 2001). Irony and empathy appear to develop over the ages of 6–13. Early in development, children do not understand the concept of saying one thing while meaning another, so that 6-year-old children cannot use or detect white lies, and misinterpret irony as "honest errors" (Demorest *et al.*, 1984). Young children understand a speaker's statement as literal evidence of belief and purpose, so that a literal statement represents an internal state or an error. Later in development, children can recognize deliberate falsehoods and take into consideration both the facts of the situation and, to a limited extent, what they believe the speaker believes (Demorest *et al.*, 1984). When what the speaker says does not match the situation, children interpret the utterance as deceitful. Recognizing a protosocial function of deceit may foster the understanding of empathy; certainly, by 9 years of age, children begin to correctly interpret white lies (Demorest *et al.*, 1984). Another developmental advance is marked by the ability to understand a nondeceitful speaker saying what she does not believe as in ironic criticism. At this point in development, children can discriminate ironic from deceptive intent (Demorest *et al.*, 1984). The ability to understand ironic criticism is well established by 13 years of age (Winner, 1988).

8.3.2 Atypical development

Irony and empathy engage complex theory of mind processes concerned with affective evaluations of one individual that manipulate the mental states and feelings of another. Children with TBI have difficulty understanding the affective valence of first- and second-order intentions in irony and empathy, even when they are able to understand the intentions of literal statements of the same form (Dennis *et al.*, 2001).

9 Prefrontal cortex lesions, personality and psychosocial function

Changes in personality and psychosocial function following prefrontal lesions have been reported from Gage to the present time. Clinically, a syndrome of developmental sociopathy following early prefrontal lesions has been identified in a series of case studies reported by Eslinger and colleagues (1992, 2004). Damage to the orbital and medial prefrontal cortex leads to emotional lability, as well as to deficits in social and emotional functioning (Eslinger *et al.*, 2004) regardless of age at injury (Kolb *et al.*, 2004). This region has also been implicated in antisocial behavior, particularly aggression, in both children and adults (Blair, 2004; Séguin, 2004).

Personality and social function are changed for the worse after childhood TBI (Yeates *et al.*, 2004), and personality changes are directly related to the presence of frontal lobe lesions. Children with closed head injury commonly have frontal lobe contusional injury, which has been shown to contribute, independent of overall injury severity, to deficits in psychosocial function (Levin *et al.*, 2004).

Prospective studies have demonstrated that the dorsal prefrontal cortex system and the frontal lobe white matter are important for effortful regulation of affective states in children. In a prospective study of personality change in 177 children in the first 6 months after TBI, Max *et al.* (2005) found that personality change occurred in nearly a quarter of the participants; and that lesions of the dorsal prefrontal cortex, specifically the superior frontal gyrus, were associated with personality change after controlling for severity of injury or for the presence of other lesions. In a longitudinal follow-up from 6 months to 24 months postinjury, these authors (Max *et al.*, 2006) found that personality change occurred in 13% of participants between 6 and 12 months after injury and 12% in the second year after injury, and that lesions of the dorsal prefrontal cortex, specifically the superior frontal gyrus (and particularly lesions of the frontal white matter) continued to be associated with personality change between 6 and 12 months after injury, after controlling for severity of injury and the presence of other brain lesions.

10 Modeling developmental frontal lobe functions

It has been proposed that development of executive function and theory of mind each reflect improvements in cognitive complexity and control involving the manipulation of embedded rules (Frye *et al.*, 1995; Happaney & Zelazo, 2003). Working memory might provide the platform for these control processes; certainly, working memory and cognitive inhibition are both components of conflict tasks for typically developing children (Kirkham & Diamond, 2003).

Recent studies have attempted to model the relations among frontal lobe resources, such as inhibitory control and working memory, and frontal lobe functions, such as theory of mind. These models test hypotheses about the directionality of the relations among resources and functions, and help delineate similarities and differences in integrated prefrontal functions in children and adults.

Dennis and coworkers (2006, submitted) performed path analyses to model the relations among frontal lobe lesions, theory of mind, and the executive functions of working memory and cognitive inhibition in a sample of children with closed head injury. Path analysis revealed two forms of relationship among the variables. The relation between cognitive inhibition and theory of mind involved a single mediated path, such that cognitive inhibition predicted theory of mind through working memory. In contrast, frontal injury had a direct impact on working memory, which then separately determined theory of mind performance, the direct single paths between frontal lesions and theory of mind being nonsignificant.

Both child and adult theory of mind require frontal lobe integrity. Unlike adult theory of mind, however, the expression of theory of mind in childhood is not modular, in that it is causally dependent on the domain general functions of working memory and inhibitory control.

The relation between executive function and theory of mind in both preschoolers and school-aged children is different from that in adults. Inhibitory control and theory of mind are each part of the broad complement of adult frontal lobe skills (e.g. Shammi & Stuss, 1999; Stuss et al., 2001), and each is associated with frontal lobe activity (Fletcher et al., 1995), although they are dissociable in empirical studies of adults with various forms of brain pathology (Fine et al., 2001; Lough et al., 2001; Bird et al., 2004). In preschoolers, there is a robust association between individual differences in performance on executive function and theory of mind tasks, typically, false belief comprehension (Hughes, 2002).

The different form of the relation in children and adults suggests that frontal lobe functions that are linked during development become more segregated in adult life, which is congruent with the venerable idea that the brain mechanisms required for developing a function are not identical to those that sustain it, once acquired (Hebb, 1942). More specifically, if executive functions are more important for the emergence and childhood expression of theory of mind than they are for adult theory of mind, then theory of mind may be disrupted in more and different ways in childhood than in adult life, which is consistent with data showing that immature frontal brain circuitry is more susceptible to interference than is adult frontal circuitry (Durston et al., 2002).

11 Conclusion

With respect to both structure and function, the development of the prefrontal cortex is intricate and protracted. Far from involving the accrual of connections, structural brain development involves an ongoing recalibration of thickness and volume between and within brain regions, including subdivisions of the frontal lobe. Functional brain development involves increased inhibitory control over behavior, and the manner in which frontal lobe resources such as working memory and inhibitory control enable prefrontal functions moves through several stable developmental states before reaching adult-like function. Brain injury to the organization or structure of the developing prefrontal cortex is associated, not only with deficits in prefrontal functions, but also with a reconfiguration of the typical developmental state at the time of the injury. What is not fully understood is how changes after prefrontal lesions vary with the known moderators of outcome in other forms of developmental brain insult: biological severity of primary and secondary injury, age at injury, time since injury, and the reserve capacity within the child, the family, and the environment.

REFERENCES

Ackerly, S. (1964). A case of paranatal bilateral frontal lobe defect observed for thirty years. In *The Frontal Granular Cortex and Behavior*, ed. J. M. Warren and K. Akert. New York, NY: McGraw-Hill, pp. 192−218.

Ackerly, S. & Benton, A. (1948). Report of a case of bilateral frontal lobe defect. *Research Publications of the Association for Nervous and Mental Diseases*, **27**, 479−504.

Allen, G., Buxton, R., Wong, E. & Courchesne, E. (1997). Attentional activation of the cerebellum independent of motor involvement. *Science*, **275**, 1940−3.

Appollonio, I., Grafman, J., Schwartz, V., Massaquoi, S. & Hallett, M. (1993). Memory in patients with cerebellar degeneration. *Neurology*, **43**, 1536−44.

Band, G. P. H., van der Molen, M. W., Overtoom, C. C. E. & Verbaten, M. N. (2000). The ability to activate and inhibit speeded responses: Separate developmental trends. *Journal of Experimental Child Psychology*, **75**, 263−90.

Barnes, M. A. & Dennis, M. (2001). Knowledge-based inferencing after childhood head injury. *Brain and Language*, **76**, 253−65.

Bechara, A. (2004). The role of emotion in decision-making: Evidence from neurological patients with orbital frontal damage. *Brain and Cognition*, **55**, 30−40.

Bibby, H. & McDonald, S. (2005). Theory of mind after traumatic brain injury. *Neuropsychologia*, **43**, 99−114.

Bird, C. M., Castelli, F., Malik, O., Frith, U. & Husain, M. (2004). The impact of extensive medial frontal lobe damage on "Theory of Mind" and cognition. *Brain*, **127**, 914−28.

Bjorklund, D. F. & Harnishfeger, K. K. (1990). The resources construct in cognitive development: Diverse sources of evidence and a theory of inefficient inhibition. *Developmental Review*, **10**, 48−71.

Blair, R. J. R. (2004). The roles of orbital frontal cortex in the modulation of antisocial behaviour. *Brain and Cognition*, **55**, 198−208.

Broca, P. (1877). Sur le cerveau à l'état foetal. Discussion. *Societé d'Anthropologie de Paris*, **2**, 217−22.

Buck, R. (1994a). Social and emotional functions in facial expression and communication: The readout hypothesis. *Biological Psychology*, **38**, 59–115.

Buck, R. (1994b). The neuropsychology of communication: Spontaneous and symbolic aspects. *Journal of Pragmatics*, **22**, 265–78.

Bunge, S. A., Ochsner, K. N., Desmond, J. E., Glover, G. H. & Gabrieli, J. D. E. (2001). Prefrontal regions involved in keeping information in and out of mind. *Brain*, **124**, 2074–86.

Cabeza, R. & Nyberg, L. (2000). Imaging cognition II: An empirical review of 275 PET and fMRI studies. *Journal of Cognitive Neuroscience*, **12**, 1–47.

Ceci, S. J. & Bronfenbrenner, U. (1985). "Don't forget to take the cupcakes out of the oven": Prospective memory, strategic time-monitoring, and context. *Child Development*, **56**, 152–164.

Chapman, S. B., Culhane, K. A., Levin, H. S., *et al.* (1992). Narrative discourse after closed head injury in children and adolescents. *Brain and Language*, **43**, 42–65.

Cowan, N. (1997). The development of working memory. In *The Development of Memory in Childhood*, ed. N. Cowan & C. Hulme. Hove, UK: Psychology Press, pp. 163–200.

Crick, N. R. & Dodge, K. A. (1994). A review and reformulation of social-information processing mechanisms in children's social adjustment. *Psychological Bulletin*, **115**, 74–101.

Crone, E. A. & van der Molen, M. W. (2004). Developmental changes in real life decision making: Performance on a gambling task previously shown to depend on the ventromedial prefrontal cortex. *Developmental Neuropsychology*, **25**, 251–79.

Culhane-Shelburne, K., Chapieski, L., Hiscock, M. & Glaze, D. (2002). Executive functions in children with frontal and temporal lobe epilepsy. *Journal of the International Neuropsychological Society*, **8**, 623–32.

Damasio, H., Graboski, T., Frank, R., Galaburda, A. M. & Damasio, A. R. (1994). The return of Phineas Gage: Clues about the brain from the skull of a famous patient. *Science*, **264**, 1102–5.

Davidson, D. (1991). Children's decision-making examined with an information-board procedure. *Cognitive Development*, **6**, 77–90.

Demetre, J. D., Lee, D. N., Pitcairn, T. K. & Grieve, R. (1992). Errors in young children's decisions about traffic gaps: Experiments with roadside simulations. *British Journal of Psychology*, **83**, 189–202.

Demorest, A., Meyer, C., Phelps, E., Gardner, H. & Winner, E. (1984). Words speak louder than actions: Understanding deliberately false remarks. *Child Development*, **55**, 1527–34.

Dempster, F. N. (1993). Resistance to interference: Developmental changes in a basic processing mechanism. In *Emerging Themes in Cognitive Development: Foundation*, Vol. 1, ed. M. L. Howe and R. Pasnak. New York, NY: Springer-Verlag, pp. 3–27.

Dennis, M. (1988). Language and the young damaged brain. In *Clinical Neuropsychology and Brain Function: Research, Measurement and Practice*, Vol. 7, ed. T. Boll and B. K. Bryant. Washington, DC: American Psychological Association, pp. 85–123.

Dennis, M. (1991). Frontal lobe function in childhood and adolescence: A heuristic for assessing attention regulation, executive control, and the intentional states important for social discourse. *Developmental Neuropsychology*, **7**, 327–58.

Dennis, M. (2000). Childhood medical disorders and cognitive impairment: Biological risk, time, development, and reserve. In *Pediatric Neuropsychology: Research, Theory, and*

Practice, ed. K. O. Yeates, M. D. Ris and H. G. Taylor. New York, NY: Guilford Press, pp. 3–22.

Dennis, M. (2003). Acquired disorders of language in children. In *Behavioural Neurology and Neuropsychology*, ed. T. E. Feinberg and M. J. Farah. New York, NY: McGraw-Hill Inc., pp. 783–99.

Dennis, M., Agostino, A., Roncadin, C., & Levin, H. (2006). Theory of mind depends on domain general executive functions of working memory and inhibitory control in children with closed head injury. Manuscript submitted for publication.

Dennis, M. & Barnes, M. A. (1990). Knowing the meaning, getting the point, bridging the gap, and carrying the message: Aspects of discourse following closed head injury in childhood and adolescence. *Brain and Language*, **39**, 428–46.

Dennis, M. & Barnes, M. A. (2000). Speech acts after mild or severe childhood head injury. *Aphasiology*, **14**, 391–405.

Dennis, M., Barnes, M. A., Donnelly, R. E., Wilkinson, M. & Humphreys, R. (1996). Appraising and managing knowledge: Metacognitive skills after childhood head injury. *Developmental Neuropsychology*, **12**, 17–34.

Dennis, M., Barnes, M. A., Wilkinson, M. & Humphreys, R. P. (1998). How children with head injury represent real and deceptive emotion in short narratives. *Brain and Language*, **61**, 450–83.

Dennis, M., Edelstein, K., Copeland, K., *et al.* (2005). Covert orienting to exogenous and endogenous cues in children with spina bifida. *Neuropsychologia*, **43**, 976–87.

Dennis, M., Edelstein, K., Hetherington, R., *et al.* (2004). Neurobiology of perceptual and motor timing in children with spina bifida in relation to cerebellar volume. *Brain*, **127**, 1293–1301.

Dennis, M., Hetherington, C. R., Spiegler, B. J. & Barnes, M. A. (1999). Functional consequences of congenital cerebellar dysmorphologies and acquired cerebellar lesions of childhood. In *The Changing Nervous System: Neurobehavioral Consequences of Early Brain Disorders*, ed. S. H. Broman and J. M. Fletcher. New York, NY: Oxford University Press, pp. 172–98.

Dennis, M., Purvis, K., Barnes, M. A., Wilkinson, M. & Winner, E. (2001). Understanding of literal truth, ironic criticism, and deceptive praise after childhood head injury. *Brain and Language*, **78**, 1–16.

Dennis, M., Spiegler, B., Riva, D. & MacGregor, D. (2004). Neuropsychological outcome. In *Brain and Spinal Tumors of Childhood*, ed. D. Walker, G. Perilongo, J. Punt and R. Taylor. New York, NY: Oxford University Press, pp. 213–27.

Dennis, M. & Whitaker, H. (1977). Hemispheric equipotentiality and language acquisition. In *Language Development and Neurological Theory*, ed. S. Segalowitz and F. Gruber. New York, NY: Academic Press, pp. 93–106.

Dennis, M., Wilkinson, M., Koski, L. & Humphreys, R. P. (1995). Attention deficits in the long term after childhood head injury. In *Traumatic Head Injury in Children*, ed. S. Broman and M. E. Michel. New York, NY: Oxford University Press, pp. 165–187.

Derrfuss, J., Brass, M. & Yves von Cramon, D. (2004). Cognitive control in the posterior frontolateral cortex: Evidence from common activations in task coordination, interference control, and working memory. *NeuroImage*, **23**, 604–12.

D'Esposito, M., Postle, B. R., Ballard, D. & Lease, J. (1999). Maintenance versus manipulation of information held in working memory: An event-related fMRI study. *Brain and Cognition*, **41**, 66–86.

Dews, S. & Winner, E. (1997). Attributing meaning to deliberately false utterances: The case of irony. In *The Problem of Meaning: Behavioral and Cognitive Perspectives*, ed. C. Mandell and A. McCabe. New York, NY: Elsevier Science, pp. 377–414.

Diamond, A. (1996). Evidence for the importance of dopamine for prefrontal cortex functions early in life. *Philosophical Transactions of the Royal Society of London B*, **351**, 1483–94.

Diamond, A. (2000). Close interrelation of motor development and cognitive development and of the cerebellum and prefrontal cortex. *Child Development*, **71**, 44–56.

Diamond, A., Briand, L., Fossella, J. & Gehlback, L. (2004). Genetic and neurochemical modulation of prefrontal cognitive functions in children. *The American Journal of Psychiatry*, **161**, 125–32.

Diamond, A. & Taylor, C. (1996). Development of an aspect of executive control: Development of the abilities to remember what I said and to "Do as I say, not as I do". *Developmental Psychobiology*, **29**, 315–34.

Dowsett, S. M. & Livesey, D. J. (2000). The development of inhibitory control in preschool children: Effects of 'executive skills' training. *Developmental Psychobiology*, **36**, 161–74.

Dufresne, A. & Kobasigawa, A. (1989). Children's spontaneous allocation of study times: Differential and sufficient aspects. *Journal of Experimental Child Psychology*, **47**, 274–96.

Dunn, R. P. & Strick, P. L. (2003). An unfolded map of the cerebellar dentate nucleus and its projections to the cerebral cortex. *Journal of Neurophysiology*, **89**, 634–39.

Durston, S., Thomas, K. M., Yang, Y., *et al.* (2002). A neural basis for the development of inhibitory control. *Developmental Science*, **5**, 9–16.

Ekman, P. & Friesen, W. V. (1978). *The facial action coding system: A technique for the measurement of facial action*. Palo Alto, CA: Consulting Psychologists Press.

Engle, R. W., Conway, A. R. A., Tuholski, S. W. & Shisler, R. J. (1995). A resource account of inhibition. *Psychological Science*, **6**, 122–5.

Eslinger, P. J., Flaherty-Craig, C. V. & Benton, A. L. (2004). Developmental outcomes after early prefrontal cortex damage. *Brain and Cognition*, **55**, 84–103.

Eslinger, P. J., Grattan, L., Damasio, H. & Damasio, A. R. (1992). Developmental consequences of childhood frontal lobe damage. *Archives of Neurology*, **49**, 764–9.

Fiez, J., Petersen, S., Cheney, M. & Raichle, M. (1992). Impaired non-motor learning and error detection associated with cerebellar damage. *Brain*, **115**, 155–78.

Fine, C., Lumsden, J. & Blair, J. R. (2001). Dissociation between 'theory of mind' and executive functions in a patient with early left amygdala damage. *Brain*, **124**, 287–98.

Fivush, R. & Hamond, N. R. (1990). Autobiographical memory across the preschool years: Towards reconceptualizing childhood amnesia. In *Knowing and Remembering in Young Children. Emory Symposium in Cognition*, Vol. 3, ed. J. A. Hudson. New York: Cambridge University Press, pp. 223–48.

Flavell, J. H., Green, F. L. & Flavell, E. R. (1985). The road not taken: Understanding the implications of initial uncertainty in evaluating spatial directions. *Developmental Psychology*, **21**, 207–16.

Fletcher, J. M., Copeland, K., Frederick, J., *et al.* (2005). Spinal lesion level in spina bifida: A source of neural and cognitive heterogeneity. *Journal of Neurosurgery,* 102, 268–79.

Fletcher, P., Happé, F., Frith, U., *et al.* (1995). Other minds in the brain: A functional imaging study of the 'theory of mind' in story comprehension. *Cognition,* 57, 109–28.

Fletcher, P. C. & Henson, R. N. A. (2001). Frontal lobes and human memory. *Brain,* 124, 849–81.

Fodor, J. (1983). *The Modularity of Mind.* Cambridge MA: MIT Press.

Friedman, N. P. & Miyake, A. (2004). The relations among inhibition and interference control executives: A latent-variable analysis. *Journal of Experimental Psychology: General,* 133, 101–35.

Frye, D., Zelazo, P. D. & Palfai, T. (1995). Theory of mind and rule-based reasoning. *Cognitive Development,* 10, 483–527.

Fuster, J. (2000). The prefrontal cortex of the primate. A synopsis. *Psychobiology,* 28, 125–31.

Garrity, L. I. (1975). An electromyographical study of subvocal speech and recall in preschool children. *Developmental Psychology,* 11, 274–81.

Gazzeley, A., Cooney, J., McEvoy, K., Knight, R. & D'Esposito, M. (2005). Top-down enhancement and suppression of the magnitude and speed of neural activity. *Journal of Cognitive Neuroscience,* 17, 507–17.

Gerstadt, C. L., Hong, Y. J. & Diamond, A. (1994). The relationship between cognition and action: Performance of children 3.5–7 years old on a Stroop-like day-night test. *Cognition,* 53, 129–53.

Gogtay, N., Giedd, J. N., Lusk, L., *et al.* (2004). Dynamic mapping of human cortical development during childhood through early adulthood. *Proceedings of the National Academy of Sciences USA,* 101, 8174–9.

Goldman-Rakic, P. S., Bourgeois, J.-P. & Rakic, P. (1997). Synaptic substrate of cognitive development: Life-span analysis of synaptogenesis in the prefrontal cortex of the nonhuman primate. In *Development of the Prefrontal Cortex: Evolution, Neurobiology, and Behavior,* ed. N. A. Krasnegor, G. R. Lyon & P. S. Goldman-Rakic. Baltimore, MD: Paul H. Brookes, pp. 27–47.

Goldman-Rakic, P. S. & Leung, H.-C. (2002). Functional architecture of the dorsolateral prefrontal cortex in monkeys and humans. In *Principles of Frontal Lobe Function,* ed. D. T. Stuss and R. T. Knight. New York, NY: Oxford University Press, pp. 31–50.

Grafman, J. (1989). Plans, actions, and mental sets: Managerial knowledge units in the frontal lobes. In *Integrative Theory and Practice in Neuropsychology,* ed. E. Perecman. Hillsdale, NJ: Lawrence Erlbaum Associates, Inc., pp. 93–138.

Grafman, J. (2002). The structured event complex and the human prefrontal cortex. In *Principles of Frontal Lobe Function,* ed. D. T. Stuss and R. T. Knight. New York, NY: Oxford University Press, pp. 209–35.

Grafman, J., Litvan, I., Massaquoi, S., *et al.* (1992). Cognitive planning deficit in patients with cerebellar atrophy. *Neurology,* 42, 1493–6.

Grattan, L. & Eslinger, P. J. (1992). Long-term psychological consequences of childhood frontal lobe lesion in patient D. T. *Brain and Cognition,* 20, 185–95.

Hall, W. S. & Nagy, W. E. (1986). Theoretical issues in the investigation of the words of internal report. In *From Models to Modules: Studies in Cognitive Science from the McGill Workshops*, ed. A. Gopnik and M. Gopnik. Norwood, NJ: Ablex, pp. 26–65.

Hanten, G., Dennis, M., Zhang, L., Barnes, M. & Robertson, G. (2004). Childhood head injury and metacognitive processes in language and memory. *Developmental Neuropsychology*, **25**, 85–106.

Hanten, G., Levin, H. S. & Song, J. X. (1999). Working memory and metacognition in sentence comprehension by severely head-injured children: A preliminary study. *Developmental Neuropsychology*, **16**, 393–414.

Happaney, K. & Zelazo, P. D. (2003). Inhibition as a problem in the psychology of behavior. *Developmental Science*, **6**, 468–70.

Happé, F., Malhi, G. S. & Checkley, S. (2001). Acquired mind-blindness following frontal lobe surgery? A single case study of impaired "theory of mind" in a patient treated with stereotactic anterior capsulotomy. *Neuropsychologia*, **39**, 83–90.

Harlow, J. M. (1868). Recovery after severe injury to the head. *Publication of the Massachusetts Medical Society*, **2**, 327–46.

Harnishfeger, K. K. & Bjorklund, D. F. (1994). The ontogeny of inhibition mechanisms: A renewed approach to cognitive development. In *Emerging Themes in Cognitive Development: Foundations*, Vol. 1, ed. M. L. Howe and R. Pasnak. New York, NY: Springer-Verlag, pp. 28–49.

Harnishfeger, K. K. & Pope, R. S. (1996). Intending to forget: The development of cognitive inhibition in directed forgetting. *Journal of Experimental Child Psychology*, **62**, 292–315.

Haverkate, H. (1990). A speech act analysis of irony. *Journal of Pragmatics*, **14**, 77–109.

Hayes-Roth, B. & Hayes-Roth, F. (1979). A cognitive model of planning. *Cognitive Science*, **3**, 275–310.

Hebb, D. O. (1942). The effect of early and late brain injury upon test scores, and the nature of normal adult intelligence. *Proceedings of the American Philosophical Society*, **85**, 275–92.

Houghton, G. & Tipper, S. P. (1994). A model of inhibitory mechanisms in selective attention. In *Inhibition Processes in Attention, Memory, and Language*, ed. D. Dagenbach and T. H. Carr. San Diego, CA: Academic Press, pp. 53–112.

Hughes, C. (2002). Executive functions and development: Why the interest? *Infant and Child Development*, **11**, 69–71.

Hulme, C. & Roodenrys, S. (1995). Practitioner review: Verbal working memory development and its disorders. *Journal of Child Psychology and Psychiatry*, **36**, 373–98.

Huttenlocher, P. R. (1979). Synaptic density in human frontal cortex– developmental changes and effects of aging. *Brain Research*, **163**, 195–205.

Ivry, R. & Keele, S. (1989). Timing functions of the cerebellum. *Journal of Cognitive Neuroscience*, **1**, 136–52.

Janusz, J. A., Kirkwood, M. W., Yeates, K. O. & Taylor, H. G. (2002). Social problem-solving skills in children with traumatic brain injury: Long-term outcomes and prediction of social competence. *Child Neuropsychology*, **8**, 179–94.

Karttunen, L. (1971). Implicative verbs. *Language*, **47**, 340–58.

Kates, W. R., Frederikse, M., Mostofsky, S. H., *et al.* (2002). MRI parcellation of the frontal lobe in boys with attention deficit hyperactivity disorder or Tourette syndrome. *Psychiatry Research Neuroimaging*, **116**, 63–81.

Kennard, M. A. (1938). Reorganization of motor function in the cerebral cortex of monkeys deprived of motor and premotor areas in infancy. *Journal of Neurophysiology*, **1**, 477–96.

Kennard, M. (1940). Relation of age to motor impairment in man and in subhuman primates. *Archives of Neurology and Psychiatry*, **44**, 377–97.

Kennard, M. & Fulton, J. (1942). Age and reorganization of central nervous system. *Mount Sinai Hospital Journal*, **9**, 594–606.

Kennard, M., Spencer, S. & Fountain, G. (1941). Hyperactivity in monkeys following lesions of the frontal lobes. *Journal of Neurophysiology*, **4**, 512–24.

Kerr, A. & Zelazo, P. D. (2004). Development of "hot" executive function: The children's gambling task. *Brain and Cognition*, **55**, 148–57.

Kim, S., Ugurbil, K. & Strick, P. (1994). Activation of a cerebellar output nucleus during cognitive processing. *Science*, **265**, 949–51.

Kiparsky, P. & Kiparsky, C. (1970). Fact. In *Progress in Linguistics*, ed. M. Bierwisch and K. Heidolph. The Hague: Mouton, pp. 143–73.

Kirkham, N. & Diamond, A. (2003). Sorting between theories of perseveration: Performance in conflict tasks requires memory, attention, and inhibition. *Developmental Science*, **6**, 474–6.

Kochanska, G., Murray, K., Jacques, T. Y., Koenig, A. L. & Vandegeest, K. A. (1996). Inhibitory control in young children and its role in emerging internalization. *Child Development*, **67**, 490–507.

Kolb, B., Pellis, S. & Robinson, T. E. (2004). Plasticity and functions of the orbital frontal cortex. *Brain and Cognition*, **55**, 104–15.

Konrad, K., Gauggel, S., Manz, A. & Scholl, M. (2000). Lack of inhibition: a motivational deficit in children with attention deficit/hyperactivity disorder and children with traumatic brain injury. *Child Neuropsychology*, **6**, 286–96.

Kreutzer, M. A., Leonard, C. & Flavell, J. H. (1975). Prospective remembering in children. In *Memory Observed: Remembering in Natural Contexts*, ed. U. Neisser. San Francisco: Freeman, pp. 343–8.

Kvavilashvili, L. & Ellis, J. (1996). Varieties of intentions: Some distinctions and classifications. In *Prospective Memory: Theory and Application*, ed. M. A. Brandimonte, G. O. Einstein and M. A. McDaniel. Mahwah, NJ: Lawrence Erlbaum Associates, Inc., pp. 23–51.

Kvavilashvili, L., Messer, D. L. & Ebdon, P. (2001). Prospective memory in children: The effects of age and task interruption. *Developmental Psychology*, **37**, 418–30.

Lee, Z. I., Byun, W. M., Jang, S. H., *et al.* (2003). Diffusion tensor magnetic resonance imaging of microstructural abnormalities in children with brain injury. *American Journal of Physical Medicine and Rehabilitation*, **82**, 556–9.

Levin, H. S., Benavidez, D., Verger-Maestre, K., *et al.* (2000). Reduction of corpus callosum growth after severe traumatic brain injury in children. *Neurology*, **54**, 647–53.

Levin, H. S., Culhane, K. A., Hartman, J., *et al.* (1991). Developmental changes in performance on tests of purported frontal lobe functioning. *Developmental Neuropsychology*, **7**, 377–95.

Levin, H. S., Culhane, K. A., Mendelsohn, D., *et al.* (1993). Cognition in relation to MRI in head injured children and adolescents. *Archives of Neurology*, **50**, 897–905.

Levin, H. S., Fletcher, J. M., Kusnerik, L., *et al.* (1996). Semantic memory following pediatric head injury: Relationship to age, severity of injury, and MRI. *Cortex*, **32**, 461–78.

Levin, H. S., Mendelsohn, D., Lilly, M., *et al.* (1994). Tower of London performance in relation to magnetic resonance imaging following closed head injury in children. *Neuropsychology*, **8**, 171–9.

Levin, H. S., Song, J., Ewing-Cobbs, L. & Robertson, G. (2001). Porteus maze performance following traumatic brain injury in children. *Neuropsychology*, **15**, 557–67.

Levin, H. S., Zhang, L., Dennis, M., *et al.* (2004). Psychosocial outcome of TBI in children with unilateral frontal lesions. *Journal of the International Neuropsychological Society*, **10**, 305–16.

Levine, B. (2004). Autobiographical memory and the self in time: Brain lesion effects, functional neuroanatomy, and lifespan development. *Brain and Cognition*, **55**, 54–68.

Levisohn, L., Cronin-Golomb, A. & Schmahmann, J. D. (2000). Neuropsychological consequences of cerebellar tumour resection in children: cerebellar cognitive affective syndrome in a paediatric population. *Brain*, **123**, 1041–50.

Livesey, D. J. & Morgan, G. A. (1991). The development of response inhibition in 4- and 5-year-old children. *Australian Journal of Psychology*, **43**, 133–7.

Lough, S., Gregory, C. & Hodges, J. R. (2001). Dissociation of social cognition and executive function in frontal variant frontotemporal dementia. *Neurocase*, **7**, 123–30.

McCauley, S. R. & Levin, H. S. (2000). Prospective memory deficits in children and adolescents sustaining severe closed-head injury. Presentation at the *Annual Meeting of the Cognitive Neuroscience Society*, San Francisco, CA.

McCauley, S. R. & Levin, H. S. (2001). Prospective memory and executive function in children with severe traumatic brain injury. Presentation at the *3rd International Conference on Memory (ICOM-3)*, Valencia, Spain.

McCauley, S. R. & Levin, H. S. (2004). Prospective memory in pediatric traumatic brain injury: A preliminary study. *Developmental Neuropsychology*, **25**, 5–20.

Macmillan, M. (2000). *An Odd Kind of Fame: Stories about Phineas Gage*. Cambridge, MA: MIT Press.

Manly, T., Robertson, I. H., Anderson, V. & Nimmo-Smith, I. (1999). *Test of Everyday Attention for Children*. Bury St. Edmunds: Thames Valley.

Marlowe, W. B. (1992). The impact of a right prefrontal lesion on the developing brain. *Brain and Cognition*, **20**, 205–13.

Matsuzawa, J., Matsui, M., Konishi, T., *et al.* (2001). Age-related volumetric changes of brain gray and white matter in healthy infants and children. *Cerebral Cortex*, **11**, 335–42.

Max, J. E., Levin, H. S., Landis, J., *et al.* (2005). Predictors of personality change due to traumatic brain injury in children and adolescents in the first six months after injury. *Journal of the American Academy of Child and Adolescent Psychiatry*, **44**, 435–42.

Max, J. E., Levin, H. S., Schachar, R., *et al.* (2006). Predictors of personality change due to traumatic brain injury in children and adolescents 6 to 24 months after injury. *Journal of Neuropsychiatry and Clinical Neurosciences*. **18**, 21–32.

Mazzoni, G. & Nelson, T.O. (Eds.). (1998). *Metacognition and Cognitive Neuropsychology: Monitoring and Control Processes*. Mahwah, NJ: Lawrence Erlbaum Associates, Inc.

Mendelsohn, D., Levin, H.S., Bruce, D., *et al.* (1992). Late MRI after head injury in children: Relationship to clinical features and outcome. *Child's Nervous System*, **8**, 445–52.

Middleton, F. & Strick, P. (2001). Cerebellar projections to the prefrontal cortex of the primate. *Journal of Neuroscience*, **21**, 700–12.

Miller, E.K. (2000). The prefrontal cortex and cognitive control. *Nature Reviews: Neuroscience*, **1**, 59–65.

Miller, E.K. & Cohen, J.D. (2001). An integrative theory of prefrontal cortex function. *Annual Review of Neuroscience*, **24**, 167–202.

Mize, J. & Ladd, G.W. (1988). Predicting preschoolers' peer behaviour and status from their interpersonal strategies: A comparison of verbal and enactive responses to hypothetical social dilemmas. *Developmental Psychology*, **24**, 782–8.

Montgomery, J.W. (1995). Sentence comprehension in children with specific language impairment: The role of phonological working memory. *Journal of Speech and Hearing Research*, **33**, 187–99.

Moses, L.J. (2001). Executive accounts of theory of mind development. *Child Development*, **72**, 688–90.

Oberauer, K. & Suess, H.M. (2001). Individual and developmental differences in working memory across the life span: Comment. *Psychonomic Bulletin and Review*, **7**, 727–33.

O'Donnell, S., Noseworthy, M., Levine, B., Brandt, M. & Dennis, M. (2005). Cortical thickness of the frontopolar area in typically developing children and adolescents. *Neuroimage*, **24**, 948–54.

Pascual-Leone, J. (2001). If the magical number is 4, how does one account for operations within working memory? *Brain and Behavioral Sciences*, **24**, 136–8.

Passolunghi, M.C., Brandimonte, M.A. & Cornoldi, C. (1995). Encoding modality and prospective memory in children. *International Journal of Behavioural Development*, **18**, 631–48.

Paus, T. (2005). Mapping brain maturation and cognitive development during adolescence. *Trends in Cognitive Sciences*, **9**, 60–8.

Perner, J., Lang, B. & Kloo, D. (2002). Theory of mind and self-control: More than a common problem of inhibition. *Child Development*, **73**, 752–67.

Petrides, M., Alivisatos, B., Meyer, E. & Evans, A.C. (1993). Functional activation of the human frontal cortex during the performance of verbal working memory tasks. *Proceedings of the National Academy of Sciences*, **90**, 878–82.

Petrides, M. & Pandya, D.N. (2002). Association pathways of the prefrontal cortex and functional observations. In *Principles of Frontal Lobe Function*, ed. D.T. Stuss and R.T. Knight. New York, NY: Oxford University Press, pp. 31–50.

Pfefferbaum, A., Mathalon, D.H., Sullivan, E.V., *et al.* (1994). A quantitative magnetic resonance imaging study of changes in brain morphology from infancy to late adulthood. *Archives of Neurology*, **51**, 874–87.

Porteus, S.D. (1959). *Porteus Maze Test: Fifty Years' Application*. Palo Alto, CA: Pacific Books.

Purvis, K. & Schachar, R. (2001). Inhibitory deficit and ADHD following closed head injury. *Journal of the International Neuropsychological Society*, **7**, 165.

Rabinowicz, T. (1986). The differentiate maturation of the human cerebral cortex. In *Human Growth*, Vol. 3, ed. F. Falkner and J. M. Tanner. New York, NY: Plenum Publishing Corporation, pp. 97–123.

Ratterman, M., Spector, L, Grafman, J., Levin, H. & Harwood, H. (2001). Partial and total-order planning: evidence from normal and prefrontally damaged populations. *Cognitive Science*, **25**, 941–75.

Reiman, E., Raichle, M., Robins, E., *et al.* (1989). Neuroanatomical correlates of a lactate-induced anxiety attack. *Archives of General Psychiatry*, **46**, 493–500.

Reiss, A. L., Abrams, M. T., Singer, H. S., Ross, J. L. & Denckla, M. B. (1996). Brain development, gender and IQ in children. *Brain*, **119**, 1763–74.

Richards, J. E. (2003). The development of visual attention and the brain. In *The Cognitive Neuroscience of Development*, ed. M. de Haan and M. H. Johnson. Hove, UK: Psychology Press, pp. 73–98.

Riva, D. & Giorgi, C. (2000). The cerebellum contributes to higher functions during development. Evidence from a series of children surgically treated for posterior fossa tumours. *Brain*, **123**, 1051–61.

Roberts, W. A. (2002). Are animals stuck in time? *Psychological Review*, **128**, 473–89.

Rogoff, B., Newcombe, N. E. & Kagan, J. (1974). The development of knowledge concerning the effect of categorization upon free recall. *Child Development*, **44**, 238–46.

Roncadin, C., Guger, S., Archibald, J., Barnes, M. & Dennis, M. (2004). Working memory after mild, moderate, or severe childhood head injury. *Developmental Neuropsychology*, **25**, 21–36.

Roncadin, C., Rich, J. B., Pascual-Leone, J. & Dennis, M. (2003). Working memory and inhibitory control after early childhood closed head injury. *Journal of the International Neuropsychological Society*, **9**, 141.

Rudolph, K. & Heller, T. (1997). Interpersonal problem solving, externalizing behavior, and social competence in preschoolers: A knowledge-performance discrepancy? *Journal of Applied Developmental Psychology*, **18**, 107–17.

Rypma, B. & D'Esposito, M. (2000). Isolating the neural mechanisms of age-related changes in human working memory. *Nature Neuroscience*, **3**, 509–15.

Saarni, C. (1999). *The Development of Emotional Competence*. London, UK: Guilford Press.

Sadeh, M. & Cohen, I. (2001). Transient loss of speech after removal of posterior fossa tumors – one aspect of a larger neuropsychological entity: the cerebellar cognitive affective syndrome. *Pediatric Hematology and Oncology*, **18**, 423–6.

Schachar, R., Levin, H. S., Max, J. E., Purvis, K. & Chen, S. (2004). Attention deficit hyperactivity disorder symptoms and response inhibition after closed head injury in children: Do preinjury behavior and injury severity predict outcome? *Developmental Neuropsychology*, **25**, 179–98.

Scheibel, R. S. & Levin, H. S. (1997). Frontal lobe dysfunction following closed head injury in children: Findings from neuropsychology and brain imaging.

In *Development of the Prefrontal Cortex: Evolution, Neurobiology, and Behavior*, ed. N. A. Krasnegor, G. R. Lyon and P. S. Goldman-Rakic. Baltimore, MD: Paul H. Brookes, pp. 241–60.

Schmahmann, J. & Pandya, D. (1995). Prefrontal cortex projections to the basilar pons in rhesus monkey: implications for the cerebellar contributions to higher function. *Neuroscience Letters*, **199**, 175–8.

Schmahmann, J. & Pandya, D. (1997). Anatomic organization of the basilar pontine projections from prefrontal cortices in rhesus monkey. *Journal of Neuroscience*, **17**, 438–58.

Schmahmann, J. D. & Sherman, J. C. (1998). The cerebellar cognitive affective syndrome. *Brain*, **121**, 561–79.

Schneider, W. (1998). The development of procedural metamemory in childhood and adolescence. In *Metacognition and Cognitive Neuropsychology: Monitoring and Control Processes*, ed. G. Mazzoni and T. O. Nelson. Mahwah, NJ: Lawrence Erlbaum Associates, Inc., pp. 1–21.

Segalowitz, S. J. & Davies, P. L. (2004). Charting the maturation of the frontal lobe: An electrophysiological strategy. *Brain and Cognition*, **55**, 116–33.

Séguin, J. R. (2004). Neurocognitive elements of social antisocial behaviour: Relevance of an orbitofrontal cortex account. *Brain and Cognition*, **55**, 185–97.

Shammi, P. & Stuss, D. T. (1999). Humor appreciation. A role for the right frontal lobe. *Brain*, **122**, 657–66.

Shimamura, A. P. & Squire, L. R. (1986). Memory and metamemory: A study of feeling of knowing phenomenon in amnesic patients. *Journal of Experimental Psychology: Learning Memory Cognition*, **12**, 452–60.

Shum, D. (2005). Prospective memory following traumatic brain injury in children and adolescents. Presentation at the *Joint Mid-Year Meeting of the International Neuropsychology Society*, Dublin, Ireland.

Silveri, M., Leggio, M. & Molinari, M. (1994). The cerebellum contributes to linguistic production: A case of agrammatic speech following a right cerebellar lesion. *Neurology*, **44**, 2047–50.

Sommerville, S. C., Wellman, H. M. & Cultice, J. C. (1983). Young children's deliberate reminding. *The Journal of Genetic Psychology*, **143**, 87–96.

Sowell, E. R., Delis, D., Stiles, J. & Jernigan, T. L. (2001). Improved memory functioning and frontal lobe maturation between childhood and adolescence: a structural MRI study. *Journal of the International Neuropsychological Society*, **7**, 312–22.

Sowell, E. R. & Jernigan, T. L. (1998). Further MRI evidence of late brain maturation: Limbic volume increases and changing asymmetries during childhood and adolescence. *Developmental Neuropsychology*, **14**, 599–617.

Sowell, E. R., Thompson, P. M., Holmes, C. J., *et al.* (1999). Localizing age-related changes in brain structure between childhood and adolescence using statistical parametric mapping. *NeuroImage*, **9**, 587–97.

Sowell, E. R., Trauner, D. A., Gamst, A. & Jernigan, T. L. (2002). Development of cortical and subcortical brain structures in childhood and adolescence: A structural MRI study. *Developmental Medicine and Child Neurology*, **44**, 4–16.

Steinberg, L. (2005). Cognitive and affective development in adolescence. *Trends in Cognitive Sciences*, **9**, 69–74.

Stuss, D. T. & Anderson, V. (2004). The frontal lobes and theory of mind: Developmental concepts from adult focal lesion research. *Brain and Cognition*, **55**, 69–83.

Stuss, D. T., Gallup, G. G. & Alexander, M. P. (2001). The frontal lobes are necessary for 'theory of mind'. *Brain*, **124**, 279–86.

Thatcher, R. W. (1997). Human frontal lobe development: A theory of cyclical cortical reorganization. In *Development of the Prefrontal Cortex: Evolution, Neurobiology, and Behavior*, ed. N. A. Krasnegor, G. R. Lyon and P. S. Goldman-Rakic. Baltimore, MD: Paul H. Brookes, pp. 85–113.

Tranel, D. (2002). Emotion, decision making, and the ventromedial prefrontal cortex. In *Principles of Frontal Lobe Function*, ed. D. T. Stuss and R. T. Knight. New York, NY: Oxford University Press, pp. 338–53.

Tulving, E. (2002). Chronesthesia: Conscious awareness of subjective time. In *Principles of Frontal Lobe Function*, ed. D. T. Stuss and R. T. Knight. New York, NY: Oxford University Press, pp. 311–25.

Turkstra, L., McDonald, S. & DePompei, R. (2001). Social information processing in adolescents: Data from normally developing adolescents and preliminary data from their peers with traumatic brain injury. *Journal of Head Trauma Rehabilitation*, **16**, 469–83.

Warschausky, S., Cohen, E. H., Parker, J. G., Levendosky, A. A. & Okun, A. (1997). Social problem-solving skills of children with traumatic brain injury. *Pediatric Rehabilitation*, **1**, 77–81.

Wichman, H. & Oyasato, A. (1983). Effects of locus of control and task complexity on prospective remembering. *Human Factors*, **25**, 583–91.

Wilde, E. A., Hunter, J. V., Newsom, M. R., *et al.* (2005). Frontal and temporal morphometric findings on MRI in children after moderate to severe traumatic brain injury. *Journal of Neurotrauma*, **22**, 333–44.

Williams, B. R., Ponesse, J. S., Schachar, R. J., Logan, G. D. & Tannock, R. (1999). Development of inhibitory control across the life span. *Developmental Psychology*, **35**, 205–13.

Winner, E. (1988). *The Point of Words: Children's Understanding of Metaphor and Irony.* Cambridge, MA: Harvard University Press.

Wood, J. & Grafman, J. (2003). Human prefrontal cortex: Processing and representational perspectives. *Nature Reviews Neuroscience*, **4**, 139–47.

Yakovlev, P. I. & Lecours, A. R. (1967). The myelogenetic cycles of regional maturation of the brain. In *Regional Development of the Brain in Early Life*, ed. A. Minkowski. Oxford, England: Blackwell, pp. 3–70.

Yeates, K. O., Schultz, L. H. & Selman, R. L. (1990). Bridging the gaps in child-clinical assessment: Toward the application of social-cognitive development theory. *Clinical Psychology Review*, **10**, 567–88.

Yeates, K. O., Swift, E., Taylor, H. G., *et al.* (2004). Short and long-term social outcomes following pediatric traumatic brain injury. *Journal of the International Neuropsychological Society*, **10**, 412–26.

Figure 2.2 Projections from visual cortices to some lateral and orbitofrontal cortices. Neurons projecting to area 8 at the confluence of the upper and lower limbs of the arcuate sulcus (center, red area) originate in posterior visual association cortices (red dots); neurons projecting to the posterior part of ventral area 46 (center, green area) originate in posterior inferior temporal cortices (green triangles); neurons projecting to orbitofrontal area 11 (bottom, blue area) originate in anterior inferior temporal cortices (blue squares). Abbreviations: A, arcuate sulcus; AMT, anterior middle temporal dimple; C, central sulcus; Ca, calcarine fissure; Cg, cingulate sulcus; IO, inferior occipital sulcus; IP, intraparietal sulcus; LF, lateral fissure; MO, medial orbital sulcus; MPO, medial parietooccipital sulcus; P, principal sulcus; PO, parietooccipital sulcus.

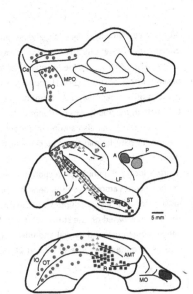

Figure 2.7 Neuronal density profile in different types of prefrontal cortices. Three-dimensional graphs showing differences in neuronal density (Y axis), laminar thickness by layer (X axis), and number of neurons under 1 mm² of cortical surface (Z axis) in: (A), agranular; (B), dysgranular; (C), eulaminate I; (D), eulaminate II cortices. Dotted lines for x axis demarcate extent of cortical layers, and solid lines indicate 500-mm intervals of cortical thickness. The density of neurons in the upper layers (IV–II) increases progressively from agranular to eulaminate II areas. (From Dombrowski et al. [2001].)

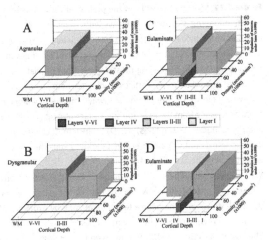

Figure 2.8 The pattern of connections predicted by the structural model. A, top: projections between areas that differ markedly in laminar structure originate predominantly in the deep layers of areas with fewer layers or lower cell density, and their axons terminate mostly in the upper layers of areas with more layers of higher cell density. A, bottom: the opposite pattern is seen for the reciprocal projections. B, top: a less extreme version of the above pattern is predicted in the interconnections of areas that differ moderately in laminar structure, such as when a cortex with lower cell density projects to a cortex with higher cell density. B, bottom: when a cortex with higher cell density projects to a cortex with lower cell density. The bottom panels show a cartoon of laminar features that form the basis for grouping areas into cortical types. The number of types used for parcellling schemes can vary, as areas show gradual changes in neuronal density within layers. (Adapted from Barbas & Rempel-Clower [1997].)

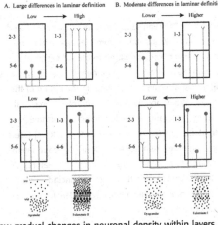

Figure 2.10 Pathways originating and terminating in different layers encounter a different microenvironment with respect to inhibitory control. Hypothetical scheme for prefrontal to temporal pathways based on rules of corticocortical connections. Pyramidal projection neurons originating in layer 3 of prefrontal cortex (dark blue) terminate in the middle layers of temporal cortex among excitatory neurons (green), but also among inhibitory neurons that are positive for parvalbumin (solid black), which are most prevalent in

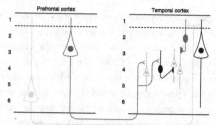

the middle layers of the cortex. Parvalbumin neurons innervate the proximal dendrites or axon initial segment of pyramidal neurons locally. Pyramidal projection neurons from the deep layers of prefrontal cortex (light blue) terminate in layer 1 of temporal cortex among the distal dendrites of other pyramidal neurons, but also around calbindin inhibitory neurons which are most prevalent in layers 2–upper 3 of the cortex. Calbindin neurons innervate the distal dendrites of pyramidal neurons locally. The model is based on the structural model for connections (Barbas & Rempel-Clower, 1997), the pattern of connections between prefrontal and medial and inferior (Rempel-Clower & Barbas, 2000) and superior temporal (Barbas et al., 1999) cortices, and the prevalence of PV and CB neurons in superior temporal cortices (Barbas et al., 2005b).

Figure 2.11 Serial pathways from the prefrontal cortex reach central autonomic structures. Pathways were mapped after injection of the bidirectional tracer BDA in the lateral (LA) hypothalamic area. (A) The first pathway is marked by projection neurons (blue dots) originating most densely from medial prefrontal and orbitofrontal cortices leading to the injection site (brown area in B); (B) the second pathway is marked by labeled axons emanating from the injection site and terminating in several autonomic nuclei (brown lines); (C, D) brainstem nuclei; (E) the thoracic spinal cord; (F) a bidirectional pathway links the amygdala with the same hypothalamic nuclei. The shaded areas in the amygdala show the specific termination zones of axons from orbitofrontal cortex (yellow), which originate from the deep layers (mainly layer 5), and the diffuse termination zone by axons from medial prefrontal cortex (light brown), as described by Ghashghaei & Barbas (2002). (Reproduced from Barbas et al. [2003].)

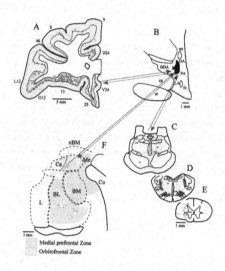

Figure 3.1 The representational forms of the SEC and their proposed localization within the prefrontal cortex. All subcomponents can contribute to the formation of an SEC, with the different subcomponents being differentially weighted in activation depending on the nature of the represented SEC and moment-by-moment behavioral demands. For example, the left anterior ventromedial prefrontal cortex (PFC) would be expected to represent a long multievent sequence of social information with specialized processing of the meaning and features of the single events within the sequence, including the computation of their sequential dependencies and primary meaning.

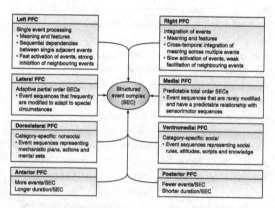

Figure 4.2 Working memory maintained by a spatially tuned network activity pattern (a "bump attractor"). Top: model architecture. Excitatory pyramidal cells are labeled by their preferred locational cues (0° to 360°). Pyramidal cells of similar preferred cues are connected through local E-to-E connections. Interneurons receive inputs from excitatory cells and send feedback inhibition by broad projections. Middle: a network simulation of delayed oculomotor response experiment. C: cue period; D: delay period; R: response period. Pyramidal neurons are labeled along the y-axis according to their preferred cues. The x-axis represents time. A dot in the rastergram indicates a spike of a neuron whose preferred location is at y, at time x. Note the enhanced and localized neural activity that is triggered by a transient cue stimulus and persists during the delay period. The population firing profile, averaged over the delay period, is shown on the right. Bottom left: firing activities of a single cell when the cue was shown in one of the eight locations indicated in the center diagram. This neuron exhibits an elevated persistent activity in the delay only for one direction (270°), and is suppressed relative to intertrial spontaneous activity in the upper visual field. Bottom right: the delay period tuning curve shows the average discharge rate during the delay period (circles), together with a Gaussian fit of the data. The horizontal line indicates average intertrial spontaneous activity. Data provided by A. Compte.

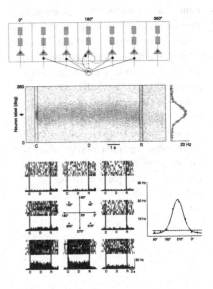

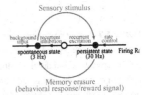

Figure 4.3 Schematic illustration of the biophysics underlying an attractor dynamics. An attractor is a neural firing state that is stable to perturbations: when a small input perturbs the network to a lower or higher activity level, there is a "restoring force" to bring the network back to the attractor state. In this case, the spontaneous state is stabilized from below by background inputs, and from above by feedback synaptic inhibition. A sufficiently powerful sensory stimulus can drive a cell assembly to "escape" from the spontaneous state, and after the stimulus is withdrawn the system settles in one of the active memory states at an elevated firing rate. The persistent activity state is stabilized from below by excitatory reverberation, and from above by various negative feedback "rate control" mechanisms. Finally, a behavioral response or reward signal can turn the network off and erase the memory. (Adopted from Wang [2001] with permission.)

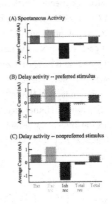

Figure 4.4 Balanced excitation and inhibition in the spatial working memory model (same as in Figure 4.2). Various components of synaptic current in a single cell during spontaneous activity (top), during delay activity following presentation of a preferred stimulus (middle), and during delay activity following presentation of a nonpreferred stimulus (bottom). The dotted line indicates the value of excitatory synaptic currents needed to reach the (deterministic) firing threshold. In the two lower panels, the dotted boxes indicate the value of the corresponding component during spontaneous activity, to show the differences between delay and spontaneous activity. Background external inputs are superthreshold. Recurrent circuit is dominated by inhibition (brown) over excitation (orange) in the spontaneous state, so that the net recurrent synaptic current is hyperpolarizing (blue). During delay activity both recurrent excitation and inhibition are larger and dynamically balance each other, in such a way that the overall synaptic excitation becomes slightly larger following a preferred stimulus (leading to persistent activity at an elevated rate) than after a nonpreferred stimulus.

Figure 4.5 Gamma oscillations during working memory. (A) Spatiotemporal firing pattern of a spatial working memory model same as in Figure 4.2 (with slightly different parameters) except that firing rates are color-coded. (B) 500 ms blowup of (A) to show synchronous oscillations in the spatiotemporal activity pattern (top), the local field potential (middle) and membrane potential of a single neuron (bottom). On the right is shown the power spectrum of the local field, demonstrating a large peak at about 40 Hz. (Adopted from Compte *et al.* [2000] with permission.)

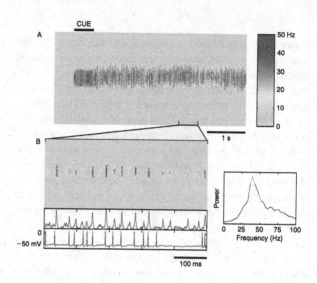

Figure 4.7 A spatial working memory model, with single neurons endowed with three compartments (soma, proximate and distal dendrites) and a number of voltage-gated ion channels. (A) Left: schematic single pyramidal cell model; right: spatiotemporal network activity (top) and membrane potential of a single cell (bottom) in a simulation of the delayed oculomotor experiment. Data provided by J. Tegnér (2002). (B) Electroresponsiveness of an isolated pyramidal cell model with a nonselective cation current ICan. The calcium-dependent activation of ICan is slow, leading to a ramping-up time course of the neural response. A few action potentials are still fired after stimulus extinction, in parallel with a slow deactivation of ICan. Notice that the neuron is not bistable; it returns to stable resting state. (C) Slow ionic currents (here ICan) reduce the minimum level of NMDAR that is required for sustained delay activity. Further increase in gCan renders the neuron intrinsically bistable (not shown). (Adopted from Tegnér *et al.* [2002] with permission.)

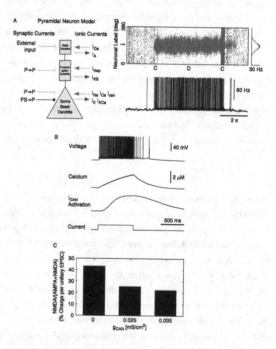

Figure 4.8 Resistance against distractors. (A) In the spatial working memory model, the initial cue (upper arrow on the left) triggers persistent activity centered at 180°. During the delay, a second cue (distractor) is shown briefly (lower arrow on the left). When the distractor is close to the initial stimulus, the network performs a vector sum so that the final remembered cue is half-way between the two (arrow on the right). On the other hand, when the distractor is far away from the initial stimulus, the network operates in a winner-take-all regime, so that the final remembered cue is either the initial stimulus or the distractor, depending on the strength of the stimuli. (B) Behavior of an object working memory model as function of dopamine modulation of NMDAR-mediated recurrent excitation and GABA$_A$R inhibition (x-axis) and amplitude of cue stimulation (y-axis). A very weak stimulus (initial cue) cannot elicit persistent activity (lower left region), whereas a powerful stimulus (distractor) can override recurrent dynamics and disrupt delay activity (upper left region). The desirable behavior (robust persistent activity in spite of distractors) (middle right region) is sensitive to dopamine modulations. (Adopted from Brunel & Wang [2001] with permission.)

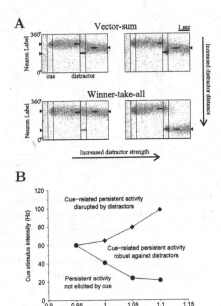

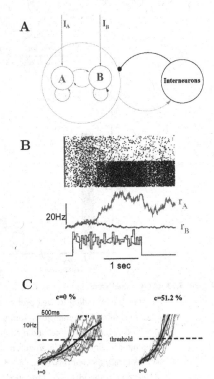

Figure 4.9 (A) A simple model for two-alternative forced-choice tasks. There are two pyramidal cell groups, each of which is selective to one of the two directions (A=left, B=right) of random moving dots in a visual motion discrimination experiment. Within each pyramidal neural group there are strong recurrent excitatory connections which can sustain persistent activity triggered by a transient preferred stimulus. The two neural groups compete through feedback inhibition from interneurons. The motion coherence is expressed as c = (μ A−μ B)/(μ A+μ B), where μ A and μ B are the mean values of inputs IA and IB. (B) A network simulation with zero coherence. Top to bottom: network spiking raster, population firing rates rA and rB, stochastic inputs IA and IB. Note the initial slow ramping (time integration) and eventual divergence of rA and rB (categorical choice). (C) In reaction time simulations, when one of the two neural groups reaches a fixed threshold (15 Hz) of population firing activity, the decision is made and the deliberation or decision time is read out. The decision time is longer and more variable at low coherence (left) than at high coherence (right). (Adopted from Wang [2002] with permission.)

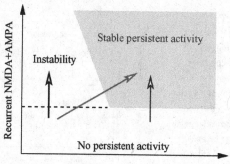

Figure 4.11 Schematic depiction of the dependence of stable persistent activity on both sufficiently strong recurrency (y-axis) and large NMDA/AMPA ratio at local excitatory synapses (x-axis). A circuit that does not exhibit persistent activity may be endowed with this ability by strengthening excitatory connections while preserving a relatively large NMDA/AMPA ratio (blue arrow). However, an enhancement of recurrency at a low NMDA/AMPA ratio can lead to network dynamical instability (black arrow), in which case the NMDA/AMPA ratio needs to be increased simultaneously (red arrow).

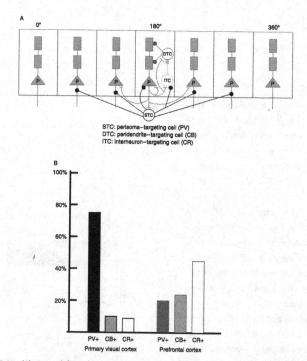

Figure 4.13 (A) A spatial working memory model with three subclasses of GABAergic interneurons. Pyramidal (P) neurons are arranged according to their preferred cues (0 – 360°). There are localized recurrent excitatory connections, and broad inhibitory projections from perisoma-targeting (parvalbumin-containing, PV) fast-spiking neurons to P cells. Within a column, calbindin-containing (CB) interneurons target the dendrites of P neurons, whereas calretinin-containing (CR) interneurons preferentially project to CB cells. Excitation of a group of pyramidal cells recruits locally CR neurons, which sends enhanced inhibition to CB neurons, leading to dendritic disinhibition of the same pyramidal cells. (Adopted from Wang *et al.* [2004] with permission.) (B) Proportional distribution of PV, CB and CR expressing GABAergic cells in primary visual cortex and prefrontal cortex. See text for details.

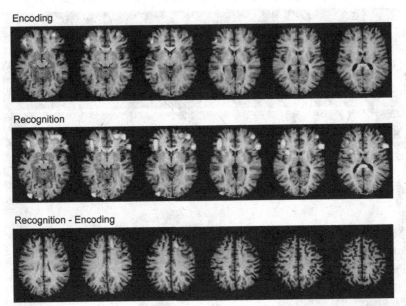

Encoding

Recognition

Recognition - Encoding

Figure 7.1 ControlSPM map showing areas activated by word encoding (top), recognition (middle), and recognition minus encoding (bottom) after averaged baseline subtraction. Displayed on a sagittal 4-mm MRI standardized into Talairach space (left is left). Colored areas exceed a corrected cluster-level value of $p < 0.05$.

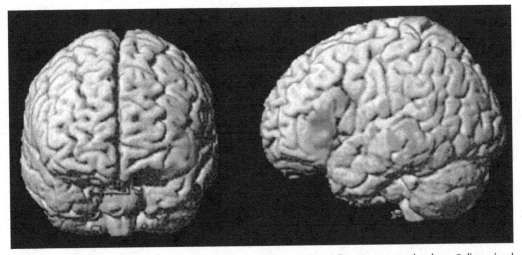

Figure 7.3 SPMmap showing areas activated by deep minus shallow word encoding. Maps are rendered on a 3-dimensional brain to show similarity of activation in the left ventrolateral prefrontal cortex in controls (green) and patients with schizophrenia (red). Overlapping activation in yellow. Colored areas exceed a corrected cluster-level value of $p < 0.05$.

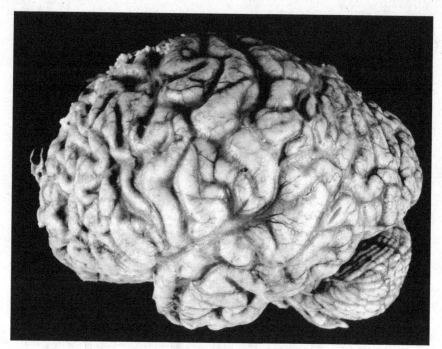

Figure 8.1 FLDwith marked frontal atrophy but preserved and wide central sensory motor cortex.

Case studies of focal prefrontal lesions in Man

David W. Loring and Kimford J. Meador

1 Introduction

Against the nineteenth century backdrop of the tension between Franz Joseph Gall and Johann Spurzheim's *phrenology* versus Marie-Jean-Pierre Flourens' *equipotentiality*, Paul Broca and subsequently Carl Wernicke demonstrated cortical localization of expressive and receptive language functions and their descriptions were soon embraced by the larger medical and scientific community. As additional evidence of hemispheric specialization, John Hughlings Jackson described difficulty with "memory for persons, objects, and places" associated with posterior right hemisphere lesions which led him to introduce the term "imperception" (Finger, 1994). Interest in the frontal lobe was largely restricted to language characteristics associated with lesions of Broca's area as contrasted against those associated with more posterior lesions involving Wernicke's area.

Despite the advances of understanding brain function in the second half of the nineteenth century, the tension between the localizationist versus anti-localizationist camps continued to be present. Current interest in the frontal lobe extends far beyond expressive speech, and involves its role in executive functioning, perseveration, judgment, attention, emotional behavior, and motor programming and regulation, with regional specialization within the frontal system increasingly appreciated for unique contributions to complex human behavior. Thus, localization and antilocalization approaches are able to coexist within a functional system framework. In the present chapter, we will present important cases demonstrating the behavioral impairments associated with prefrontal lobe lesions that have greatly contributed to our understanding of neuropsychological functions of these regions. The prefrontal regions are those anterior and mesial to those subserving motor function (i.e. primary motor cortex and frontal eye fields) and expressive speech (i.e. Broca's area) (Benton, 1991).

Because lesions of these frontal lobe regions often result in recognizable and distinct frontal lobe syndromes, the entire frontal lobe is often regionalized into lateral (dorsolateral), mesial, and orbital frontal areas. Dorsolateral frontal syndrome (executive dysfunction syndrome) consists of difficulty generating hypotheses and flexibly maintaining or shifting sets, and may be assessed with neuropsychological tests including Card Sorting Test, generative fluency, poor organizational strategies, and motor programming deficits.

The mesial frontal/anterior cingulate syndrome is characterized by reduced spontaneous activity that ranges from *akinetic mutism* to transient abulic hypokinesia (hypokinesia from "loss of will"). Patients are typically apathetic, do not speak spontaneously, will answer questions in monosyllables if at all, move little, eat and drink only if fed, show little or no emotion, and may be incontinent. If able to cooperate with neuropsychological testing, these patients may be able to perform adequately on many neuropsychological tests but have more difficulty on tests of response inhibition such as go/no-go tasks.

Orbital frontal syndrome, which is the primary topic of the cases presented in this chapter, is characterized by prominent personality changes. These changes may include emotional lability, impulsivity, irritability, becoming more outspoken and less worried, and occasionally showing imitation and utilization behaviors (enslavement to environmental cues). Orbital-frontal syndrome is caused by lesions of the orbital region (undersurface) of the frontal lobes. This area is also sometimes referred to as the limbic frontal lobe because of its extensive connectivity to limbic structures such as the amygdala.

Antecedents of current clinical interest in the frontal lobe lesions can be traced to the early nineteenth century during the heyday of phrenology, which postulated that cerebral specialization of complex human behaviors not only existed, but that they could be detected through examining the overlying skull, which reflected the size of the regions of behavioral specialization of underlying brain anatomy. It was also at this time that the pattern of convolutions began to become recognized as defining more or less consistent patterns of anatomy (e.g. Rolando, 1831), thereby allowing specific function to be more easily ascribed to underlying brain structure. By 1870, the gross morphology of the brain and its landmarks were well described (Benton, 1991). Gall and Spurzheim's (1809) view of brain function was that the brain contained discrete mental faculties and functioned as an assemblage of "organs." In contrast, Flourens proposed "mass action" of the brain in which a threshold of volume loss was necessary prior to the appearance of clinical symptoms.

Flourens derived support for his position by many reports of brain injuries without any associated functional impairment.

2 Phineas Gage

Against this backdrop of whether there existed a differentiation of function in the brain or whether the brain operated as a more holist unit emerges Phineas Gage, one of the most famous cases in behavioral neurology, neuro-psychiatry, and neuropsychology. A review reveals how the initial report of Gage's injury was first used as evidence to support an antilocalizationist inter-pretation of brain—behavior relationships after a follow-up report 20 years later detailing Gage's behavioral deficits. In short, it is an early case study in the philosophy of science.

Gage's injury involved the projection of a large tamping iron, which was used to pack sand over an explosive charge to excavate rock during railway construction, through the left side of his skull. That this magnitude of injury did not immediately cause death was of great surprise, and the early characteriza-tion of this case focused upon Gage's surprising survival. The local newspaper report reflected the early belief that the injury caused no significant behavioral effect. "The most singular circumstance connected with this melancholy affair is, that he was alive at two o'clock this afternoon, and in full possession of his reason, and free from pain" *Free Soil Union* (Ludlow, Vermont) (Macmillan, 2000a). Using contemporary computational methods, the lesion likely involved bilateral anterior orbital frontal cortex, polar and anterior mesial frontal cortices, and the rostral anterior cingulate (Damasio *et al.*, 1994). The underlying white matter was more greatly involved in the left hemisphere. Gage developed epilepsy many years later, and died following status epilepticus in 1861 over 12 years following his accident.

John M. Harlow, MD was primarily responsibile for Gage's medical care following the accident. Harlow's physiology professor at Jefferson Medical School was Robley Dunglison. Dunglison was not a "phrenologist," but consid-ered the approach of phrenology as a potentially valid approach to characterize human brain function. Although Dunglison described phrenological theory in his 1832 text entitled *Human Physiology*, he also cautioned that "the views of Gall (Franz Joseph Gall) are by no means established. They require numerous and careful experiments, which is not easy for every one to institute" (Barker, 1995). This background likely provided the perspective needed to characterize the behavioral deficits when they were finally described in detail approximately 20 years later. It is likely that it was this exposure to phrenology that permitted Harlow to recognize and appreciate the fractionalization of behavior through this unfortunate "experiment," although Harlow did not report Gage's behavioral changes in any detail until 20 years later (Harlow, 1868).

Harlow's initial report emphasized Gage's surprising physical recovery (Harlow, 1848, 1999). Despite this emphasis, however, there are several hints of significant behavioral change. Harlow stated that Gage "does not estimate size or money accurately, though he has memory as perfect as ever. He would not take $1000 for a few pebbles which he took from an ancient river bed where he was at work." He is also described as being "very childish," exercising poor judgment (e.g. walking a long distance in cold and damp without an overcoat) and not following recommended activity levels during his recovery. Gage "appears to be in a way of recovering if he can be controlled," and Harlow concludes by stating, "the mental manifestations of the patient, I reserve for a future communication."

Because the behavioral changes were not explicitly described in Harlow's 1848 report, Gage's initial notoriety involved his remarkable recovery despite the significant damage to the brain, and this recovery was met with initial skepticism. Gage was subsequently examined by one of those skeptics, Henry Bigelow, MD from Harvard Medical School. As a historical aside, Bigelow was a pioneer in introducing ether anesthesia for surgery (Wheeler, 1997) as well as being a prominent antivivisectionist (Barker, 1995).

Bigelow wrote to Harlow requesting details of the case and subsequently arranged for Gage to travel to Boston and be examined (Macmillan, 2000a). Bigelow reported that Gage was "quite recovered in faculties of body and mind," "A physician who holds in his hand a crowbar . . . will not readily believe that it has been driven . . . through the brain of a man who is still able to walk off . . . Being at first wholly skeptical, I have been personally convinced . . ." (Bigelow, 1850). Because Harlow always referred to the tamping iron by its proper name, Bigelow's use of "crowbar" helps to trace the greater influence of Bigelow's report compared to Harlow's in subsequent citations of Gage, and there are multiple references to the "American crowbar case" (Barker, 1995).

In contrast to Harlow, who was exposed to phrenology during his training, Bigelow's background was antilocalizationist and included F. A. Longet, the French physiologist who stated that "one healthy cerebral hemisphere may suffice for the exercise of intelligence . . . observations of severe wound of the brain: loss of cerebral substance affecting various regions of the cerebrum, with intact intelligence" (Barker, 1995). In Bigelow's description of Gage, he states "it is well known that a considerable portion of the brain has been in some cases abstracted without impairing its functions. Atrophy of an entire cerebral hemisphere has also been recorded" (Bigelow, 1850). Thus, Bigelow's description of Gage as being "quite recovered in his faculties of body and mind" is consistent with this approach to understanding brain function.

The majority of references to the "crowbar" case cited Bigelow emphasizing complete mental recovery as evidence for the antilocalizationalist approach refuting phrenology, and this view of the case was widely reported in texts of that era (Barker, 1995). Of the 14 Gage citations in American medical journals prior to the 1868 report, 11 refer to Bigelow's version and none describe a behavioral impairment alluded to in Harlow's initial report (Barker, 1995).

Bigelow's description of complete recovery was widely cited until 1868 when Harlow published another report on Gage, at which time the significant behavioral changes associated with the injury were detailed.

"His contractors, who regarded him as the most efficient and capable foreman in the employ previous to his injury, considered the change in his mind so marked that he could not give him his place again. The equilibrium, or balance, so to speak, between his intellectual faculties and animal propensities, seems to have been destroyed. He is fitful, irreverent, indulging at times in the grossest profanity (which was not previously his custom) ... manifesting but little deference for his fellows, impatient of restraint or advice when it conflicts with his desires, at time pertinaceously obstinate, yet capricious and vacillating, devising many plans for future operation, which are no sooner arranged than they are abandoned in turn for others appearing more feasible."

Indeed, Gage "was no longer Gage."

Harlow's (1868) descriptions of Gage were quickly incorporated into American texts, but less quickly in Europe (Barker, 1995). David Ferrier reported in the mid 1870s that Gage had no change in intellectual function. However, after reading a reprint of Harlow's 1868 paper sent to him by H. P. Bowditch, a physiology professor at Harvard, Ferrier wired for copies of the now famous woodcuts illustrating Gage's injury. These were subsequently used in his Goulstonian lectures on cerebral localization in which focal mapping of cerebral function was used as an example of how frontal lobe injury could be associated with personality changes in the absence of sensory or motor deficits (Neylan, 1999). The importance of Gage is evident in the continuing citation of this case involving multiple recent articles and books (Damasio *et al.*, 1994; Macmillan, 2000a, 2000b; Haas, 2001; Mataro *et al.*, 2001; Fleischman, 2002; Ratiu & Talos, 2004; Wagar & Thagard, 2004).

In Ferrier's reply to Bowditch, he states initially that "I think your proposal to imitate the lesion with the brain in situ would be a most desirable experiment" and later commented "I hope—Bigelow notwithstanding—that Putnam and you will really carry out your proposed investigation. I can do no experimental work now.... All that is done away with as I cannot work under the accursed antivivisection laws" (Barker, 1995). Thus, Bigelow's antivivisectionist activism likely contributed additional tension to the localization versus antilocalizationist debate on Gage's recovery.

Interestingly, Ferrier's observations about how the same data can be interpreted in vastly different lights continue to be applicable today.

"In investigation the reports on diseases and injuries of the brain I am constantly being amazed at the inexactitude and distortion to which they are subjected by men who have some pet theory to support. The facts suffer so frightfully that I feel obliged always to go to the fountain-head—dirty and muddy though this frequently turns out."

3   Patient K.M.

The beneficial effect of extensive frontal lobe resection on cognition and behavior is detailed in the case of K.M., a 27-year-old man who underwent bilateral frontal lobe resection for poorly controlled posttraumatic epilepsy (Hebb & Penfield, 1940; Hebb, 1945). This is an important case, not only for understanding the contribution of the prefrontal region to cognition and behavior, but also because it demonstrates an important distinction between an active or irritative lesion associated with an ongoing seizure focus compared to that associated with a destructive lesion, as well as how there may be negative behavioral effects of abnormal tissue on normal tissue such that pathological tissue may interfere with normal brain function. As noted by Hebb (1945), "the small and diffuse region of partial necrosis can have a greater effect in the production of symptoms than a larger area of complete destruction and clean cut removal of tissue."

K.M. sustained a skull fracture with significant brain injury when he was 16 years old, resulting in damage to both frontal lobes. After his injury, he developed severe posttraumatic epilepsy with significant behavioral changes. The significant behavioral changes included poor judgment (e.g. going outside in winter without proper clothing) or forgetting to perform an errand for which he originally set out to perform (e.g. mailing a letter). In this context, he appeared behaviorally very similar to Gage. More importantly, however, was a significant change in K.M.'s temperament in which he became violent, stubborn and destructive, a problem made more significant by his large physical size and strength. He even appeared to enjoy scaring his neighbors, acting as though he was in one of his violent moods even when he was not.

Because of the medical intractability of K.M.'s seizures, he underwent epilepsy surgery by Dr. Wilder Penfield at the Montreal Neurological Institute removing "one third of the mass of the frontal lobes" bilaterally. K.M. was tested with the Stanford-Binet and McGill revision of the Army Beta tests both pre- and postoperatively. When tested 2 months after surgery, K. M.'s Stanford-Binet IQ increased from 83 to 94. It is unclear if this improvement occurred at least in part as a function of the different forms of the Stanford-Binet being used for pre- and postoperative assessments (Form L preoperatively and Form M postoperatively). Form M did not contain a vocabulary test (Sattler, 1974), and higher scores tended to be associated with Form M in subsequent postoperative evaluations. Nevertheless, it is clear from these data that no significant decline in overall function was present. In addition to the changes on the Stanford-Binet, a postoperative improvement on the McGill revision of the Army Beta test was described from 63 to 71. Although it is likely that practice effects contributed to the improvement from pre- to postoperative scores since Army Beta contained many of the subtests that Wechsler incorporated into the WAIS (Boake, 2002) and the performance tests tend to be more affected by practice than verbal subtests (Lezak *et al.*, 2004), as with the Stanford-Binet, these data indicate the absence of a significant cognitive decline following surgery. Good postoperative performances were also described for Kohs blocks, backward digit span, and category sorting. Thus, surgical resection of the frontal lobes in K. M. did not apparently produce any significant neuropsychological impairment.

A significant postoperative behavioral improvement in personality and temperament was described. "The patient has now a pleasant personality. He is no longer facetious or vulgar ... but is considerate of the other patients and has acquired a pleasant sense of humor." The negative behaviors developed after K. M.'s brain injury. Six years after the operation, K. M. was described as being "one of the more popular persons in the village." Thus, even in the absence of formal diagnostic evaluation, there is evidence of significant behavioral improvement following surgery with a return to premorbid behavioral tendencies. In fact, he was described years later by his relatives as being his "old self" (Hebb, 1945).

As real-world evidence of both his behavioral normalization as well as the absence of developing significant neuropsychological impairment is his military service that was performed following the surgery, K. M. enlisted in the army without apparent difficulty for either cognitive or behavior reasons. He continued to serve without incident until he had a seizure following significant physical exertion, at which time he was medically discharged from the service. K. M. had no difficulty finding work, although a labor shortage associated with World War II may have contributed in part to that ease. He was able to manage his money without significant difficulty and, although not "saving" money for the future, always had money on hand when it was needed. Of course, not planning for the distant future financially is characteristic of many individuals without bilateral prefrontal injury, and is hardly diagnostic.

An important contribution of this case is the demonstration that extensive frontal resection is not necessarily associated with a loss of psychometric intelligence. "For the effect of lesions of the frontal lobe on human intelligence, it seems that one will have to look elsewhere than to clinical observation or ratings by intelligence tests such as are now available." Further, normal performances were noted on several tests that are presently commonly associated with "frontal lobe function" including backward digit span and category sorting.

More important, however, is that K. M.'s lesion (s) was very different from that of Gage; K. M. had significant preexisting damage to the region that was resected, and further, this area was associated with significant and active seizure focus. The negative effect associated with the epileptogenic region (i.e. nociferous cortex) is described explicitly. "It becomes evident that human behavior and mental activity may be more greatly impaired by the positive action of an abnormal area of brain than by the negative effect of its complete absence." As later noted by Hebb, "the question ... of whether (frontal lobe) behavioral defects are the result of the surgical removal or whether they are due to the presence of pathological changes in the remaining part of the brain" continues to be appropriate for clinical correlates of brain function, even in the present days of sophisticated neuroimaging.

4   More recent "classics": patient E. V. R.

E. V. R. was a 35-year-old man and a successful accountant and comptroller before developing personality changes, which led to the discovery of a large orbital frontal meningioma compressing both frontal lobes (Eslinger & Damasio, 1985). After successful surgical resection, the lesion was described as involving both orbital and lower mesial frontal cortices. Although E. V. R. returned to work after 3 months, his performance and overall behavior changed dramatically. He quit his job to invest in a building partnership with a previous coworker who had been fired, and subsequently lost his entire savings. E. V. R. was then fired from multiple jobs, generally due to being late for work and being disorganized. Nevertheless, E. V. R.'s basic skills, manners, and temper were appropriate. His wife of many years left him, and E. V. R. moved in with his parents. He remarried, was again divorced, and subsequently was considering marriage to a woman 14 years his senior (a "semiprominent socialite") who he was trying to convince to support the establishment of a "luxury travel business" to drive "wealthy people" on vacation around the country in a motor home.

Much of his behavior was ritualistic and compulsive, with some days consumed entirely by shaving and hair-washing. Purchasing small items required in-depth consideration of brands, prices, and the best method of purchase. He refused to part with dead houseplants, old phone books, six broken fans, five broken television sets, three bags of empty orange juice concentrate cans, 15 cigarette lighters, and countless stacks of old newspapers.

Despite these behavioral changes, neuropsychological testing was normal. Two years after surgery, E. V. R.'s WAIS verbal IQ was 120, performance IQ was 108, and Wechsler Memory Scale MQ was 140. All MMPI scales were in the normal range. One evaluation concluded that "adjustment problems are not the result of organic problems or neurological dysfunction ... instead they reflect emotional and psychological adjustment problems and therefore are amenable to psychotherapy." In a separate neuropsychological assessment, E. V. R. obtained all six categories on the Wisconsin Card Sorting Test in only 70 sorts, and had normal memory performance using the Brown-Peterson interference procedure, an approach that has been reported to be sensitive to frontal lobe lesions (Stuss & Levine, 2002).

E. V. R. has maintained an interest in world events and could discuss complex social issues as well as the economy and financial matters. In contrast to his personal behavior in which he continually made errors in judgment, his social judgment for problems presented to him during testing was good. For example, when given a vignette about a psychiatrist refusing to provide treatment to a patient after the psychiatrist found out that the patient was forced to engage in cannibalism to stay alive, E. V. R. replied, "The psychiatrist's duty is to treat a patient for whatever his mental ills may be, not to judge whether he should have or shouldn't have treatment."

5   More recent "classics": imitation, utilization, and environmental dependency

The contrast between the ability to make good abstract judgments to verbal scenarios and his poor real-time judgments in his personal life is the most valuable contribution of this case. This dissociation contrasts with patients with "acquired sociopathy" in which the approach to real-life social problems and hypothetical social problems tend to be the same (see next section). As the authors note: "He had learned and used normal patterns of social behavior before his brain lesion, and although he could recall such patterns when he was questioned about their applicability, *real life situations failed to evoke them.*"

The issue of behavior being elicited by real-life situations was described in two papers in which behavioral response was directly dependent upon the environment (Lhermitte, 1986; Lhermitte *et al.*, 1986). Imitation behavior occurs when a patient imitates the imitation of the examiner's gestures without being instructed to do so and is considered to be a form of utilization behavior in which objects in the environment elicit behavioral response. Both are symptoms of the same behavioral disorder.

The inferior portion of frontal lobes (unilateral or bilateral) tends to be associated with imitation or utilization behavior. Types of behavior that may elicit imitation include sudden hand clapping or saluting, thumbing one's nose, folding a piece of paper, or simply tapping the leg with various rhythms. Patients with imitation or utilization behavior tend to have additional neuro-psychological impairment in both memory and intelligence, poor performance on the Wisconsin Card Sorting Test, and not surprisingly, motor perseveration on Luria figures.

Patients demonstrating imitation behavior believe it to be volitional and report that they thought the examiner had meant for them to imitate. In that sense, imitation behavior differs from echolalia or echopraxia. As discussed by the authors, the parietal lobes process a constant stream of incoming sensory information forming a constant link between the subject and external world. Frontal lobe impairment removes inhibitory influences such that the behavioral dependence is affected more by the quality of the external stimulus field and less by internal factors.

Two cases are described in detail who demonstrated behaviors that were not only dependent on the physical environment, but also reflected more complex social factors such as the socioeconomic background of the patients and their gender. Lhermitte introduced the term "environmental dependency" to describe the behaviors. The first case was a 51-year-old male engineer with a high socioeconomic background who developed a left frontal oligodendrog-lioma that was resected, and then treated with chemotherapy and radiation therapy. The second patient was a 52-year-old woman with an astrocytoma of the basal left frontal lobe that was resected, which was followed by radiation therapy. She came from an average background and had been employed doing domestic work.

Both of these patients were exposed to a variety of social situations, and at times, responded very differently to the identical setting. For example, when entering a room with a buffet table and approximately 20 people present, the male patient helped himself to food and orange juice while the female patient unstacked chairs, arranged glasses on the serving table, and offered to serve food to Lhermitte (including port!). The male patient from a higher socioeconomic background acted like a guest, whereas the female patient who had been employed providing domestic help acted like a hostess.

A similar pattern was seen when the patients sat down next to a table that contained a variety of items including makeup and handguns. After sitting down next to a table, the male patient first frowned when seeing the makeup items until he saw the handguns, which he picked up and examined. The female patient, in contrast, immediately picked up the makeup products and began to apply them to her face.

In an apartment, the male started examining the paintings that were hanging on the wall as if he were in an art gallery after the author quietly uttered the word "museum." The female patient started to walk though the apartment after hearing "museum," but she did not study the paintings systemically; instead she paid a great deal of attention to the curios on the table. In both these and other examples, behavior was elicited through cues in the environment (environmental dependency), which was modulated by the patient's personality and prior experiences. The patients thought that they had reacted in a naturally volitional way toward the environment. This call to action can even be observed to a less degree in healthy subjects as observed by behavior when a bowl of popcorn or potato chips is placed on a table.

Lhermitte described environmental dependency syndrome as a physical adherence to external stimuli resulting from a loss of autonomy from the environment. There is a reciprocal relationship between the frontal and parietal regions. In the healthy brain, the prefrontal lobe has an inhibitory influence on more basic behaviors that arise from sensory stimulation in the environment. In addition, the prefrontal regions (particularly the dorsolateral region) allows the elaboration of goal-directed and adaptive behavior, based upon both environmental contingencies as well as the subject's internal state from limbic information received through the paralimbic orbital frontal region. When the prefrontal region is damaged, the normal interaction is disturbed and the behaviors triggered by sensory stimulation in the partial lobes are "released" without inhibitory control. In this case, sensory stimulation (visual or tactile) may result in utilization of imitation behavior.

6 Early prefrontal injury

All of the cases described above sustained their injuries as adults. A small series of two patients (called only A and B in the report) who sustained prefrontal injuries before 16 months of age illustrate how age of injury affects behavioral outcome.

Patient A was a 20-year-old woman who was run over by a vehicle when she was 15 months and apparently recovered fully within days. MRI performed as an adult indicated bilateral frontal lobe involvement involving polar and ventro-medial areas. Patient B was a 23-year-old man who had a right frontal lobe tumor resected when he was 3 months of age. As an adult, MRI revealed unilateral right frontal injury of the medial and dorsal pole.

The first patient's behavioral difficulties did not emerge until she was 3 years old when she did not respond normally to punishment. In adolescence, she was disruptive, verbally and physically abusive, and would steal from family and from stores. She became pregnant at 18 years old, but after birth, she displayed no sensitivity to her baby's needs. She was unable to hold down a job due to lack of dependability and gross work infractions.

The second patient was not as disruptive at school, but generally lacked normal motivation. He, too, could not hold down a job, and fathered a child but failed to fulfill any paternal obligation. He engaged in petty planned thievery and would threaten and occasionally physically assault others. He also lied frequently, often with no known motivation.

According to the authors, the magnitude of these behaviors is more severe than in comparably lesioned adults. In contrast to adults such as E. V. R., these patients did not retrieve the complex socially relevant knowledge when queried, presumably because it was never acquired. In addition, unlike adult patients sustaining similar injures, these two subjects displayed antisocial behavior such as violence against others and repeatedly stealing items (i.e. "acquired sociopathy"), although much of the behavior did not seem to be goal-directed, appearing more impulsive in character.

7   Concluding remarks

The cases reported in this chapter were selected based upon their historical importance, their relevance to demonstrating different behavioral effects based upon specific lesion characteristics, as well as their demonstration of some inhibitory control over behaviors elicited by environmental cues or imitation. Although the story of Phineas Gage is often cited, it is typically not described in great detail. In addition, the fact that Gage's behavioral outcome was used for approximately 20 years as evidence that significant frontal lobe damage could be present without pronounced behavioral change is almost without exception not included.

There is often times a tendency to treat all lesions as equivalently disruptive to cognition and behavior. K. M. demonstrated a much improved behavioral outcome following surgical resection of an existing lesion despite the fact that the surgical lesion involved a much greater volume of brain tissue compared to the original epileptogenic lesion. In present nomenclature, the disruptive effect of the "active" lesion is termed "nociferous."

The cases of K. M. and E. V. R. demonstrate an absence of neuropsychological impairment following extensive frontal lobe damage, despite multiple assessments using comprehensive batteries with tests commonly used to assess frontal lobe function. Interesting here was the dissociation between the ability of E. V. R. to provide "correct" answers to social and ethical situations when presented to him in the laboratory setting and his ability to implement "correct" behaviors in the real world. In particular, E. V. R.'s desire to make a living by driving "rich people" around in a mobile home is an example that certain types of poor social skills are unlikely to be fully captured by formal tests or questionnaires.

Lhermitte's report of imitation and utilization behavior, and his case reports of two patients with environmental dependency syndrome, depicts a different facet of frontal inhibitory control over behavior since it provides details of a nonemotional response to environmental cues rather than an alteration of behavior in which either poor judgment is seen or a "coarsening" of personality develops. The reciprocal relationship between the frontal and parietal regions illustrates the constant dynamic interaction between various brain regions and systems, and helps to illustrate how normal frontal lobe function exerts selective control of response to both simple items in the environment as well as orchestrated, complex, and individually specific response to different social contexts. The contribution of frontal lobe function to human behavior ranges from the personality changes of Phineas Gage to the blurring of "free will" associated with environmental dependency disorder, illustrating why much of our understanding of frontal lobe function has been derived from carefully described case studies.

REFERENCES

Barker, F. G., 2nd. (1995). Phineas among the phrenologists: the American crowbar case and nineteenth-century theories of cerebral localization. *Journal of Neurosurgery*, **82**, 672–82.

Benton, A. L. (1991). The prefrontal region: its early history. In *Frontal Lobe Function and Dysfunction*, eds. H. S. Levin, H. M. Eisenberg and A. L. Benton. New York: Oxford University Press, pp. 3–32

Bigelow, H. J. (1850). Dr. Harlow's case of recovery from the passage of an iron bar through the head. *American Journal of Medical Science*, **20**, 1–22.

Boake, C. (2002). From the Binet-Simon to the Wechsler-Bellevue: tracing the history of intelligence testing. *Journal of Clinical and Experimental Neuropsychology*, **24**, 383–405.

Damasio, H., Grabowski, T., Frank, R., Galaburda, A. M. & Damasio, A. R. (1994). The return of Phineas Gage: clues about the brain from the skull of a famous patient. *Science*, **264**, 1102–5.

Eslinger, P. J. & Damasio, A. R. (1985). Severe disturbance of higher cognition after bilateral frontal lobe ablation: patient EVR. *Neurology*, **35**, 1731–41.

Finger, S. (1994). *Origins of Neuroscience: A History of Explorations into Brain Function.* New York: Oxford University Press.

Fleischman, J. (2002). *Phineas Gage: A Gruesome but True Story about Brain Science.* New York: Houghton Mifflin.

Haas, L. F. (2001). Phineas Gage and the science of brain localisation. *Journal of Neurology, Neurosurgery, and Psychiatry*, **71**, 761.

Harlow, J. M. (1848). Passage of an iron rod through the head. *Boston Medical and Surgical Journal*, **39**, 389–93.

Harlow, J. M. (1999). Passage of an iron rod through the head. *Journal of Neuropsychiatry and Clinical Neuroscience*, **11**, 281–3.

Hebb, D. O. (1945). Man's frontal lobes: a critical review. *Archives of Neurology and Psychiatry*, **54**, 10–24.

Hebb, D. O. & Penfield, W. (1940). Human behavior after extensive bilateral removal from the frontal lobes. *Archives of Neurology and Psychiatry*, **43**, 421–38.

Lezak, M. D., Howieson, D. B. & Loring, D. W. (2004). *Neuropsychological Assessment*, 4th ed. New York: Oxford University Press.

Lhermitte, F. (1986). Human autonomy and the frontal lobes. Part II: Patient behavior in complex and social situations: the "environmental dependency syndrome". *Annals of Neurology*, **19**, 335–43.

Lhermitte, F., Pillon, B. & Serdaru, M. (1986). Human autonomy and the frontal lobes. Part I: Imitation and utilization behavior: a neuropsychological study of 75 patients. *Annals of Neurology*, **19**, 326–34.

Macmillan, M. (2000a). *An Odd Kind of Fame: Stories of Phineas Gage.* Cambridge, MA: MIT Press.

Macmillan, M. (2000b). Restoring Phineas Gage: a 150th retrospective. *Journal of the History of the Neurosciences*, **9**, 46–66.

Mataro, M., Jurado, M. A., Garcia-Sanchez, C., *et al.* (2001). Long-term effects of bilateral frontal brain lesion: 60 years after injury with an iron bar. *Archives of Neurology*, **58**, 1139–42.

Neylan, T. C. (1999). Frontal lobe function: Mr. Phineas Gage's famous injury. *Journal of Neuropsychiatry and Clinical Neuroscience*, **11**, 280–1.

Ratiu, P. & Talos, I.-F. (2004). The tale of Phineas Gage, digitally remastered. *The New England Journal of Medicine*, **351**, e21.

Rolando, L. (1831). Della struttura degli emisferi cerebrali. *Memorie della Reale Academia di Scienze di Torino*, **35**, 103–46.

Sattler, J. M. (1974). *Assessment of Children's Intelligence.* Philadelphia: W. B. Saunders.

Stuss, D. T. & Levine, B. (2002). Adult clinical neuropsychology: lessons from studies of the frontal lobes. *Annual Review of Psychology*, **53**, 401–33.

Wagar, B. M. & Thagard, P. (2004). Spiking Phineas Gage: a neurocomputational theory of cognitive-affective integration in decision making. *Psychological Reviews*, **111**, 67–79.

Wheeler, H. B. (1997). The 1996 Bigelow Award of the Boston Surgical Society: Henry Jacob Bigelow and David C. Sabiston, Jr. *Annals of Surgery*, **226**, 146–52.

7

Left prefrontal function and semantic organization during encoding and retrieval in healthy and psychiatric populations

Daniel Ragland

1 Introduction

Memory makes learning and cognition possible as it bridges temporal gaps between behavior and outcome. Given the fundamental importance of this function it is not surprising that it is subject to prefrontal control. To facilitate its study, memory has been subdivided into different categories and stages of processing. The chapter will begin with a review of this taxonomy to illustrate how lesion models evolved from a primary focus on the hippocampus to a growing appreciation of the prefrontal cortex. Presentation of more recent neuropsychological and imaging data will describe the role of the left and right prefrontal cortex in word encoding and retrieval. These data will show how the left inferior prefrontal cortex mediates semantic organizational processing and contributes to efficient encoding and retrieval. A discussion of schizophrenia will illustrate how psychiatric disorders that disrupt prefrontal function also compromise strategic memory processes and impair episodic memory performance. The chapter will close with preliminary data demonstrating how providing patients with organizational strategies may help to reengage their prefrontal cortex and improve task performance. A discussion of cognitive remediation implications will end the chapter.

2 Memory systems and effects of focal lesions

As the "father" of psychology, William James was probably the first to realize the importance of developing operational definitions of different memory functions to facilitate scientific study. He made an initial distinction between short-term memory and long-term memory that remains relevant today. Short-term memory was defined as something, "...that comes to us as belonging to the rearward position of the present space of time, and not to the genuine past" (James, 1890). A hallmark measure of short-term memory is the digit-span task in which a subject is asked to repeat a series of digits immediately after they have been presented by an examiner. Successful completion of this task requires active rehearsal and directed attention. It is a limited capacity (e.g. 7–9 digits) single modality (i.e. phonological) temporary storage process that is essential for online information processing. Early neurological studies of patients with focal brain lesions found that amnesic patients with damage to the hippocampus or diencephalon could perform digit-span tasks successfully, whereas patients with frontal lobe lesions had reduced digit spans (see Shimamura, 1990 for review).

Short-term memory was subsequently developed into a three-component working memory model (Baddeley, 1992). Working memory refers to a multi-modality limited capacity system for the temporary maintenance and manipulation of information. Maintenance of auditory information is accomplished through verbal rehearsal within the "articulatory loop," and visual information is maintained within the "visuo-spatial sketch pad." Manipulation of information and allocation of attentional resources is managed by the "central executive" (Baddeley & Hitch, 1974). This central executive component of working memory is particularly sensitive to the effects of frontal lobe lesions, and a large body of human and primate lesion studies and functional imaging research has established the important role of the prefrontal cortex in working memory. These issues are thoroughly discussed in Chapters 2, 3 and 4 of this book and are not a focus of the current chapter.

Long-term memory is the other primary division of memory function. It was initially defined as, "the knowledge of a former state of mind after it has already once dropped from consciousness" (James, 1890). Long-term memory does not have a limited capacity, and is not dependent upon active rehearsal. These differences were initially demonstrated by presenting subjects with increasingly long digit-span tasks that exceeded the short-term memory span capacity. With repeated administrations healthy subjects were able to learn up to 16 digits. Although there were no differences between healthy subjects and amnesic patients on shorter spans, patients with amnesia were unable to demonstrate supra-span learning (Drachman & Arbit, 1966).

Examination of the serial position effect was another way that short-term memory and long-term memory were dissociated. The serial position effect occurs when subjects are asked to recall a long list of items that exceed their short-term span. During recall, subjects tend to retrieve more items from the beginning of the list (primacy effect) and from the end of the list (recency effect) than from the middle of the list. Primacy effects occur because items at the beginning of the list receive increased rehearsal and, therefore, enter the long-term memory store. In contrast, primacy effects reflect short-term working memory processes. Early studies demonstrated that there were no differences in recency effects between healthy controls and patients with amnesia. However, primacy effects were dramatically reduced in amnesic patients, leading to the conclusion that intact hippocampal function is essential to long-term memory processes (Warrington & Weiskrantz, 1970).

The effect of hippocampal lesions in human and primate studies led to a further subdivision of long-term memory processes. Larry Squire and colleagues made a distinction between two primary types of long-term memory: procedural and declarative. Procedural memory was defined as information that cannot be accessed as specific facts and is not associated with a specific time and place. Procedural memory comprises motor skill learning, classical conditioning, implicit memory (priming), and other nonassociative forms of memory. It is not affected by hippocampal lesions and is spared in patients with amnesia (Squire, 1987). In contrast, declarative memory was defined as, "Information that is directly accessible to conscious recollection. It can be declared. It deals with the facts and data that are acquired through learning." (Squire, 1987). Declarative memory received a further subdivision into episodic and semantic memory, with semantic memory referring to our general knowledge about objects and concepts (Tulving, 1972), and episodic memory referring to a multicomponent process allowing recall of previously experienced personal events (Tulving, 2002). A series of lesion studies of nonhuman primates confirmed that it was this episodic aspect of long-term declarative memory that was selectively impaired by mesial temporal lesions to the hippocampus, amygdala and surrounding rhinal and peri-rhinal cortex (Zola-Morgan & Squire, 1986; Mishkin & Appenzeller, 1987; Squire, 1992).

This differential effect of hippocampal damage on episodic memory was also documented in clinical studies of humans with focal brain damage. Patient H. M. became amnesic in 1953 as the result of a bilateral resection of his hippocampus to treat intractable epilepsy. Although H. M. could remember events from earlier in his life, he had difficulty remembering events from the 2 years prior to surgery (retrograde amnesia), and was incapable of remembering any new events occurring after surgery (anterograde amnesia). Despite this dense anterograde amnesia, H. M. had intact short-term memory, unimpaired procedural learning of motor skills, and normal performance on implicit memory tasks such as lexical priming. These combined clinical and focal lesion results provided further evidence that long-term storage of episodic memory is dependent upon the hippocampus and surrounding mesial temporal cortex.

Although episodic memory was initially equated with the hippocampus, there was growing evidence in the clinical literature that amnesia could also occur due to damage to other parts of the brain. This included findings that Korsakoff's dementia could produce dense anterograde amnenesia as a result of damage to the diencephalon due to chronic alcohol abuse. Similar episodic memory impairments were documented in patients with Parkinson's dementia and Huntington's dementia who had suffered degeneration of frontal and striatial brain regions. The presence of these "other amnesias" was reviewed by Victor and colleagues (1989) who noted high rates of amnesia in patients with damage to the mammillary bodies, the hypothalamus, the thalamus, the cerebral cortex and cerebellum as well as to the hippocampus.

Primate lesion studies also contributed to the notion that other brain regions outside of the hippocampus were important to successful episodic memory performance. This research was based on several memory paradigms. In delayed response tasks primates were visually presented with two food wells, one of which was baited. An opaque screen was then lowered and was subsequently raised after a varying delay interval. To receive the food reward the primate had to remember which food well had been baited. A variant of this task was the delayed alternation task. It followed the same procedure, with the exception that the animal had to go to the food well that had not been previously baited to receive the food reward. Although hippocampal lesions impaired performance on both versions of this task, primates with thalamic lesions also demonstrated performance impairments at longer delay intervals (Zola-Morgan & Squire, 1985). The effect of frontal lobe lesions on these tasks was variable. In some, but not all cases, delayed response was disrupted and, more frequently, there were deficits in delayed alternation performance. In reviews of the literature, Fuster (1985) noted that patients with frontal lesions could perform delayed response tasks correctly with even long delays as long as there were no distracting events to disrupt their focused attention. Frontal cortex was, thus, associated with the ability to avoid interference effects and to sustain directed attention. Deficits in delayed alternation task performance following dorsolateral prefrontal (DPFC) lesions were also attributed to problems mediating cross-temporal contingencies in order to bridge the gap between perception and action (Fuster, 1985).

Because humans can use language to rehearse and maintain short-term memory traces during delay intervals, standard delayed recognition and alternation tasks were not appropriate for assessing long-term episodic memory in human participants. This problem was resolved by developing tasks that either exceeded the short-term memory span, had longer delay intervals, or filled the delay interval with other tasks to prevent rehearsal.

The three most widely used tests of long-term episodic memory in humans have been free recall, cued recall, and recognition tasks. For each task subjects are first presented with a list of target items (commonly words, faces, or drawings of visual objects) that they are asked to remember over a 20–30-minute filled delay. During free recall, subjects are asked to recall as many target items as they can in any order. During cued recall they are provided with a retrieval cue that is somehow related to the target item (e.g. semantic or phonemic similarity to a target word) and are asked to generate the associated target item. During recognition tasks target items are mixed with new items that were not included in the learning list and subjects are asked to determine whether or not each item was presented on the original learning list.

Although hippocampal damage clearly disrupted performance on each one of these tasks, the effect of frontal lobe lesions varied from study to study. Therefore Wheeler and colleagues (1995) performed a meta-analysis of all existing free recall, cued recall, and recognition studies and confirmed that frontal damage disrupted performance on all three types of tasks, with the greatest impairment found in free recall, followed by cued recall, and recognition. During this period, investigators also found that individuals with frontal lobe lesions had difficulty encoding information semantically (Moscovitch, 1982), identifying the source of the encoded information (Janowsky et al., 1989), and determining the temporal order of remembered events (Shimamura, 1990).

These combined results helped to identify the aspects of episodic memory that were dependent upon intact frontal lobe function. A general consensus formed that the frontal lobe is not responsible for consolidation, storage, and retention of new information (Petrides, 2000; Winocur et al., 2001). However, the frontal cortex appears crucial for the organizational and strategic aspects of episodic memory necessary for efficient encoding, guiding retrieval, and verifying memory output (Winocur et al., 2001). Therefore, although the hippocampus appears sufficient for long-term storage and retrieval of episodic information, the prefrontal cortex is necessary for organizing that information in a relational and temporal context to facilitate encoding and subsequent retrieval. An appreciation of the complementary nature of these different brain regions leads to the acknowledgement that all cortical regions are involved both in information processing and memory storage (Squire, 1987).

3 Functional imaging of episodic memory in healthy populations

With the advent of functional imaging it became possible to assess brain behavior relationships without the need for focal lesions. Positron emission tomography (PET) and [133]Xenon clearance studies of regional cerebral blood flow (CBF), and functional magnetic resonance imaging (fMRI) studies of blood oxygen level dependent (BOLD) signal change allowed the simultaneous examination of multiple brain regions while individuals were engaged in different aspects of episodic encoding and retrieval. Contrasts between active task conditions and low-level baseline conditions allowed investigators to identify candidate brain regions. Initial PET studies of episodic retrieval were divided between those finding evidence of hippocampal and mid-temporal activation versus those finding more diffuse activation effects in prefrontal and other cortical and subcortical regions (see Heiss *et al.*, 1992; Perani *et al.*, 1992; Roskies, 1994 for reviews). With the development of fMRI more consistent evidence of prefrontal effects was obtained across verbal and nonverbal stimuli, examining both encoding and retrieval stages of episodic memory (Buckner & Petersen, 1996; Desgranges *et al.*, 1998; Nyberg, 1998).

Unanticipated asymmetries in prefrontal activation gave rise to the "hemispheric encoding-retrieval asymmetry" (HERA) model (Tulving *et al.*, 1994). The HERA model states that left prefrontal cortex is responsible for encoding information into episodic memory and retrieving information from semantic memory, whereas right prefrontal cortex is responsible for retrieving information from episodic memory. In the original formulation of the model, left prefrontal activation was proposed in the absence of homologous right prefrontal activation. Right prefrontal activation was described as frequently occurring without comparable left prefrontal activation. This model provided a valuable heuristic, and its broad assertions have been generally well supported (Kapur *et al.*, 1994; Shallice *et al.*, 1994; Grady *et al.*, 1995; Haxby, 1996; Kapur *et al.*, 1996). However, evidence of bilateral prefrontal activation during encoding (Roland & Gulyas, 1995), and retrieval (Grasby *et al.*, 1993; Andreasen *et al.*, 1995a, 1995b; Kapur *et al.*, 1995; Petrides *et al.*, 1995; Roland & Gulyas, 1995; Schacter *et al.*, 1996), has led to several modifications.

In modifying the HERA model, most investigators have made hemispheric and regional distinctions between anterior and inferior portions of the prefrontal cortex. Petrides *et al.* (1995) examined PET CBF during verbal free recall and paired associate tasks. They concluded that the anterior mid-dorsolateral frontal cortex (Brodmann areas [BA] 9 and 46) is involved in online performance monitoring in relation to current plans. Activation of the posterior ventrolateral frontal cortex (BA 45 and 47) was attributed to strategic encoding and active retrieval of specific information from association cortices. Based on reviews of the literature and their own word stem completion studies, Buckner and colleagues (Buckner, 1996; Buckner & Petersen, 1996) suggested a similar division between anterior (area 10) and inferior prefrontal cortex (BA 44/45), and proposed different hemispheric functions for these two regions. The authors found that left inferior frontal activation occurs during episodic encoding, semantic retrieval, and episodic retrieval tasks using word stimuli, and concluded that the left inferior frontal gyrus is required for accessing and maintaining a verbal representation. In contrast they found that the right inferior frontal gyrus is responsible for nonverbal representations, and occurs during episodic retrieval tasks only when spatial stimuli are processed. The authors placed less emphasis than Petrides *et al.* (1995) on the necessity of strategic encoding or active retrieval, and reported evidence of LIFG activation across both strategic free recall and nonstrategic recognition tasks. Regarding the right anterior prefrontal region, Buckner and colleagues (Buckner, 1996; Buckner & Petersen, 1996) agreed with previous conclusions that right hemispheric activation of BA 10 is uniquely related to episodic retrieval, and occurs with both verbal and nonverbal stimuli.

In a review of nine verbal recognition studies, Nyberg (1998) also proposed a subdivision between anterior and posterior prefrontal areas, and concluded that right hemispheric prefrontal activation is specific to episodic retrieval regardless of modality or stimulus type. Our own PET results (Figure 7.1) generally corresponded with Nyberg's view of the HERA model (Ragland *et al.*, 2000). Verbal encoding was found to produce a focal unilateral activation of left inferior prefrontal cortex (BA 45) in the absence of significant right prefrontal activation. However, activation in this region was not specific to encoding, as it was also seen during the recognition task, and did not differ in magnitude during the two stages of memory performance. In contrast, activation of a right anterior prefrontal region (BA 9 and 10) was specific to word recognition and showed greater activation during recognition than during encoding. Differential activation during recognition was also less isolated, extending to the anterior cingulate, right superior temporal gyrus, and bilateral visual association cortices. These findings were subsequently replicated in an fMRI study of the same word encoding and recognition protocol (Ragland *et al.*, 2004). Thus, it appears that the right anterior prefrontal cortex plays a selective role in episodic retrieval across stimulus modalities and retrieval tasks. However, the left prefrontal cortex can be engaged in both stages of memory performance, and is involved in strategic control and monitoring of episodic encoding and retrieval.

4   Semantic processing and prefrontal function during episodic memory

Neuropsychological and functional imaging studies of verbal episodic memory have identified a central role of frontally mediated semantic organization

Encoding

Recognition

Recognition - Encoding

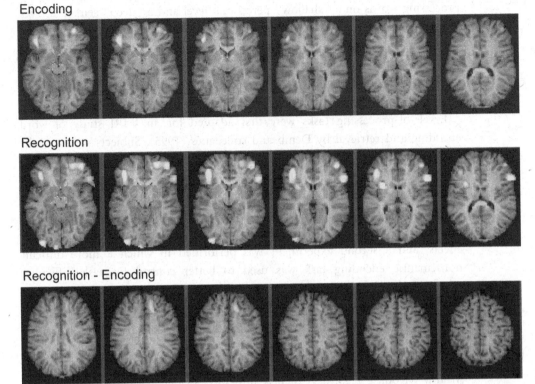

Figure 7.1 Control SPM map showing areas activated by word encoding (top), recognition (middle), and recognition minus encoding (bottom) after averaged baseline subtraction. Displayed on a sagittal 4-mm MRI standardized into Talairach space (left is left). Colored areas exceed a corrected cluster-level value of p<0.05. (For a color version of this figure, please see the color plate section.)

in successful encoding and retrieval. Early studies showed that, as information encoding moves from shallow perceptual processing to more elaborative semantic-associative encoding, the strength of the memory trace increases (Kintsch, 1968; Craik & Lockhart, 1972). The benefit of semantic organization is reflected by better recall of semantically related word lists that can be categorized (Gold *et al.*, 1992; Brebion *et al.*, 1997). When presented with word lists that can be semantically related in either blocked or unblocked formats, healthy subjects tend to group words by semantic category, resulting in better subsequent performance on recall and recognition tasks.

The effect of semantic processing on regional brain function has been examined with functional imaging using levels-of-processing (Craik & Lockhart, 1972) paradigms. During levels-of-processing tasks subjects alternate between processing words on a "shallow" perceptual level and a "deep" semantic level. Subsequent word retrieval is faster and more accurate for words that underwent deep versus shallow processing. Imaging studies employing levels-of-processing paradigms have linked deep versus shallow processing with activation of left inferior prefrontal cortex in healthy subjects (Demb et al., 1995; Buckner et al., 1998a, 1998b; Wagner et al., 1998; McDermott et al., 1999).

Levels-of-processing tasks were first adapted for an fMRI study of word encoding and retrieval by Demb and colleagues (1995). Subjects were visually presented with two lists of 20 words each that were previously rated as concrete or abstract and were printed in uppercase or lowercase letters. In the shallow encoding condition, subjects were asked to make an uppercase/lowercase decision, and in the deep encoding condition they made a concrete/abstract decision. Each condition was repeated twice to examine repetition priming effects, and a second experiment was performed in which a more difficult nonsemantic encoding task was used to better control for task difficulty. After the fMRI recordings, a recognition task was administered in which half of the shallow and half of the deep target words were combined with 20 novel words, and the subject was required to decide whether each word had been previously presented. Subjects recalled more words following deep encoding, and produced a larger left inferior frontal response for deep versus shallow encoding regardless of task difficulty. Evidence of repetition priming (i.e. decreased left inferior frontal response with word repetition) was also found for deep encoding.

This initial experiment was followed by several studies by Buckner and colleagues who employed the same paradigm, and examined fMRI change during recognition rather than during encoding. In the first study (Buckner et al., 1998a), two low success and two high success recognition blocks were alternated in an A-B-A-B design. Low recognition success blocks (high retrieval effort) consisted of words that had undergone shallow encoding, and high recognition success blocks (low retrieval effort) included words that had undergone deep encoding. The investigators found that bilateral orbital frontal and left inferior frontal activation was greater for words that had undergone shallow encoding (high effort, low success), whereas right prefrontal activation was greater for recognition of words that had undergone deep encoding (low effort, high success). The second study by this group employed event-related fMRI procedures to further test the hypothesis that right prefrontal activity is involved in retrieval success (Buckner et al., 1998b). This study employed the deep encoding condition only, and used an event-related recognition paradigm in which target words that were previously encoded were randomly intermixed with novel words. The right prefrontal cortex was activated both by correct identification of targets, and correct rejection of foils. The investigators concluded that the right prefrontal region has a role in high-level monitoring and is not dependent upon retrieval success as previously suggested (Rugg *et al.*, 1996).

Our own levels-of-processing study (Ragland *et al.*, 2005) examined fMRI effects during both word encoding and retrieval. As in previous studies, healthy control subjects were faster and more accurate at recognizing words that had undergone deep versus shallow processing. During the encoding stage, deep versus shallow processing resulted in focal activation of the left ventro-lateral prefrontal cortex (BA 47), which is a region believed to be involved in semantic working memory. Correct recognition of deep versus shallow words resulted in greater activation of right dorsolateral prefrontal cortex (BA 9) and visual association areas. Thus, it appeared that the levels-of-processing effect on recognition performance was related to increased activation of semantic processing areas in the left prefrontal cortex during encoding and to greater activation of episodic retrieval areas in the right prefrontal cortex during word recognition. We subsequently investigated whether these same results would be obtained in patients with schizophrenia.

5 Effect of schizophrenia on semantic processing, episodic memory and prefrontal function

Schizophrenia is a devastating neurodevelopmental disorder occurring in about 1% of the world population. Although its most remarkable features are positive symptoms such as delusions, thought disorder and auditory hallucinations, it also produces a constellation of negative symptoms such as loss of interest and social withdrawal. In addition to these clinical symptoms, schizophrenia causes generalized dysfunction across cognitive domains. A recent meta-analysis of neuropsychological studies (Heinrichs & Zakzanis, 1998) found that the largest effect sizes of schizophrenia are for verbal learning and memory, supporting the conclusion that schizophrenia tends to produce a differential deficit in learning and memory against a background of generalized cognitive dysfunction (Rund, 1989; McKenna *et al.*, 1990; Saykin *et al.*, 1991; Gold *et al.*, 1992; Tamlyn *et al.*, 1992; Gur *et al.*, 1999). This differential memory impairment is not explained by demographic variables such as education or sex (Seidman *et al.*, 1998), or by clinical variables including medication, duration and severity of illness (Aleman *et al.*, 1999). The cognitive profile is similar for unmedicated first episode and previously treated patients (Saykin *et al.*, 1994), and remains stable over time (Censits *et al.*, 1997). Memory also tends to better predict patients' functional outcome (e.g. ability to hold a job) than either clinical symptoms or other cognitive or demographic variables (Green, 1996).

The pattern of memory deficits in patients with schizophrenia is similar to what is seen in patients with dementing disorders that affect fronto-striatal function such as Huntington's or Parkinson's dementia. As in these other disorders episodic memory is impaired more during encoding and retrieval than during long-term storage (Gold et al., 1992; Heinrichs & Awad, 1993; Paulsen et al., 1995). Patients with schizophrenia do not show the pattern of rapid forgetting and storage deficits characteristic of cortical dementias such as Alzheimer's disease. During retrieval, deficits are more consistently noted on recall tests than on recognition tasks, leading some to emphasize the importance of information encoding over episodic retrieval (McClain, 1983; Heaton et al., 1994). However, a recent meta-analysis (Aleman et al., 1999) found moderate effects on recognition performance and large effects on recall performance. Moreover, nonrelational recognition tasks can be accomplished based on feelings of familiarity (noetic) as well as actual recall of the encoding event (autonoetic). Recognition may appear less impaired because patients rely more on familiarity effects. When autonoetic knowledge is directly assessed (e.g. source monitoring) patients are impaired even when their initial recognition performance was intact (Danion et al., 1999). Thus, schizophrenia appears to be producing prominent encoding rather than storage difficulties with less marked evidence of retrieval difficulties.

During verbal episodic memory tasks patients tend not to semantically categorize words to facilitate encoding and retrieval (Koh et al., 1973; Koh & Peterson, 1978; Gold et al., 1992; Paulsen et al., 1995; Iddon et al., 1998). A likely reason for this encoding problem is that patients have difficulty self-generating organizational strategies (Brébion et al., 1997; Iddon et al., 1998; Stone et al., 1998). This "strategic memory" explanation is supported by findings that patients can benefit from being trained in semantic organizational strategies (McClain, 1983), and from being provided with blocked versus unblocked lists of words (Gold et al., 1992; Brébion et al., 1997). In an earlier study we directly manipulated encoding strategies using the previously described levels-of-processing task (Craik & Lockhart, 1972) in which subjects alternated between processing words on a "shallow" perceptual level (uppercase/lowercase) and a "deep" semantic level (concrete/abstract). Patients were slower and less accurate in classifying words during encoding. However, they showed a normal levels-of-processing effect on recognition accuracy (Ragland et al., 2003). Both patients and controls were faster and more accurate in recognizing words that had undergone deep processing (Figure 7.2). However, patients responded more slowly and maintained a more conservative response bias despite this normal levels-of-processing effect on recognition accuracy.

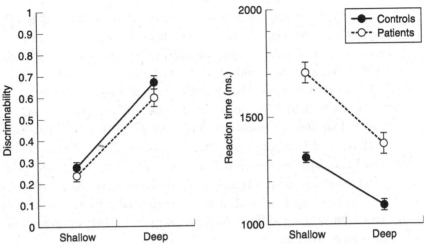

Figure 7.2   Mean (±SEM) recognition discriminability (left graph) and reaction time (right graph) for 30 healthy controls and 30 patients with schizophrenia.

These residual group differences in recognition performance suggested that simply providing patients with a semantic encoding strategy did not fully remediate their episodic memory. Residual retrieval problems were also detected when source monitoring was tested (Ragland *et al.*, 2006). During source monitoring, subjects were presented with target items that were on the original learning list as well as novel words that had not been previously presented. Rather than simply being asked whether each word was "new" or "old" (as in recognition testing), they were asked to identify the source of the old words. If the subject thought that the stimulus was an old word they had to specify whether that word had been presented during a shallow or a deep condition during the initial encoding task. By requiring retrieval of the encoding event patients could not rely on familiarity effects and had to utilize autonoetic knowledge.

When source memory was examined, we found that controls had significantly better source identification following deep encoding. However, this effect occurred only at a trend level in patients. These difficulties in source retrieval provided additional evidence that providing patients with a semantic encoding strategy can restore recognition performance, but does not fully normalize the strength of their memory trace.

The effect of schizophrenia on brain function during episodic memory tasks was initially studied with PET and [133]xenon clearance methods. These early studies focused on retrieval and found evidence of reduced blood flow and atypical asymmetries in frontal and temporal cortex (Wood & Flowers, 1990; Gur et al., 1994; Ganguli et al., 1997; Ragland et al., 1998). In a series of PET studies of prose recall, Andreasen et al. (1996, 1997) and Crespo-Facorro et al. (1999) extended these findings to the thalamus and cerebellum and supported a distributed dysfunction ("cognitive dysmetria") model. Fewer studies examined encoding. Both SPECT (Nohara et al., 2000) and PET studies (Hazlet et al., 2000) found that impaired semantic organization during encoding was associated with reduced frontotemporal activation. In the first PET study to examine both word encoding and retrieval (Ragland et al., 2001), we found evidence of left frontotemporal dysfunction during both memory stages. Whereas retrieval success was associated with focal left prefrontal activation in controls, patients relied on a more diffuse "compensatory" network of motor and posterior association regions.

These results were subsequently replicated with fMRI (Ragland et al., 2004). In that study we utilized the same word encoding and recognition paradigm, and again found evidence of bilateral reductions in prefrontal activation in patients with schizophrenia during word encoding. Patients also showed reduced left dorsolateral prefrontal activation and intact right anterior prefrontal activation during word retrieval. With the improved temporal resolution of fMRI we also found evidence of group differences in hippocampal regions. During word encoding patients produced greater activation than controls in parahippocampal regions. This finding of prefrontal cortex underactivation and parahippocampal overactivation suggested that the functional connectivity of dorsolateral prefrontal and temporal-limbic structures is disrupted by schizophrenia. During this study we also found that patients were less likely than controls to report semantic associative processing strategies (e.g. relating one word to another) during word encoding and were more likely to rely on simple rehearsal. We suspected that this less efficient encoding strategy may have contributed to the reduced prefrontal activation.

Encoding strategies have been manipulated during fMRI through the use of levels-of-processing tasks. A series of word-stem completion studies (Heckers et al., 1998; Weiss et al., 2003) found that retrieval of deep versus shallow words was associated with greater right hippocampal activation in controls and greater prefrontal activation in patients. Hippocampal response was blunted because of patient overactivation during baseline and shallow retrieval conditions. However a subsequent study measuring fMRI during encoding found that patients had decreased left prefrontal and increased left superior temporal activation for deep versus shallow words (Kubicki et al., 2003).

Our own levels-of-processing study (Ragland et al., 2005) examined word encoding and retrieval. As previously noted, patients showed the same improvement in recognition speed and accuracy as healthy controls for words that had undergone deep versus shallow processing. During deep versus shallow encoding, patients also successfully activated their left ventrolateral prefrontal cortex (BA 47; Figure 7.3). Thus, it appeared that providing patients with a semantic encoding strategy not only remediated their recognition performance, but also allowed them to engage their left prefrontal cortex. However, once patients' left prefrontal cortex was engaged, they showed a much less efficient pattern of brain response than healthy controls. Although controls did not show any areas of greater activity than patients during deep versus shallow encoding, patients had greater activation than controls in left hippocampus, left thalamus and left lingual gyrus. Evidence of patient overactivation was also seen during recognition of deep versus shallow words. Although there was no group difference in activation of right anterior prefrontal retrieval areas, patients produced greater activation than controls in the left frontal pole (BA 10). Thus, although providing patients with semantic encoding strategies can help to remediate word recognition deficits and can reengage prefrontal function, this intervention does not fully normalize brain function as patients continue to produce a more diffuse and less efficient pattern of regional activation. Nevertheless, these and other imaging findings have increased interest in remediation efforts.

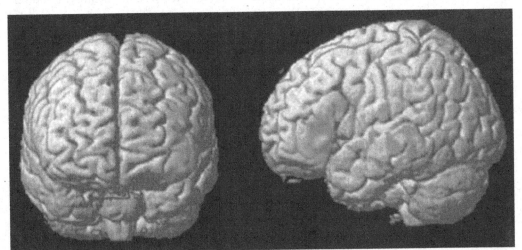

Figure 7.3   SPM map showing areas activated by deep minus shallow word encoding. Maps are rendered on a 3-dimensional brain to show similarity of activation in the left ventrolateral prefrontal cortex in controls (green) and patients with schizophrenia (red). Overlapping activation in yellow. Colored areas exceed a corrected cluster-level value of p<0.05. (For a color version of this figure, please see the color plate section.)

Recent schizophrenia research has related verbal memory deficits to a variety of community outcome measures including daily function and occupational performance (Lysaker *et al.*, 1995; Green, 1996; Velligan *et al.*, 2000). This has led to a renewed interest in cognitive remediation as a way to improve functional outcome (Bellack *et al.*, 1999). A recent meta-analysis of the rehabilitation literature (Kurtz *et al.*, 2001) found medium to large effect sizes for executive function, attention and memory, suggesting that the severity of these cognitive difficulties can be lessened with appropriate remediation efforts. Combining remediation interventions with functional imaging will make it possible to test effects on both cognitive performance and brain function.

6 Concluding remarks

This chapter reviewed the progress that cognitive neuroscience has made in understanding the role of the prefrontal cortex in episodic memory. Early clinical studies of patients with focal brain lesions helped to form a taxonomy of memory systems, and successfully dissociated forms of short-term and long-term memory. These initial studies clarified that the prefrontal cortex was important to short-term and working memory, and that the hippocampus was essential for long-term declarative and episodic memory. These observational studies were greatly advanced by primate lesion studies that further clarified the hippocampal and mesial temporal brain structures important to episodic memory. However, these studies also began to identify individuals with episodic memory impairments whose brain damage was not restricted to the hippocampus. Both human and animal lesion studies and functional imaging research demonstrated that the prefrontal cortex is necessary for maintaining attention during delayed response tasks, mediating cross-temporal contingencies during delayed alternation tasks, generating successful semantic and associative encoding strategies, identifying encoding sources, and monitoring output during episodic retrieval. Thus, although the hippocampus is necessary for storage of long-term memories, it is not sufficient, as prefrontal functions are necessary to facilitate encoding and retrieval in most learning situations. Like patients with Huntington's and Parkinson's dementia, patients with schizophrenia are a good illustration of what happens to episodic memory when frontal and striatal brain regions are compromised. Patients with schizophrenia have trouble initiating effective encoding strategies during initial learning. This results in a weaker memory trace, resulting in retrieval deficits that are most obvious when recall or source identification is tested. Neuropsychological and functional imaging studies that have manipulated encoding strategies have shown that providing patients with semantic encoding strategies can help to reengage prefrontal function and improve memory performance. These combined remediation and functional imaging studies are a promising area for future research in schizophrenia and other brain disorders that affect memory performance.

REFERENCES

Aleman, A., Hijman, R., de Haan, E. H. F. & Kahn, R. S. (1999). Memory impairment in schizophrenia: A meta-analysis. *American Journal of Psychiatry*, **156**, 1358–66.

Andreasen, N. C., O'Leary, D. S., Arndt, S., *et al.* (1995a). Short-term and long-term verbal memory: A positron emission tomography study. *Proceedings of the National Academy of Sciences*, **92**, 5111–15.

Andreasen, N. C., O'Leary, D. S., Arndt, S., *et al.* (1995b). PET studies of memory: I. Novel and practiced free recall of complex narratives, *NeuroImage*, **2**, 284–95.

Andreasen, N. C., O'Leary, D. S., Cizadlo, T., *et al.* (1996). Schizophrenia and cognitive dysmetria: A positron emission tomography study of dysfunctional prefrontal-thalamic-cerebellar circuitry. *Proceedings of the National Academy of Sciences*, **93**, 9985–90.

Andreasen, N. C., O'Leary, D. S., Flaum, M., *et al.* (1997). Hypofrontality in schizophrenia: Distributed dysfunctional circuits in neuroleptic-naïve patients. *Lancet*, **349**, 1730–4.

Baddeley, A. D. (1992). Working memory. *Science*, **255**, 556–9.

Baddeley, A. D. & Hitch, G. J. (1974). Working memory. In *The Psychology of Learning and Motivation*, Vol. 8, ed. G. A. Bower. New York: Academic Press, pp. 47–89.

Bellack, A. S., Gold, J. M. & Buchanan, R. W. (1999). Cognitive rehabilitation for schizophrenia: problems, prospects, and strategies. *Schizophrenia Bulletin*, **25**, 257–74.

Brébion, G., Amador, X., Smith, M. J. & Gorman, J. M. (1997). Mechanisms underlying memory impairment in schizophrenia. *Psychological Medicine*, **27**, 383–93.

Buckner, R. L. (1996). Beyond HERA: Contributions of specific prefrontal brain areas to long-term memory retrieval. *Psychonomic Bulletin and Review*, **3**, 149–58.

Buckner, R. L., Koutstaal, W., Schacter, D. L., *et al.* (1998a). Functional-anatomic study of episodic retrieval using fMRI II. Selective averaging of event-related fMRI trials to test the retrieval success hypothesis. *NeuroImage*, **7**, 163–75.

Buckner, R. L., Koutstaal, W., Schacter, D. L., Wagner, A. D. & Rosen, B. F. (1998b). Functional-anatomic study of episodic retrieval using fMRI I. Retrieval effort versus retrieval success. *NeuroImage*, **7**, 151–62.

Buckner, R. L. & Petersen, S. E. (1996). What does neuroimaging tell us about the role of prefrontal cortex in memory retrieval? *Seminars in Neuroscience*, **8**, 47–55.

Censits, D. M., Ragland, J. D., Gur, R. C. & Gur, R. E. (1997). Neuropsychological evidence supporting a neurodevelopmental model of schizophrenia: A longitudinal study. *Schizophrenia Research*, **24**, 289–98.

Craik, F. & Lockhart, R. (1972). Levels of processing: a framework for memory research. *Journal of Verbal Learning and Verbal Behavior*, **11**, 671–84.

Crespo-Facorro, B., Paradiso, S., Andreasen, N. C., et al. (1999). Recalling word lists reveals "cognitive dysmetria" in schizophrenia: A positron emission tomography study. *American Journal of Psychiatry*, **156**, 386–92.

Danion, J. M., Rizzo, L. & Bruant, A. (1999). Functional mechanisms underlying impaired recognition memory and conscious awareness in patients with schizophrenia. *Archives of General Psychiatry*, **56**, 639–44.

Demb, J. B., Desmond, J. E., Wagner, A. D., et al. (1995). Semantic encoding and retrieval in the left inferior prefrontal cortex: a functional MRI study of task difficulty and process specificity. *Journal of Neuroscience*, **15**, 5870–8.

Desgranges, B., Baron, J. C. & Eustache, F. (1998). The functional neuroanatomy of episodic memory: the role of the frontal lobes, the hippocampal formation, and other areas. *NeuroImage*, **8**, 198–213.

Drachman, D. A. & Arbit, J. (1966). Memory and the hippocampal complex. II. Is memory a multiple process? *Archives of Neurology*, **15**, 52–61.

Fuster, J. M. (1985). The prefrontal cortex, mediator of cross-temporal contingencies. *Human Neurobiology*, **4**, 169–79.

Ganguli, R., Carter, C., Mintun, M., et al. (1997). PET brain mapping study of auditory verbal supraspan memory versus visual fixation in schizophrenia. *Biological Psychiatry*, **41**, 33–42.

Gold, J. M., Randolf, C., Carpenter, C. J., Goldberg, T. E. & Weinberger, D. R. (1992). Forms of memory failure in schizophrenia. *Journal of Abnormal Psychology*, **101**, 487–94.

Grady, C. L., McIntosh, A. R., Horwitz, B., et al. (1995). Age-related reductions in human recognition memory due to impaired encoding. *Science*, **269**, 218–21.

Grasby, P. M., Frith, C. D., Friston, K., et al. (1993). Functional mapping of brain areas implicated in auditory-verbal memory function. *Brain*, **116**, 1–20.

Green, M. F. (1996). What are the functional consequences of neurocognitive deficits in schizophrenia? *American Journal of Psychiatry*, **153**, 321–30.

Gur, R. C., Moelter, S. T. & Ragland, J. D. (1999). Learning and memory in schizophrenia. In *Cognition in Schizophrenia*, ed. T. Sharma and P. Harvey. Oxford: Oxford University Press, pp. 73–91.

Gur, R. C., Ragland, J. D., Resnic, S. M., et al. (1994). Lateralized increases in cerebral blood flow during performance of verbal and spatial tasks: Relationship with performance level. *Brain and Cognition*, **24**, 244–58.

Haxby, J. V. (1996). Medial temporal lobe imaging. *Nature*, **380**, 669–70.

Hazlet, E. A., Buchsbaum, M. S., Jeu, L. A., et al. (2000). Hypofrontality in unmedicated schizophrenia patients studied with PET during performance of a serial verbal learning task. *Schizophrenia Research*, **43**, 33–46.

Heaton, R., Paulsen, J. S., McAdams, L. A., et al. (1994). Neuropsychological deficits in schizophrenics: relationship to age, chronicity and dementia. *Archives of General Psychiatry*, **51**, 469–76.

Heckers, S., Rauch, S. L., Goff, D., et al. (1998). Impaired recruitment of the hippocampus during conscious recollection in schizophrenia. *Nature Neuroscience*, **1**, 318–23.

Heinrichs, R. W. & Awad, A. G. (1993). Neurocognitive subtypes of chronic schizophrenia. *Schizophrenia Research*, **9**, 49–58.

Heinrichs, R. W. & Zakzanis, K. K. (1998). Neurocognitive deficit in schizophrenia: A quantitative review of the evidence. *Neuropsychology*, **12**, 426–45.

Heiss, W. D., Pawlik, G., Holthoff, V., Kessler, J. & Szelies, B. (1992). PET correlates of normal and impaired memory functions. *Cerebrovascular Brain Metabolism Reviews*, **4**, 1–27.

Iddon, J. L., McKenna, P. J., Sahakian, B. J. & Robbins, T. W. (1998). Impaired generation and use of strategy in schizophrenia: evidence from visuospatial and verbal tasks. *Psychological Medicine*, **28**, 1049–62.

James, W. (1890/1918). *The Principles of Psychology*. New York: Henry Holt & Co.

Janowsky, J. S., Shimamura, A. P. & Squire, L. R. (1989). Source memory impairment in patients with frontal lobe lesions. *Neuropsychologia*, **27**, 1043–56.

Kapur, S., Craik, F. I. M., Jones, C., *et al.* (1995). Functional role of the prefrontal cortex in retrieval of memories: A PET study. *NeuroReport*, **6**, 1880–4.

Kapur, S., Craik, F. I. M., Tulving, E., *et al.* (1994). Neuroanatomical correlates of encoding in episodic memory: Levels of processing effect. *Proceedings of the National Academy of Sciences*, **91**, 2008–11.

Kapur, S., Tulving, E., Cabeza, R., *et al.* (1996). The neural correlates of intentional learning of verbal materials: A PET study in humans. *Cognitive Brain Research*, **4**, 243–9.

Kintsch, W. (1968). Recognition and free recall of organized lists. *Journal of Experimental Psychology General*, **78**, 481–7.

Koh, S., Kayton, L. & Berry, R. (1973). Mnemonic organization in young nonpsychotic schizophrenics. *Journal of Abnormal Psychology*, **81**, 299–310.

Koh, S. & Peterson, R. (1978). Encoding orientation and the remembering of schizophrenic young adults. *Journal of Abnormal Psychology*, **87**, 303–13.

Kubicki, M., McCarley, R. W., Nestor, P. G., *et al.* (2003). An fMRI study of semantic processing in men with schizophrenia. *NeuroImage*, **20**, 1923–33.

Kurtz, M. M., Moberg, P. J., Gur, R. C. & Gur, R. E. (2001). Approaches to cognitive remediation of neuropsychological deficits in schizophrenia: a review and meta-analysis. *Neuropsychology Review*, **11**, 197–210.

Lysaker, P., Bell, M. & Beam-Goulet, J. (1995). Wisconsin Card Sorting Test and work performance in schizophrenia. *Schizophrenia Research*, **56**, 45–51.

McClain, L. (1983). Encoding and retrieval in schizophrenia free recall. *Journal of Nervous and Mental Disease*, **171**, 471–9.

McDermott, K. B., Ojemann, J. G., Petersen, S. E., *et al.* (1999). Direct comparison of episodic encoding and retrieval of words: and event-related fMRI study. *Memory*, **7**, 661–78.

McKenna, P. J., Tamlyn, D., Lund, C. E., *et al.* (1990). Amnesic syndrome in schizophrenia. *Psychological Medicine*, **20**, 967–72.

Mishkin, M. & Appenzeller, T. (1987). The anatomy of memory. *Scientific American*, **256**, 80–9.

Moscovitch, M. (1982). Multiple dissociations of function in amnesia. In *Human Memory and Amnesia*, ed. L. Cermak. Hillsdale, NJ: Erlbaum, pp. 337–370.

Nohara, S., Suzuki, M., Kurach, M., et al. (2000). Neural correlates of memory organization deficits in schizophrenia: a single photon emission computed tomography study with 99mTc-ethyl-cysteinate dimer during a verbal learning task. *Schizophrenia Research*, **42**, 209–22.

Nyberg, L. (1998). Mapping episodic memory. *Behavioral Brain Research*, **90**, 107–14.

Paulsen, J. S., Heaton, R. K., Sadek, J. R., et al. (1995). The nature of learning and memory impairments in schizophrenia. *Journal of the International Neuropsychological Society*, **1**, 88–99.

Perani, D., Gilardi, M. C., Cappa, S. F. & Fazio, F. (1992). PET studies of cognitive functions: A review. *Journal of Nuclear and Biological Medicine*, **36**, 324–36.

Petrides, M. (2000). Dissociable roles of mid-dorsolateral prefrontal and anterior inferotemporal cortex in visual working memory. *Journal of Neuroscience*, **20**, 7496–503.

Petrides, M., Alivisatos, B. & Evans, A. C. (1995). Functional activation of the human ventrolateral frontal cortex during the mnemonic retrieval of verbal information. *Proceedings of the National Academy of Sciences*, **92**, 5803–7.

Ragland, J. D., Gur, R. C., Glahn, D. C., et al. (1998). Frontotemporal cerebral blood flow change during executive and declarative memory tasks in schizophrenia: a positron emission tomography study. *Neuropsychology*, **12**, 399–413.

Ragland, J. D., Gur, R. C., Lazarev, M. G., et al. (2000). Hemispheric activation of anterior inferior prefrontal cortex during verbal encoding and recognition. *NeuroImage*, **11**, 624–33.

Ragland, J. D., Gur, R. C., Raz, J., et al. (2001). Effect of schizophrenia on fronto-temporal activity during word encoding and recognition: A PET cerebral blood flow study. *American Journal of Psychiatry*, **158**, 1114–25.

Ragland, J. D., Gur, R. C., Valdez, J. N., et al. (2005). Levels-of-processing effect on frontotemporal function in schizophrenia during word encoding and recognition. *American Journal of Psychiatry*, **162**, 1783–4.

Ragland, J. D., Gur, R. C., Valdez, J., et al. (2004). Event-related fMRI of frontotemporal activity during word encoding and recognition in schizophrenia. *American Journal of Psychiatry*, **161**, 1004–15.

Ragland, J. D., McCarthy, E., Valdez, J., et al. (2006). Levels-of-processing effect on internal source monitoring in schizophrenia. *Psychological Medicine*, **36**, 1–8.

Ragland, J. D., Moelter, S. T., McGrath, C., et al. (2003). Levels-of-processing effect on word recognition in schizophrenia. *Biological Psychiatry*, **54**, 1154–61.

Roland, P. E. & Gulyas, B. (1995). Visual memory, visual imagery, and visual recognition of large field patterns by the human brain: Functional anatomy by positron emission tomography. *Cerebral Cortex*, **1**, 79–93.

Roskies, A. L. (1994). Mapping memory with positron emission tomography. *Proceedings of the National Academy of Sciences*, **91**, 1980–91.

Rugg, M. D., Fletcher, P. C., Frith, C. D., Frackowiak, R. S. J. & Dolan, R. J. (1996). Differential response of the prefrontal cortex in successful and unsuccessful memory retrieval. *Brain*, **119**, 2073–83.

Rund, B. R. (1989). Distractibility and recall capability in schizophrenics: A four year longitudinal study of stability in cognitive performance. *Schizophrenia Research*, **2**, 265–75.

Saykin, A. J, Gur, R. C., Gur, R. E., *et al.* (1991). Neuropsychological function in schizophrenia: Selective impairment in memory and learning. *Archives of General Psychiatry*, **48**, 618–24.

Saykin, A. J., Shtasel, D. L., Gur, R. E., *et al.* (1994). Neuropsychological deficits in neuroleptic naive patients with first-episode schizophrenia. *Archives of General Psychiatry*, **51**, 124–31.

Schacter, D. L., Alpert, N. M., Savage, C. R., Rauch, S. L. & Albert, M. S. (1996). Conscious recollection and the human hippocampal formation: Evidence from positron emission tomography. *Proceedings of the National Academy of Sciences*, **93**, 321–5.

Seidman, L. J., Stone, W. S., Jones, R., Harrison, R. H. & Mirsky, A. F. (1998). Comparative effects of schizophrenia and temporal lobe epilepsy on memory. *Journal of the International Neuropsychological Society*, **4**, 342–52.

Shallice, T., Fletcher, P., Frith, C. D., *et al.* (1994). Brain regions associated with acquisition and retrieval of verbal episodic memory. *Nature*, **368**, 633–5.

Shimamura, A. P. (1990). Memory and amnesia. *Western Journal of Medicine*, **152**, 177–8.

Squire, L. R. (1987). *Memory and Brain*. New York: Oxford University Press.

Squire, L. R. (1992). Memory and the hippocampus: a synthesis from findings with rats, monkeys, and humans. *Psychological Review*, **99**, 195–231.

Stone, M., Gabrieli, J. D. E., Stebbins, G. T. & Sullivan, E. V. (1998). Working and strategic memory deficits in schizophrenia. *Neuropsychology*, **12**, 278–88.

Tamlyn, D., McKenna, P. J., Mortimer, A. M., *et al.* (1992). Memory impairment in schizophrenia: Its extent, affiliations, and neuropsychological character. *Psychological Medicine*, **22**, 101–15.

Tulving, E. (1972). Episodic and semantic memory. In *Organization of Memory*, ed. E. Tulving and W. Donaldson. New York: Academic Press, pp. 381–403.

Tulving, E. (2002). Episodic memory: From mind to brain. *Annual Review of Psychology*, **53**, 1–25.

Tulving, E., Kapur S., Craik, F. I. M., Moscovitch, M. & Houle, S. (1994). Hemispheric encoding/retrieval asymmetry in episodic memory: Positron emission tomography findings. *Proceedings of the National Academy of Sciences*, **91**, 2016–20.

Velligan, D. I., Bow-Thomas, C. C., Mahurin, R. K., Miller, A. L. & Halgunseth, B. A. (2000). Do specific neurocognitive deficits predict specific domains of community function in schizophrenia? *Journal of Nervous and Mental Disease*, **188**, 518–24.

Victor, M., Adams, R. D. & Collins, G. H. (1989). *The Wernicke-Korsakoff Syndrome and Related Neurological Disorders due to Alcoholism and Malnutrition*, 2nd ed. Philadelphia: F. A. Davis.

Wagner, A. D., Schacter, D. L., Rotte, M., *et al.* (1998). Building memories: remembering and forgetting of verbal experiences as predicted by brain activity. *Science*, **281**, 1188–91.

Warrington, E. K. & Weiskrantz, L. (1970). The amnesic syndrome: Consolidation or retrieval? *Nature*, **228**, 628–30.

Weiss, A.P., Schacter, D.L., Goff, D.C., *et al.* (2003). Impaired hippocampal recruitment during normal modulation of memory performance in schizophrenia. *Biological Psychiatry,* **53**, 48–55.

Wheeler, M.A., Stuss, D.T. & Tulving, E. (1995). Frontal lobe damage produces episodic memory impairment. *Journal of the International Neuropsychological Society,* **1**, 525–36.

Winocur, G., McDonald, R.M. & Moscovitch, M. (2001). Anterograde and retrograde amnesia in rats with large hippocampal lesions. *Hippocampus,* **11**, 18–26.

Wood, F.B. & Flowers, D.L. (1990). Hypofrontal vs. hypo-sylvian blood flow in schizophrenia. *Schizophrenia Bulletin,* **16**, 413–24.

Zola-Morgan, S. & Squire, L.R. (1985). Medial temporal lesions in monkeys impair memory on a variety of tasks sensitive to human amnesia. *Behavioral Neuroscience,* **99**, 22–34.

Zola-Morgan, S. & Squire, L.R. (1986). Memory impairment in monkeys following lesions of the hippocampus. *Behavioral Neuroscience,* **100**, 155–60.

8

Clinical symptoms and neuropathology in organic dementing disorders affecting the frontal lobes

Arne Brun and Lars Gustafson

1 Introduction

Historically the clinical importance of localized cortical atrophy within the frontal and the temporal lobes was first described by Arnold Pick, who pointed out the relationship between these lesions and aphasia and behavioral changes, "thereby bringing neuropathology and psychiatry into closer union...so that the latter may be brought nearer to understanding" (Pick, 1892). Pick's first cases showed mainly temporal lobe involvement and the association with frontal lobe atrophy appeared in later publications. The histopathology of this lobar atrophy was given by Alzheimer (1911) and the clinico-pathological entity of Pick's disease (PiD) was established in the 1920s (Onari & Spatz, 1926; Stertz, 1926). Van Mansvelt (1954) reviewed 196 published cases and found an important variation of the distribution of pathology with frontotemporal atrophy in 54%, mainly frontal atrophy in 25% and mainly temporal atrophy in 17% of the cases. Moreover, the cortical atrophy was asymmetric with left-sided predominance in 46% and right-sided predominance in 17%. The different degenerative patterns were also revealed as variations of the clinical manifestations. Since then there has been an increasing interest in brain disorders specifically affecting the frontal lobes and their often devastating effects on a variety of mental functions.

In this chapter we will first discuss some possible explanations why the frontal lobes are such frequent targets for a variety of damaging processes. After that some general mechanisms of importance for understanding the relationship between symptoms and brain changes will be described. This will be followed by a description of neuropathological findings and clinical symptoms in some of the most common dementing disorders affecting the frontal lobes.

2   Vulnerability of the frontal lobes

The selective vulnerability of the frontal lobes might be explained by a couple of different principles. One is the phylogenesis, younger structures being selectively more vulnerable than older ones. According to a general consensus this concerns especially the prefrontal cortical areas since they represent the latest addition to the brain, in humans reaching their largest relative size after a most protracted maturational period. In contrast the motor and sensory gyri are characterized by their relative robustness in line with their higher phylogenetic age and short and early maturation. Arne Brun has, as a matter of fact, proposed the label "central lobe" for this part of the cortex, based on the markedly different developmental course and structural and vulnerability properties compared to the bordering prefrontal and parietal regions (Brun, 1999). Further, in the prefrontal cortex recent phylogenetic cellular novelties are especially marked, such as the addition of a new, narrow and elongated nerve cell named spindle neuron in the cingulate and insular cortex (Nimchinsky et al., 1995). Another new feature is the fetal subpial granular layer (Brun, 1965), consisting of small round immature cells in the molecular layer just beneath the pial membrane. It is well represented only in humans, where it becomes prominent prefrontally and resolves the latest of all neocortical fields. In rat it is only faintly expressed (Jimenez et al., 2003). These vulnerability principles may also be valid for cellular, nuclear or laminar entities such as more superficial cortical neuronal layers compared to deeper ones. The superficial layers are established latest during ontogeny, most likely with a contribution from the subpial granular layer, according to Corbin and coworkers (2001) in the shape of cortical interneurons. These developmental features seem to represent the latest steps in the evolution of the brain.

Another factor beyond the high frequency of the frontal lobe damage is the sensitivity to skull trauma. The damage is predominantly found on the basal frontal surfaces. Also circulatory insufficiency is commonly playing on the weak points inherent in the frontal and especially the white matter irrigation system. These circumstances all form a plausible background for the frontal preference for degenerative, vascular, traumatic, metabolic and other forms of brain damage.

3   The relationship between symptoms and brain changes

Basically the location of changes in the brain decides the symptoms of dysfunction and thereby the clinical picture, whereas the type of changes has more impact on the course of the disease in terms of speed and progression or type of debut such as an acute or insidious start. Some lesions may be "silent" due to their discreteness or because of compensatory functions in the same or other areas of the brain. If symmetrically bilateral the same lesion may, however, produce symptoms. Symptoms may also emerge if a previously silent lesion becomes supplemented with additional silent lesions. More intense or widespread lesions give symptoms related to the severity. Thus a degenerative initially silent process might cause symptoms when it becomes profound enough by involving an increasing number of neurons and/or a reduction of the number of synapses. What seems to be the debut of the disease thus only marks the time when the reserve capacity is consumed, as also shown on metabolic imaging. The degenerative disease often started years before. Further, strategic lesions, even small, may cause dysfunction by destroying critical centers, the loss of which cannot be compensated for. Examples are small and usually bilateral infarcts in thalamic or striate nuclei, causing frontal dysfunction since they connect to and influence the frontal cortex.

The clinical manifestations of brain damage and dysfunction in frontal regions are related to the localization, type, severity and combination of lesions, but may also be influenced by other factors. In organic dementia the symptoms are mainly caused by degenerative and/or vascular lesions, but also influenced by other concomitant brain disease and somatic disorder, the premorbid personality, previous mental and physical health, current medication and socioeconomical conditions. In spite of this complexity it might be possible to learn about general principles for clinicopathological correlates based on detailed clinical, neuropathological and neuroimaging assessments (Risberg et al., 1993).

We will now review clinical and neuropathological findings in patients with dementing disorders affecting the frontal lobes such as primary degenerative disease and cerebrovascular lesions in frontal and frontal-subcortical brain regions, excluding trauma, toxic and infectious agents and aging. The focus will be upon frontotemporal dementia (FTD), as outlined clinically and neuropathologically by the Lund-Manchester research group (Brun et al., 1994; Neary et al., 1998), including Motor Neuron Disease with Dementia (MNDD) and Huntington's disease. Alzheimer's disease (AD) with frontal predominance and vascular dementia (VaD) with a predominant frontal or frontal-subcortical involvement, such as progressive subcortical vascular encephalopathy, also called Binswanger's disease (Binswanger, 1894) will also be covered.

Our experience is based on consecutively included and followed up patients with dementia with predominantly frontal lobe type of clinical features. So far more than 150 cases have been included (Gustafson et al., 2001), 60 of which have been verified postmortem, 50 have been followed up until deceased but without postmortem examination, and the remaining cases are still alive and studied prospectively.

4 Frontotemporal dementia forms

4.1 Neuropathological characteristics

The Lund-Manchester consensus document on FTD (Brun *et al.*, 1994) was based on findings in the following disease entities: frontal lobe degeneration of non-Alzheimer type (FLD), Pick's disease (PiD), semantic dementia, progressive nonfluent aphasia and motor neuron disease with dementia (MNDD). Figure 8.1 shows a macroscopic view of a brain with the FLD form of FTD. When describing the typical neuropathology of the different FTD forms it might be convenient to appoint FLD a basic model. This disease is characterized by synaptic and neuronal loss with microvacuolation and gliosis in the superficial cortical layers of the frontal and/or the anterior portion of the temporal lobe as well as in the striatum. In advanced stages is it also spreading to the parietal lobe, but sparing the central areas. Also spared is the posterior portion of the cingulate gyrus but not the anterior (Brodmann area 24), with interesting bearings on the symptomatology. This pattern is reversed in AD (Brun & Gustafson, 1976). There are no protein deposits, neither of tau nor others, save for deposits of the degradation protein ubiquitin within immunopositive threads and bodies in some cases (FTD-U). A mild loss of substantia nigra neurons may also be found.

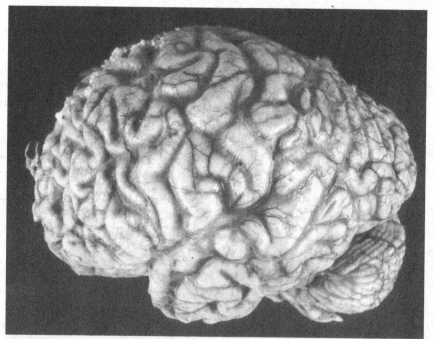

Figure 8.1   FLD with marked frontal atrophy but preserved and wide central sensory motor cortex. (For a color version of this figure, please see the color plate section.)

In the white matter there is a mild gliosis. In spite of these rather discrete changes, mainly in the superficial portion of the neuronal cortical column, this form goes with symptoms of a severe progressive frontal dysfunction as described below. The disease is sometimes claimed to be unilateral, especially in the forms with mainly speech disturbances. Pathologically this is, however, rarely the case but there may be asymmetries as to the severity or distribution of changes, further underscoring the correlation between damage and dysfunction. Clinical heterogeneity of FTD is sometimes claimed on the basis of different frontal dysfunctional symptom constellations but they all are expressions of the same disorder, the variation being explained by differences in location including starting point, mode of spread or intensity of changes.

The form FTD and Parkinsonism linked to a mutation on chromosome 17 (FTDP-17) is rare and yet dominates the FTD literature, necessitating a brief note here. In this form the FLD basic type is supplemented by degenerative changes, above all in the substantia nigra and the amygdalar nucleus. There are a number of subforms, some with tau deposits. Behavioral and cognitive manifestations would here relate to the frontotemporal cortical engagement whereas motor disturbances are extra pyramidal and nigral (Foster *et al.*, 1997).

PiD is here defined as frontotemporal degeneration with, besides the less specific inflated neurons, also the typical but not pathognomonic neuronal Pick body inclusions (European Concerted Action on Pick's Disease Consortium, 1998). These are tau and ubiquitin positive and contain either three or four repeat tau-isoforms or both though with little consequence for the clinical and pathological picture (Zhukareva *et al.*, 2002). Basically, the FLD types of cortical changes are present but they are more profound or lobar and involve in large areas also the deeper layers including a loss of synapses. This goes with wasting and gliosis of the underlying white matter. Also involved are the striate body and, especially in later stages, the amygdala and hippocampus, often in an asymmetric way, whereas the parietal lobes and in particular the sensorymotor gyri for long remain unaffected. This is reflected in the symptomatology, which will be described in detail below.

In the two forms of dementia with prominent aphasia, semantic dementia and progressive nonfluent aphasia, the changes are mainly located in the left temporal lobe. In the latter form also anterior frontal and parietal areas are affected, predominantly on the left side. They usually go without inclusions although some reports mention either tau or ubiquitin positive inclusions.

In MNDD, the neuropathology repeats that of FLD, but with the addition of the pathology of MND, regarding motor neuron degeneration and neuronal ubiquitin inclusions. Such inclusions may also be found in cases with pure FTD symptoms and pathology but without further signs of MND, something that may strengthen the bond between FTD and MND. Further, a large proportion of FTD cases have all or some MND features and FTD-MND may start with symptoms of either disease (Lomen-Hoerth *et al.*, 2002). Others even consider FLD, FLD with MND and MNDD as belonging to the same clinicopathological spectrum (Floel *et al.*, 2002; Mackenzie & Feldman, 2003).

4.2 Clinical characteristics

The core diagnostic features of FTD are presented in Table 8.1. The symptoms are strongly related to the characteristic pattern of degeneration. There is, however, an important clinical variability within the FTD group, which can be explained by differences in histopathology, topography and genetics of the degenerative process (Wilhelmsen *et al.*, 1994; Neary *et al.*, 2005; Passant *et al.*, 2005b). It is often claimed that the clinical picture of FTD may be differentiated from that of other common types of dementia such as AD and VaD, although individual cases may show a striking clinical similarity to

Table 8.1 Clinical features of frontotemporal dementia (Brun *et al.*, 1994)

The Lund-Manchester consensus statement

CORE DIAGNOSTIC FEATURES
Behavioral disorder
- Insidious onset and slow progression
- Early loss of personal awareness (neglect of personal hygiene and grooming)
- Early loss of social awareness (lack of social tact, misdemeanours such as shoplifting)
- Early loss of disinhibition (such as unrestrained sexuality, violent behavior, inappropriate jocularity, restless pacing)
- Mental rigidity and inflexibility
- Hyperorality (oral/dietary changes, overeating, food fads, excessive smoking and alcohol consumption, oral exploration of objects)
- Stereotyped and preservative behavior (wandering, mannerisms such as clapping, singing, dancing, ritualistic preoccupation such as hoarding, toileting, and dressing)
- Utilization behavior (unrestrained exploration of objects in the environment)
- Distractibility, impulsivity, and impersistence
- Early loss of insight into the fact that the altered condition is due to a pathological change of own mental state
Affective symptoms
- Depression, anxiety, excessive sentimentality, suicidal and fixed ideation, delusion (early and evanescent)
- Hyperchondriasis, bizarre somatic preoccupation (early and evanescent)
- Emotional unconcern (emotional indifference and remoteness, lack of empathy and sympathy, apathy)
- Amimia (inertia, aspontaneity)

(continued)

Table 8.1 Contd

The Lund-Manchester consensus statement

Speech disorder
- Progressive reduction of speech (aspontaneity and economy of utterance)
- Stereotypy of speech (repetition of limited repertoire of words, or themes)
- Echolalia and perseveration
- Late mutism

Spatial orientation and praxis preserved (intact abilities to negotiate the environment)

Physical signs
- Early primitive reflexes
- Early incontinence
- Late akinesia, rigidity, tremor
- Low and labile blood pressure

Investigations
- Normal EEG despite clinically evident dementia
- Brain imaging (structural or functional, or both): predominant frontal or anterior temporal abnormality, or both
- Neuropsychology (profound failure on "frontal lobe" tests in the absence of severe amnesia, aphasia, or perceptual spatial disorder)

SUPPORTIVE DIAGNOSTIC FEATURES
- Onset before 65
- Positive family history of similar disorder in a first-degree relative
- Bulbar palsy, muscular weakness and wasting, fasciculations (motor neuron disease)

DIAGNOSTIC EXCLUSION FEATURES
- Abrupt onset with ictal events
- Head trauma related to onset
- Early severe amnesia
- Early spatial disorientation, lost in surrounding, defective localization of objects
- Early severe apraxia
- Logoclonic speech with rapid loss of train of thought
- Myoclonus
- Cortical bulbar and spinal deficits
- Cerebellar ataxia
- Choreo-athetosis
- Early, severe, pathological EEG
- Brain imaging (predominant postcentral structural or functional deficit. Multifocal cerebral lesions on CT or MRI)
- Laboratory tests indicating brain involvement or inflammatory disorder (such as multiple sclerosis, syphilis, AIDS and herpes simplex encephalitis)

RELATIVE DIAGNOSTIC EXCLUSION FEATURES
- Typical history of chronic alcoholism
- Sustained hypertension
- History of vascular disease (such as angina, claudication)

FTD (Gustafson, 1987; Miller *et al.*, 1997; Pasquier *et al.*, 2004). PiD has not yet been possible to distinguish with certainty from FLD on pure clinical grounds (Gustafson, 1993). Thus the clinical characteristics described below also pertain to PiD.

FTD starts and develops slowly, usually without any obvious cause or dramatic variation of the clinical state. The age of onset is usually between 40 and 65 years (Gustafson, 1987; Neary *et al.*, 1988; Knopman *et al.*, 1990; Miller *et al.*, 1991), although cases above 70 years have been reported by several groups (Miller *et al.*, 1991; Gregory & Hodges, 1996; Passant *et al.*, 2005b). The early stage is dominated by changes and dissolution of personality, behavior and speech rather than by cognitive deterioration, although memory failures, lack of concentration and executive dysfunctions often are reported. The relatives usually have a strong feeling of an ongoing strange change of the patient's attitudes and emotional responses, but it may still be very difficult to decide when the first signs of a mental deterioration appeared. The duration of the disease is therefore easily underestimated and the symptoms are misinterpreted as expressions of psychosocial stress, conflicts or a nonorganic mental disease.

The early symptoms in FTD must be judged against information about the patient's premorbid personality, mental capacity, education and professional experience. The changes of habitual personality traits in FTD are described as emotional leveling and unconcern, lack of empathy, aspontaneity and impaired judgment. The patient becomes self-centered, emotionally cold and less concerned about his family and friends, work and own appearance. A main problem is that the patients no longer understand that his or her present condition, difficulties and conflicts are due to changes of their own mental condition. This lack of awareness and insight may strongly disturb the diagnostic process and the management and care of patients with FTD (Passant *et al.*, 2005a).

Signs of disinhibition often appear early as impulsivity, restlessness, irritability, aggressiveness, inadequate smiling and excessive sentimentality. Craving for affection and sexual contacts may be easily provoked, but usually such expressions of disinhibition are rather harmless and possible to foresee and divert. Offensive language, indecent behavior like disinhibited singing, uninvited joining of private parties and aggressive outbursts are also reported. Unrestrained stereotypical behavior such as impulsive buying, hoarding and shoplifting may, however, cause serious social and economical problems.

The changes of mood and emotional expressions may also cause differential diagnostic problems when distinguishing between FTD and nonorganic mental disorder presenting emotional, behavioral and executive dysfunction. Two contrasting subsyndromes have been described: one with disinhibition (FTD-D), distractibility and purposeless overactivity associated with atrophy of the orbitomedial frontal lobes and temporal lobes; the other syndrome (FTD-A) with apathy, inertia and loss of volition associated with widespread frontal lobe atrophy, also including the dorsolateral frontal cortex. In both syndromes the marked behavioral disorder stands in contrast to a relative preservation of practical skills (Neary et al., 1988; Snowden et al., 1996). However, when patients are studied in a longer perspective, relatively minor differences emerge between FTD-A and FTD-D. This in contrast to the marked clinical differences between FTD and semantic dementia (Snowden et al., 2001). Semantic dementia is a form of frontotemporal lobar degeneration (FTLD) more related to degeneration of the temporal lobes than frontotemporal structures. Semantic dementia is characterized by loss of conceptual knowledge. Behavioral changes occur as in FTD, emotional insight is better preserved, and repetitive behavior is more prevalent in semantic dementia compared to FTD.

Patients with FTD may appear emotionally unconcerned, at times even euphoric. Mimical movements may become tense and sparse or inadequate, often already at an early stage of FTD, which in combination with the patient's uninterest, aspontaneity, social withdrawal and reduced stereotyped speech may be misinterpreted as a nonorganic depression. Depressed mood was the tentative diagnosis in about one third of our postmortem-verified FTD cases and antidepressant agents had been tried even more frequently.

In spite of impaired insight, patients with FTD may consult a doctor about various somatic complaints, often with a bizarre hypochondriacal touch. By contrast, when elated mood is accompanied by impulsivity, increased talkativeness and confabulation, these symptoms may be difficult to differentiate from a hypomanic or manic state. Increased tearfulness and inadequate smiling may also blunt the clinical picture.

The personality changes with impaired judgment and unpredictable behavior may easily lead to conflicts in the family and in the society. The patient may be diagnosed as "psychopathic" or "criminal" in spite of a rather typical history of FTD. In contrast to the typical AD case the FTD patient's lack of judgment and insight coexist with relatively preserved practical and spatial abilities. Dangerous behavior as driver and passenger is reported, such as the patient trying to get out of the car several times on the freeway whereas another patient tried to switch off the engine when someone else was driving. Several patients continue to drive contrary to the clear advice of their doctor, and also after the driving license has been suspended. By contrast most AD patients are more self-critical and aware of their increasing perceptual and practical difficulties and therefore ready to give up driving.

Hoarding and compulsive repetitive behavior is often reported in FTD and semantic dementia, and is rather uncommon in AD (Nyatsanza et al., 2003).

A clinical scale devised to recognize stereotypical and ritualistic behaviors contains verbal stereotypes, echolalia, rigid adherence to routines/rituals, pre-occupation with counting, clock watching, repetition of the same leisure activities, hoarding or collecting obsessively, or repeatedly eating the same food. Factor analyses of symptoms in FTD result commonly in a very strong factor with stereotypic and ritualistic behavior. Patients with semantic dementia are more prone to establish behavioral routines and clock watching, which may indicate an association with temporal lobe dysfunction (Snowden *et al.*, 2001).

The psychotic features in FTD are often bizarre, badly controlled and difficult to divert with psychological techniques. The combination of bizarre, stereotyped and disinhibited features in FTD may easily give the impression of a functional psychosis, leading to a diagnosis of schizophrenia. The combination of psychotic and frontal lobe symptoms has also been described in AD and in patients with frontal subcortical white matter ischemic lesions (Brun & Gustafson, 1991; Miller *et al.*, 1991). The psychotic features in AD are more strongly related to the severity of cognitive deterioration and the temporoparietal degeneration (Gustafson & Risberg, 1993).

Changes of oral dietary behavior were early recognized as typical of damage and disease in frontotemporal regions. Various elements of a Klüver-Bucy-like syndrome, such as hyperorality, hypersexuality and the "environmental dependency syndrome" similar to the hypermetamorphosis of the Klüver-Bucy syndrome in animals, are common in FTD. These features have been related to dysfunction in frontal and frontothalamic regions (Shallice *et al.*, 1989; Eslinger *et al.*, 1991; Hashimoto *et al.*, 1995). An irresistible impulse to explore the environment is often observed at the interview. The patient stands up, moves around, touches and tries various objects in sight. This "utilization behavior" in patients with frontal lobe lesions has been described by Lhermitte *et al.* (1986). The hyperorality manifests itself in food fads, gluttony, excessive smoking and alcohol overconsumption. FTD may sometimes be misdiagnosed as alcohol-related dementia (Groen & Endtz, 1982; Gustafson, 1987). Certain types of food are preferred and the patient may also try uneatable objects, which in combination with dysphagia at a later stage may cause aspiration.

The majority of FTD cases develop a progressive dynamic aphasia first described as "Sprachverödung" (Schneider, 1927) and "dissolution du language" (Escourolle, 1958). Speech becomes aspontaneous with word-finding difficulties and frequent use of stereotyped comments and set phrases. Sometimes periods of increased unrestrained talking and singing are observed and at times also confabulation. Confabulation is more prevalent in PiD, probably related to the more severe hippocampal involvement. Imitating behavior, especially echolalia, was observed in about half of the PiD and one third of the FLD cases (van Mansfelt, 1954; Gustafson *et al.*, 2001). At a late stage more than 80% of the patients become mute, which in combination with loss of mimical movements and emotional unconcern makes communication extremely difficult. The ability to understand information may, however, be preserved comparatively late, like also the ability to write. The hand writing may, however, change in magnitude, spelling and speed of writing. The disturbances of speech and language seem strongly related to a more severe involvement of the speech-dominant hemisphere. The symptom constellation of pallilalia (stereotypy of speech), echolalia, mutism and amimia described as the PEMA-syndrome (Guiraud, 1956) is typical of FTD and rare in AD. These findings are in agreement with the impairment of motivation, attention and regulation of behavior observed in patients with damage to frontal cortical areas, especially to the premotor cortex (Luria, 1958, 1973).

There are important similarities between FTD at an early stage and the clinical spectrum of progressive aphasia (Mesulam, 1982; Neary *et al.*, 1993; Snowden & Neary, 1993; Hodges *et al.*, 2004). Progressive aphasia is clinically heterogeneous with two distinct subsyndromes: progressive nonfluent aphasia (PNA) and progressive fluent aphasia. In the latter syndrome the speech remains fluid and well articulated but becomes progressively devoid of content words reflecting a breakdown in semantic memory and is diagnostically labeled semantic dementia. PNA is dominated by language disturbances in combination with relative preservation of memory and practical abilities. At later stages many of these cases seem, however, to develop global dementia (Green *et al.*, 1990; Snowden *et al.*, 1996). Clinically there is a considerate overlap between PNA and corticobasal degeneration (Kertesz & Martinez-Lage, 1998). The behavioral changes in semantic dementia are less severe than in FTD with a brain pathology restricted to the middle and interior temporal gyri.

Cognitive impairment, mainly reduced recent memory and lack of concentration, appears early in FTD although often overshadowed by the emotional and behavioral disturbances. Temporal and spatial orientation and practical abilities are comparatively spared, but difficult to evaluate by a traditional neuropsychiatric assessment. Dyscalculia is often mentioned as an early symptom, also misspelling as an expression of sequential language dysfunction.

Neuropsychological testing is useful for the early recognition of FTD and to distinguish it from other dementias, normal aging and nonorganic mental disease. To achieve this it is important to rely not only on quantitative measures, but also on systematic evaluation of the patient's behavior in the test situation (Hagberg, 1987; Johanson *et al.*, 1990). Confabulation is more prominent in Pick's disease, probably due to more severe hippocampal degeneration (Johanson & Hagberg, 1989; Gustafson *et al.*, 2001). The early test profile in FTD is characterized by slow verbal production and relatively intact reasoning and memory, while intellectual and motor speed is reduced. By contrast, early Alzheimer patients show a relatively intact verbal ability and a simultaneous impairment of reasoning ability, verbal and spatial memory dysfunction, dysphasia and dyspraxia. AD with a later onset shows a less consistent test profile and more marked verbal memory dysfunction. Systematic evaluation of behavior qualities such as cooperation, self-criticism, distractibility, flight reactions and strategy in the test situation strongly contribute to the differentiation of FTD from AD (Johanson & Hagberg, 1989; Pachana *et al.*, 1996). Elfgren and coworkers (1993, 1996) have shown significant correlations between global impairment and verbal fluency scores and cortical blood flow of left frontal lateral, frontal medial and left temporal anterior inferior areas.

4.3   Case history: a female patient with FTD

The patient was a trained nurse, working at the general hospital. She was an only child and her mother described her as a nice, reliable person with a warm interest in her family and friends. She married early and gave birth to three children, the last one born in 1989. The patient's father died in a traffic accident at the age of 50 years. Her maternal grandfather, who suffered from a stroke at the age of 50, had a brother who became increasingly disinhibited, euphoric and careless in his sixties.

The first indication of a progressive mental change in the patient was noted in 1987 when she lost her keen interest in horseback riding. During the following year she became restless and showed a marked lack of concern for her family. This was, however, explained away by the patient's ongoing pregnancy. She lost her previous interest in cooking for her family and relied on fast food and pizzas. There was a general emotional bluntness with few expressions of joy or sadness but she was still interacting with her three children. She appeared aspontaneous, stereotypic, sometimes almost apathetic and only left her home for very short walks.

The family tried very hard to convince the patient that she needed to see a doctor but she showed no insight into her mental changes. Her speech became aspontaneous and stereotyped and the husband complained of the patient's easily aroused aggressiveness and fits of laughter. Her sleep at night was still fairly normal, but the patient was often found lying on her bed for hours during daytime. Her appetite increased with a general interest in sweets. The patient no longer managed to care for her youngest child properly. The district nurse was contacted and the patient was referred to the psychogeriatric department for diagnostic assessment and care.

At the first examination she was described as lucid and well oriented. She was slightly euphoric, disinhibited and showed no awareness and insight into her changed mental condition. She was restless and irritable, and sometimes laughed without any obvious reason. The language dysfunction was very obvious. She was aspontaneous, talking in short stereotyped phrases, sometimes also with echolalia and "baby talk." Communication became even more limited when the patient later lost her mimical movements.

The physical examination and the laboratory screening showed no indications of extracerebral somatic disease. The patient was allowed to visit her family at home, and when she returned to the hospital after such a visit she showed a rather adequate and deep sorrow. The patient developed bulimia and sometimes even tried to eat uneatable things. She was treated with neuroleptics with only limited effects.

Brain imaging with regional cerebral blood flow measurements (rCBF) showed bilateral frontal hypoperfusion. The patient further deteriorated, but in 1991 she was still oriented as to time and place, although emotionally unconcerned and apathetic. Cerebrospinal fluid analysis showed slightly increased tau and neurofilaments, indicating a neuronal degenerative process. The clinical diagnosis was FTD. The patient moved to a nursing home and stayed there until her death 2 years later. She became almost mute but obviously she was still receptive and, to some extent, remembering information and instructions. She seemed to recognize her relatives and sometimes responded by saying single words. She died suddenly and unexpectedly from acute heart failure.

The neuropathological examination showed marked frontal lobe degeneration with gliosis, microvacoulation and nerve cell loss in lamina 1−3. The cortical degeneration also involved the anterior cingulate cortex and the laterobasal and fronto-orbital regions bilaterally. The degeneration of the anterior temporal lobe was most marked on the left side. The pathological diagnosis was FLD (Brun *et al.*, 1994).

4.4   Clinical characteristics of MNDD

MNDD has been described clinically, mostly in Japan, by Mitsuyama (1984) and Morita and coworkers (1987), but also in the UK (Neary *et al.*, 1990) and other countries (Wikström *et al.*, 1982). The prevalence may be difficult to determine because of the presence of pseudobulbar emotional lability, mood disorder, dysarthria, and other neurological deficits in classical or "pure" MND. The clinical onset of mental deterioration is usually in the sixth decade and may even precede the signs of anterior horn cell involvement. The mean duration is about 30 months (Salazar *et al.*, 1983; Mitsuyama, 1984). The clinical picture is similar to that of FLD, with impaired insight, signs of disinhibition, apathy and other changes of personality. Receptive speech function, orientation and practical abilities may remain relatively untouched. The emotional changes are described as euphoria and childishness and the face becomes blunt. Fasciculations were observed in only a few of our MNDD cases, while dysphagia and muscular wasting were present in about 40% of our cases with FLD and Pick's disease (Gustafson *et al.*, 2001). The diagnosis is based on recognition of a rapidly progressive dementia of frontal lobe type in combination with physical signs of anterior horn involvement. Functional brain imaging shows predominant precentral pathology, while EEG may remain within normal range.

5   Frontal lobe features in Alzheimer's disease

5.1   Neuropathological characteristics

A frontal variant of AD has been pointed out from a clinical point of view. The prevalence is not known but suggested to be 14–17%, in our experience, more at 5%. Among the limited number of cases studied also neuropathologically some have had a combination of AD and PiD while others have shown a relative or absolute frontal preponderance of the classical AD-changes such as plaques, tangles and dystrophic neurites (Brun, 1987; Johnson *et al.*, 1999). The functional impairment implied by such pathology is here sometimes reinforced by additional frontal white matter incomplete infarcts (SIWI, discussed below), as is also often the case in AD with the regular pathology pattern.

5.2   Clinical characteristics

The predominant symptom pattern in AD with memory failure, aphasia, apraxia, agnosia and spatial disorientation is strongly related to the accentuation of degenerative changes in temporal limbic and temporoparietal cortex. Several studies have, however, shown clinical heterogeneity related to age at onset, disease duration, genetic factors and pathological correlates such as frontal lobe involvement and incomplete white matter infarctions (Chui *et al.*, 1985).

Frontal lobe symptoms such as executive dysfunction are often reported in AD (Swanberg *et al.*, 2004). Frontal lobe features, such as disinhibition and euphoria when present, seem associated with later onset and longer duration of the disease and slower rate of progression (Brun & Gustafson, 1993; Frisoni *et al.*, 1999). Most clinicopathological studies of AD, however, show a relative sparing of frontal lobe cortex and anterior cingulate gyrus (Brun & Gustafson, 1976; Brun & Englund, 1981) and there are few reports on AD with a marked frontal lobe involvement. Brun and Gustafson (1991) published data on four female AD cases with a mean duration of 9.5 years at death, all with a marked frontal lobe involvement. The Alzheimer encephalopathy in these cases was pronounced in limbic and temporoparietal areas, but even more so in the frontal lobes with accentuated widening of sulci and the ventricular system. The clinical picture was that of a rapid progressive course at an early stage in two cases. Early dysmnesia dominated in three cases, and all cases developed dysphasia, dyspraxia and dysgnosia, and in three cases also extrapyramidal signs. Loss of insight was prominent in three cases, with euphoria observed in two cases and emotional lability and inadequate laughing in two cases. These symptoms indicating a frontal lobe involvement were in good agreement with the pathology of the regional cerebral blood flow (Risberg & Gustafson, 1988; Harwood *et al.*, 2005).

6   Dementia in Huntington's disease

6.1   Neuropathological characteristics

In Huntington's disease (HD) the core pathology resides in the striatum with a main point in the caudate nucleus, early in the course involving its tail. The substantia nigra and globus pallidus are secondarily atrophied through loss of striate projections and a subthalamic nucleus, the lateral geniculate body, shows atrophy as well. Cortical engagement is widespread, but early on predominantly frontal, presumably due to striate frontal connections, also resulting in a frontal metabolic decrement. Changes consist of gliosis and neuronal loss with deposition of huntingtin, a protein encoded by an expanded HD gene producing abnormally expanded protein deposits (trinucleotide repeats). The length of the repeat relates to the severity of the disease, though other proteins may also be at play in the pathogenesis.

6.2   Clinical characteristics

Patients with Huntington's disease have in addition to the characteristic motor disturbances also dementia with predominant frontal lobe features. The average age at onset is the mid forties with a range from 25 to 50 years. This is similar to the age at onset in FTD, although large variation is seen in both disorders. Subcortical functions are affected first and dominate the picture of dementia throughout the course. The dementia starts insidiously with personality changes towards emotional blunting, self-neglect, lack of insight, apathy and depressed mood in combination with slowness of thinking and difficulties with attention, concentration and recent memory. Recognition and spatial orientation are comparatively spared. Psychotic features may predominate, sometimes already at an early stage. The clinical picture may be that of mood disorder or paranoid psychosis with bizarre and grandiose delusions, and sometimes misdiagnosed as schizophrenia. The symptom constellation may therefore be similar to that of FLD and PiD with psychotic reactions. Differential diagnosis has to rely on recognition of typical neurological features such as choreiform, clumsy and twitching movements, facial grimaces and dysarthria.

7   Vascular dementia with frontal lobe features

7.1   Neuropathological characteristics

Frontal selective incomplete white matter infarction (SIWI) and Binswanger's disease, two vascular disorders more precisely defined in what follows, show a certain preponderance for the frontal lobes, in particular their white matter. One might speculate that the reason for this relative frontal selective vulnerability to cerebrovascular affliction is the great expansion of the human frontal lobes resulting in very elongated white matter arterioli, which in addition are relatively scarce and have few shunts.

Important for SIWI is that over time these arterioli develop a special type of arteriosclerosis, fibrohyaline arteriolosclerosis, with narrowing and wall stiffening. This slows the autoregulatory adaptation to pressure falls, which paves the way for hypoperfusive episodes with tissue hypoxia. This is the contemplated pathogenesis behind selective incomplete white matter infarcts, which probably are the dominating correlate to the radiological term white matter hyper-intensities or leukoaraiosis. These infarcts are incomplete in the sense that the tissues become attenuated with partial loss of oligodendroglial cells, myelin and axons. Through accumulation, the lesions impair large areas of white matter with partial disconnection of the frontal cortex and consequent dysfunctional effects.

In Binswanger's disease hypertensive arteriolosclerosis causes occlusions with complete, lacunar infarcts, in the basal ganglia and brain stem, and also particularly in the frontal white matter. Around the latter lacunas perifocal incomplete infarctions arise within large areas, the presence of which is a more likely explanation for dysfunctional symptoms than the small lacunar infarcts.

7.2   Clinical characteristics

Vascular, frontal and frontosubcortical syndromes are often reported in vascular dementia and in mixed VaD and AD. These syndromes, which may mimic FTD, may be caused by frontal cortical infarcts, bilateral thalamic infarcts (Segarra, 1970; Poirier *et al.*, 1983; Brun, 1987; Pasquier *et al.*, 1995), bilateral caudate infarcts (Richfield *et al.*, 1987), Binswanger's disease (Jellinger & Neumayer, 1964; Janota, 1981; Tomonaga *et al.*, 1982; Fredriksson *et al.*, 1992) and incomplete white matter infarctions found in the frontal lobes only (Brun & Gustafson, 1991). The vascular lesions may thus directly involve the frontal lobe or undercut the projections to frontal structures. The clinical picture is dominated by changes of personality with signs of disinhibition, lack of insight, emotional leveling, euphoria, depressed mood and apathy. There are often a mental as well as motoric slowing, impaired attention, memory failure and executive dysfunctions, neurological gait problems, primitive reflexes and urinary incontinence. The characteristic shuffling small-stepped gait is related to lesions of basal ganglia and interruptions of thalamo-cortical and corticospinal connections. Urinary incontinence is associated with lesions in the superior frontal gyrus, anterior cingulated cortex and the connecting white matter (Andrew & Nathan, 1964; Andin et al., 2005). The combination of progressive dementia, incontinence, gait disturbance and ventricular dilatation in VaD may sometimes mimic the potentially treatable frontal type of dementia in normal pressure hydrocephalus.

The association between cerebrovascular disease and mood disorder has been shown in several clinical studies. The clinical correlations are poorly understood although the localization and severity of the brain lesion, neurotransmitter failure, the patient's age and premorbid personality have been mentioned as predisposing factors in this context. Robinson et al. (1983) analyzed the relationship between depression and the localization of the vascular lesions, finding that the severity of depression was directly correlated to the closeness of the lesion in the frontal pole irrespective of the etiology of the brain injury. Other studies confirm the strong association between depression and left hemisphere lesions. Great controversies exist, however, concerning correlations between vascular brain pathology and depression. Depression might be considered as a natural consequence of the patient's awareness of intellectual and physical disabilities. The production of a depressive syndrome probably depends on the degree of function in the better preserved cerebral structures.

Little is known about the pathological substrate of the affective syndrome of the hypomanic type, although MRI often shows white matter hyperintensities in the frontal lobes (Aylward et al., 1994). Depression in VaD and in older individuals is associated with the severity and prevalence of subcortical and/or left frontal white matter lesions (Bennett et al., 1994; Cummings, 1994; Greenwald et al., 1998; de Groot et al., 2000). White matter lesions are, however, also prevalent in healthy elderly people. Damage in white matter structures seem to play an important role in the initiation, maintenance and outcome of major depression in dementia (O'Brien et al., 1998).

8   Conclusions

Our current knowledge about the relationship between mental activity and disturbances of the complex functional systems of the brain has developed mainly on the basis of observations in patients with brain damage with different localization and type. This chapter has focused upon the clinical manifestations of frontal lobe damage caused by primary degenerative and cerebrovascular disease. Due to lack of space it has not been possible to cover frontal lobe syndromes caused by rarer hereditary disorders, head injury, infections, toxic exposure and ageing. The frontal lobes and in particular the prefrontal structures seem vulnerable to specific lesions due to developmental and structural organizational features. The impact of lesions depends not only on their localization, size and intensity but also on unrelated additional damage, on the condition of different compensating or substitutional factors as well as the brain reserve capacity.

REFERENCES

Alzheimer, A. (1911). Über eigenartige Krankheitsfälle der späteren Alters. *Zeitschrift für die Gesamte Neurologie und Psychiatrie*, **4**, 356–85.

Andin, U., Gustafson, L., Passant, U. & Brun, A. (2005). A clinico-pathological study of heart and brain lesions in vascular dementia. *Dementia and Geriatric Cognitive Disorders*, **19**, 222–8.

Andrew, J. & Nathan, P. W. (1964). Lesions on the anterior frontal lobes and disturbances of micturition and defaecation. *Brain*, **87**, 233–62.

Aylward, E. H., Roberts-Twillie, J. V., Barta, P. E., *et al.* (1994). Basal ganglia volumes and white matter hyperintensities in patients with bipolar disorder. *American Journal of Psychiatry*, **151**, 687–93.

Bennett, D. A., Gilley, D. W., Lee, S. & Cochran, E. J. (1994). White matter changes: neuronal manifestations of Binswanger's disease and clinical correlates in Alzheimer's disease. *Dementia*, **5**, 148–52.

Binswanger, O. (1894). Die Abgrenzung der allgemeinen progressiven Paralyse. *Berliner Klinische Wochenschrift*, **31**, 1103–5, 1137–9, 1180–6.

Brun, A. (1965). The subpial granular layer of the foetal cerebral cortex in man. Its ontogeny and significance in congenital cortical malformations. Thesis. *Acta Pathologica et Microbiologica Scandinavica*, **179** (Suppl.), 1–98.

Brun, A. (1987). Frontal lobe degeneration of non-Alzheimer type. 1. Neuropathology. *Archives of Gerontology and Geriatrics*, **6**, 193–208.

Brun, A. (1999). The emergence of the frontal lobe and its morbidity, as opposed to the central lobe. *Dementia and Geriatric Cognitive Disorders*, **10** (Suppl.), 3–5.

Brun, A. & Englund, E. (1981). Regional pattern of degeneration in Alzheimer's disease: neuronal loss and histopathological grading. *Histopathology*, **5**, 549–64.

Brun, A., Englund, B., Gustafson, L., *et al.* (1994). Clinical and neuropathological criteria for frontotemporal dementia. *Journal of Neurology, Neurosurgery and Psychiatry*, **57**, 416–18.

Brun, A. & Gustafson, L. (1976). Distribution of cerebral degeneration in Alzheimer's disease. A clinico-pathological study. *Archiv für Psychiatrie und Nervenkrankheiten*, **223**, 15–33.

Brun, A. & Gustafson, L. (1991). Psychopathology and frontal lobe involvement in organic dementia. In *Alzheimer's Disease: Basic Mechanisms, Diagnosis and Therapeutic Strategies*, ed. K. Iqbal, D. R. C. McLachlan, B. Winblad *et al.* London: John Wiley & Sons, pp. 27–33.

Brun, A. & Gustafson, L. (1993). I. The Lund longitudinal dementia study: A 25-year perspective on neuropathology, differential diagnosis and treatment. In *Alzheimer's Disease: Advances in Clinical and Basic Research*, ed. B. Corain, K. Iqbal, M. Nicolini *et al.* London: John Wiley & Sons, pp. 4–18.

Chui, H. C., Teng, E. L., Henderson, V. W. & Moy, A. C. (1985). Clinical subtypes of dementia of the Alzheimer type. *Neurology*, **35**, 1544–50.

Corbin, J. G., Nery, S. & Fishell, G. (2001). Telencephalic cells take a tangent: non-radial migration in the mammalian forebrain. *Nature Neuroscience*, **4**, 1177–82.

Cummings, J. L. (1994). Vascular subcortical dementias: clinical aspects. *Dementia*, **5**, 177–80.

de Groot, J. C., de Leeuw, F. E., Oudkerk, M., *et al.* (2000). Cerebral white matter lesions and depressive symptoms in elderly adults. *Archives of General Psychiatry*, **57**, 1071–76.

Elfgren, C., Passant, U. & Risberg, J. (1993). Neuropsychological findings in frontal lobe dementia. *Dementia*, **4**, 214–19.

Elfgren, C., Ryding, E. & Passant, U. (1996). Performance on neuropsychological tests related to single photon emission computerised tomography findings in frontotemporal dementia. *British Journal of Psychiatry*, **169**, 416–22.

Escourolle, R. (1958). *La Maladie de Pick. Étude Critique d'Ensemble et Synthèse Anatomo-Clinique*, Paris: R Foulon.

Eslinger, P. J., Warner, G. C., Grattan, L. M. & Easton, J. D. (1991). "Frontal lobe" utilization associated with paramedian thalamic infarction. *Neurology*, **41**, 450–2.

European Concerted Action on Pick's Disease Consortium, European Concerted Action on Pick's Disease (ECAPD) Consortium (1998). Provisional clinical and neuroradiological criteria for the diagnosis of Pick's disease. *European Neurology*, **5**, 519–20.

Floel, A. H., Lohmann, S. & Knecht, S. (2002). Neuropsychological disorders in amyotrophic lateral sclerosis. *Nervenartz*, **73**, 1144–52.

Foster, N. L., Wilhelmsen, K., Sima, A. A. F., *et al.*, and conference participants (1997). Frontotemporal dementia and parkinsonism linked to chromosome 17: A consensus conference. *Annals of Neurology*, **41**, 706–15.

Fredriksson, K., Brun, A. & Gustafson, L. (1992). Pure subcortical arteriosclerotic encephalopathy (Binswanger's disease): A clinicopathological study. Part 1: Clinical features. *Cerebrovascular Diseases*, **2**, 82–6.

Frisoni, G. B., Rozzini, L., Gozzetti, A., *et al.* (1999). Behavioral syndromes in Alzheimer's disease: description and correlates. *Dementia and Geriatric Cognitive Disorders*, **10**, 130–8.

Green, J., Morris, J. C., Sandson, J., McKeel, D. W. Jr & Miller, J. W. (1990). Progressive aphasia: a precursor of global dementia? *Neurology*, **40**, 423–9.

Greenwald, B. S., Kramer-Ginsberg, E., Krishnan, K. R., *et al.* (1998). Neuroanatomic localization of magnetic resonance imaging signal hyperintensities in geriatric depression. *Stroke*, **29**, 613–17.

Gregory, C. A. & Hodges, J. R. (1996). Clinical features of frontal lobe dementia in comparison to Alzheimer's disease. *Journal of Neural Transmission*, **47** (Suppl.), 103–23.

Groen, J. J. & Endtz, L. J. (1982). Hereditary Pick's disease: second re-examination of the large family and discussion of other hereditary cases, with particular reference to electroencephalography, and computerized tomography. *Brain*, **105**, 443–59.

Guiraud, P. (1956). *Psychiatrie Clinique*. Paris: Le Francois.

Gustafson, L. (1987). Frontal lobe degeneration of non-Alzheimer type. II. Clinical picture and differential diagnosis. *Archives of Gerontology and Geriatrics*, **6**, 209–23.

Gustafson, L. (1993). Clinical picture of frontal lobe degeneration of non-Alzheimer type. *Dementia*, **4**, 143–8.

Gustafson, L., Passant, U., Gräsbeck, A. & Brun, A. (2001). Clinical variability of frontotemporal dementia. In *Contemporary Neuropsychiatry*, ed. K. Miyoschi, C. Shapiro, M. Gavilia & Y. Morika. Tokyo: Springer-Verlag, pp. 152–7.

Gustafson, L. & Risberg, J. (1993). Deceptions and delusions in Alzheimer's disease and frontal lobe dementia. In *Delusions and Hallucinations in Old Age*, ed. C. Katona & R. Levy. London: Gaskell, pp. 216–25.

Hagberg, B. (1987). Behaviour correlates to frontal lobe dysfunction. *Archives of Gerontology and Geriatrics*, **6**, 311–21.

Harwood, D. G., Sultzer, D. L., Feil, D., *et al.* (2005). Frontal lobe hypometabolism and impaired insight in Alzheimer disease. *American Journal of Geriatric Psychiatry*, **13**, 934–41.

Hashimoto, R., Yoshida, M. & Tanaka, Y. (1995). Utilization after right thalamic infarction. *European Neurology*, **35**, 58–62.

Hodges, J. R., Davies, R. R., Xuereb, J. H., *et al.* (2004). Clinicopathological correlates in frontotemporal dementia. *Annals of Neurology*, **56**, 399–406.

Janota, I. (1981). Dementia, deep white matter damage and hypertension: 'Binswanger's disease'. *Psychological Medicine*, **11**, 39–48.

Jellinger, K. & Neumayer, E. (1964). Binswanger's progressive subcortical vascular encephalopathy. A clinico-neuropathological study. *Archiv für Psychiatrie und Nervenkrankheiten*, **205**, 523–54.

Jimenez, D., Rivera, R., Lopez-Mascaraque, L. & DeCarlos, J. A. (2003). Origin of the cortical layer 1 in rodents. *Developmental Neuroscience*, **23**, 105–15.

Johanson, A., Gustafson, L., Smith, G. J. W., *et al.* (1990). Adaptation in different types of dementia and in normal elderly subjects. *Dementia*, **1**, 95–101.

Johanson, A. & Hagberg, B. (1989). Psychometric characteristics in patients with frontal lobe degeneration of non-Alzheimer type. *Archives of Gerontology and Geriatrics*, **8**, 129–37.

Johnson, J. K., Head, E., Kim, R., Starr, A. & Cotman, C. W. (1999). Clinical and pathological evidence for a frontal variant of Alzheimer disease. *Archives of Neurology*, **56**, 1233–9.

Kertesz, A. & Martinez-Lage, P. (1998). Cognitive changes in corticobasal degeneration. In *Pick's Disease and Pick Complex*, ed. A. Kertesz and D. G. Munoz. New York: Wiley-Liss, Inc., pp. 121–128.

Knopman, D. S., Mastri, A. R., Frey, W. H., 2nd, Sung, J. H. & Rustan, T. (1990). Dementia lacking distinctive histologic features: a common non-Alzheimer degenerative dementia. *Neurology*, **40**, 251–6.

Lhermitte, F., Pillon, B. & Serdaru, M. (1986). Human autonomy and the frontal lobes. Part I: Imitation and utilization: a neuropsychological study of 75 patients. *Annals of Neurology,* **19**, 326–34.

Lomen-Hoerth, C., Anderson, T. & Miller, B. (2002). The overlap of amyotrophic lateral sclerosis and frontotemporal dementia. *Neurology,* **59**, 1077–9.

Luria, A. R. (1958). Brain disorders and language analysis. *Language and Speech,* **1**, 14–34.

Luria, A. R. (1973). *The Working Brain. An Introduction to Neuropsychology.* London: Allen Lane, The Penguin Press.

Mackenzie, I. R. & Feldman, H. (2003). Neuronal intranuclear inclusions distinguish familial FTD-MND type from sporadic disease. *Acta Neuropathologica,* **105**, 543–8.

Mesulam, M. M. (1982). Slowly progressive aphasia without generalized dementia. *Annals of Neurology,* **11**, 592–8.

Miller, B. L., Ikonte, C., Ponton, M., *et al.* (1997). A study of the Lund-Manchester research criteria for frontotemporal dementia: clinical and single-photon emission CT correlations. *Neurology,* **48**, 937–42.

Miller, B. L., Lesser, I. M., Boone, K. B., *et al.* (1991). Brain lesions and cognitive function in late-life psychosis. *British Journal of Psychiatry,* **158**, 76–82.

Mitsuyama, Y. (1984). Presenile dementia with motor neuron disease in Japan: clinico-pathological review of 26 cases. *Journal of Neurology, Neurosurgery and Psychiatry,* **47**, 953–9.

Morita, K., Kaiya, H., Ikeda, T. & Namba, M. (1987). Presenile dementia combined with amyotrophy. A review of 34 Japanese cases. *Archives of Gerontology and Geriatrics,* **6**, 263–77.

Neary, D., Snowden, J. S., Gustafson, L., *et al.* (1998). Frontotemporal lobar degeneration: a consensus on clinical diagnostic criteria. *Neurology,* **51**, 1546–54.

Neary, D., Snowden, J. S. & Mann, D. M. A. (1993). The clinical pathological correlates of lobar atrophy. *Dementia,* **4**, 154–9.

Neary, D., Snowden, J. & Mann, D. (2005). Frontotemporal dementia. *Lancet Neurology,* **4**, 771–80.

Neary, D., Snowden, J. S., Mann, D. M., *et al.* (1990). Frontal lobe dementia and motor neuron disease. *Journal of Neurology, Neurosurgery and Psychiatry,* **53**, 23–32.

Neary, D., Snowden, J. S., Northen, B. & Goulding, P. (1988). Dementia of frontal lobe type. *Journal of Neurology, Neurosurgery and Psychiatry,* **51**, 353–61.

Nimchinsky, E. A., Vogt, B. A., Morrison, J. H. & Hof, P. R. (1995). Spindle neurons of the human anterior cingulate cortex. *Journal of Comparative Neurology,* **355**, 27–37.

Nyatsanza, S., Shetty, T., Gregory, C., *et al.* (2003). A study of stereotypic behaviours in Alzheimer's disease and frontal and temporal variant frontotemporal dementia. *Journal of Neurology, Neurosurgery and Psychiatry,* **74**, 1398–402.

O'Brien, J., Ames, D., Chiu, E., *et al.* (1998). Severe deep white matter lesions and outcome in elderly patients with major depressive disorder: follow up study. *British Medical Journal,* **317**, 982–4.

Onari, K. & Spatz, H. (1926). Anatomische Beiträge zur Lehre von der Pickschen umschriebenen Grosshirnrinden-Atrophie ('Picksche Krankheit'). *Zentralblad für Neurologie,* **101**, 470–511.

Pachana, N. A., Boone, K. B., Miller, B. L., Cummings, J. L. & Berman, N. (1996). Comparison of neuropsychological functioning in Alzheimer's disease and frontotemporal dementia. *Journal of the International Neuropsychological Society*, **2**, 505–10.

Pasquier, F., Lebert, F. & Petit, H. (1995). Dementia, apathy, and thalamic infarcts. *Behavioral Neurology*, **8**, 208–14.

Pasquier, F., Richard, F. & Lebert, F. (2004). Natural history of frontotemporal dementia: comparison with Alzheimer's disease. *Dementia and Geriatric Cognitive Disorders*, **17**, 253–7.

Passant, U., Elfgren, C., Englund, E. & Gustafson, L. (2005a). Psychiatric symptoms and their psychosocial consequences in frontotemporal dementia. *Alzheimer Disease and Associated Disorders*, **19** (Suppl. 1), S15–S18.

Passant, U., Rosen, I., Gustafson, L. & Englund, E. (2005b). The heterogeneity of frontotemporal dementia with regard to initial symptoms, qEEG and neuropathology. *International Journal of Geriatric Psychiatry*, **20**, 983–8.

Pick, A. (1892). Über die Beziehungen der senilen Hirnatrophie zur Aphasie. *Prager Medizinische Wochenschrift*, **17**, 165–7.

Poirier, J., Barbizet, J., Gaston, A. & Meyrignac, C. (1983). Thalamic dementia. Expansive lacunae of the thalamo-paramedian mesencephalic area. Hydrocephalus caused by stenosis of the aqueduct of Sylvius. *Revue Neurologique (Paris)*, **139**, 349–58.

Richfield, E. K., Twyman, R. & Berent, S. (1987). Neurological syndrome following bilateral damage to the head of the caudate nuclei. *Annals of Neurology*, **22**, 768–71.

Risberg, J. & Gustafson, L. (1988). Regional cerebral blood flow in psychiatric disorders. In *Handbook of Regional Cerebral Blood Flow*, ed. S. Knezevic, V. Maximilian, Z. Mubrin, I. Prohovnik & J. Wade. Hillsdale, New Jersey: Lawrence Erlbaum, pp. 219–40.

Risberg, J., Passant, U., Warkentin, S. & Gustafson, L. (1993). Regional cerebral blood flow in frontal lobe dementia of non-Alzheimer type. *Dementia*, **4**, 186–7.

Robinson, R. G., Kubos, K. L., Starr, L. B., *et al.* (1983). Mood changes in stroke patients: relationship to lesion location. *Comprehensive Psychiatry*, **24**, 555–66.

Salazar, A. M., Masters, C. L., Gajdusek, D. C. & Gibbs, C. J., Jr. (1983). Syndromes of amyotrophic lateral sclerosis and dementia: relation to transmissible Creutzfeldt-Jakob disease. *Annals of Neurology*, **14**, 17–26.

Schneider, C. (1927). Über Picksche Krankheit. *Monatschrift für Psychiatrie und Neurologie*, **65**, 230–75.

Segarra, J. M. (1970). Cerebral vascular disease and. I. The syndrome of the mesencephalic artery (basilar artery bifurcation). *Archives of Neurology*, **22**, 408–18.

Shallice, T., Burgess, P. W., Schon, F. & Baxter, D. M. (1989). The origins of utilization behaviour. *Brain*, **112**, 1587–98.

Snowden, J. S., Bathgate, D., Varma, A., *et al.* (2001). Distinct behavioural profiles in frontotemporal dementia and semantic dementia. *Journal of Neurology, Neurosurgery and Psychiatry*, **70**, 323–32.

Snowden, J. S. & Neary, D. (1993). Progressive language dysfunction and lobar atrophy. *Dementia*, **4**, 226–31.

Snowden, J. S., Neary, D. & Mann, D. M. A. (1996). *Frontotemporal Lobar Degeneration: Fronto-Temporal Dementia, Progressive Aphasia, Semantic Dementia.* Edinburgh: Churchill Livingstone.

Stertz, G. (1926). Über die Picksche Atrophie. *Zentralblad für Neurologie*, **101**, 729–47.

Swanberg, M. M., Tractenberg, R. E., Mohs, R., Thal, L. J. & Cummings, J. L. (2004). Executive dysfunction in Alzheimer disease. *Archives of Neurology*, **61**, 556–60.

Tomonaga, M., Yamanouchi, H., Tohgi, H. & Kameyama, M. (1982). Clinicopathologic study of progressive subcortical vascular encephalopathy (Binswanger type) in the elderly. *Journal of the American Geriatric Society*, **30**, 524–9.

van Mansfelt, J. (1954). *Pick's Disease. A Syndrome of Lobar, Cerebral Atrophy; Its Clinico-Anatomical and Histopathological Types* [Thesis] Enschede, Utrecht.

Wikström, J., Pateau, A., Palo, J., Sulkava, R. & Haltia, M. (1982). Classic amyotrophic lateral sclerosis with dementia. *Archives of Neurology*, **38**, 681–3.

Wilhelmsen, K. C., Lynch, T., Pavlou, E., Higgins, M. & Nygaard, T. G. (1994). Localization of disinhibition-dementia-parkinsonism-amyotrophy complex to 17q21–22. *The American Journal of Human Genetics*, **55**, 1159–65.

Zhukareva, V., Mann, D., Pickering-Brown, S., *et al.* (2002). Sporadic Pick's disease: a tauopathy characterized by a spectrum of pathological tau isoforms in gray and white matter. *Annals of Neurology*, **51**, 730–9.

Index

action, specialized effector systems 43–8
adaptive coding model 73–4
age-based functional plasticity 130
akinetic mute syndrome 33
akinetic mutism 164
Alzheimer's disease (AD) 201, 202
    clinical characteristics 212
    frontal lobe features 212–13
    neuropathological characteristics 212
amygdala 31–3, 45, 48
anterior orbitofrontal areas 48
areal interconnections, laminar pattern 36
Attention Deficit Hyperactivity Disorder
        (ADHD) 15
Attentional control model 74–5
    Norman and Shallice's model 74
attentional processes 33
attention network 106
attractor dynamics 100
atypical prefrontal development 135–8
    brain injury 135, 151
    cerebellar lesions 136
    dentate nuclei 137
    developmental brain insult 135
    frontal lobe injury 136
auditory association area 26, 27
autism 54
autonomic homeostasis 49
axonal terminations 39

balanced excitation/inhibition 101
behavior, specialization of prefrontal cortices
        32–4
behavioral distractibility 116
behavioral symptomatology 53
big brain, advantages/disadvantages of
        4–5, 7–9
    brain diseases 5
Binswanger's disease 214
blood oxygen level dependent (BOLD) signal
        change 183
brainstem autonomic centers 45
brainstem vocalization centers 45
Brodmann areas 128, 129, 183

calbindin neurons 42
case studies
    Patient EVR 170, 175
    Patient KM 168, 175
        post-traumatic epilepsy 168
    Phineas Gage 129, 165, 174
catechol gene 136
caudal lateral areas 44
caudal orbitofrontal areas 49
CB positive neurons 41
cerebellar cognitive-affective syndrome 137
cerebellar-frontal connection 137
cerebral blood flow measurements (rCBF) 211
cognition, domains 29
connectionist model 76
    cortical system, levels 76
conscious perception of emotions 34
cortical atrophy 199
cortical sensory projections 31
cortical structure, laminar organizations of
        connections 34–43
cortical types in development, specification 53–4
corticocortical connections, laminar pattern 36
corticocortical pathways 33
corticothalamic neurons 50
confabulation 208, 209
creative explosion 1, 3

decision-correlated neural activity 109
decision-making 109–10
    associated neural networks 80
    prefrontal microcircuitry 109
delayed oculomotor task 95, 99
dendrite-targeting calbinding-containing
        interneurons 113
dendritic/somatic inhibition ratio 116
developmental frontal lobe functions, modeling
        149
    path analysis 150
    frontal lobe integrity 150
developmental psychology 131
disinhibition mechanism 113, 115
distractors, resistance against 107
disynaptic inhibition 42

dopamine 135
dorsolateral frontal syndrome 164
dynamical attractors 95

early prefrontal injury 173
early-processing sensory areas, projections 34
early-processing sensory cortices 54
electroresponsiveness 105
emotion binding 146–8
emotion messaging 147
    intentional-affective language 147
    typical/atypical development 148
emotion regulation 147. *See* emotion binding
    emotional expression 147
    emotive communication 147
    typical/atypical development 147
emotional communication 33
emotional memory 31
emotions, socially expressed 147. *See* emotion
    binding
empathy 147, 148
encoding/ retrieval, healthy and psychiatric
    populations 178
environmental dependency syndrome 172, 173, 175
epilepsy 54
epileptiform activity 43
episodic memory
    functional imaging 182. *See* memory
    semantic processing/prefrontal function 183
evolution of human brain, genetic changes 11–3
    Catechol-O-Methyltransferase (COMT)
        gene 12
    CMAH genes 11
    prefrontal cortex, evolution of 12
exchange of signals 34
excitation-inhibition balance (E-I balance) 100–3
    multistability 100
    rhythmogenesis, neural networks 102
excitatory postsynaptic currents (EPSCs) 104
executive function 150. *See also* theory of mind

feedback inhibition 104
feedback synaptic inhibition 100
feedforward inhibition 104
focal lesions' effect, memory systems 178
focal pre-frontal lesions 163
frontal eye field 28
frontal lobe 1–16, 137
    damage 117
    function, research 131
    processing model 132
    symptoms, organic dementing disorders 199, 201
    vulnerability 200
frontal lobe degeneration (non-Alzhemer type),
    FLD 202
    cortical changes 203
    frontal atrophy 202
frontal lobes Funahashi experiment 97
frontotemporal dementia (FTD) 201.
    See also Alzheimer's disease; FTD and AD,
    differences
    clinical heterogeneity 203

behavioural qualities, systematic evaluation 209
case history 210–11
clinical features 204
cognitive impairment 209
FLD form 202
forms 202
    clinical characteristics 204
    disinhibition signs 206
    early symptoms 206
    neuropathological characteristics 202
    neuropsychological testing 209
patient 207
    hand writing 209
    mimical movements 209
    personality changes 207
subsyndromes 206
    apathy (FTD-A) 207
    disinhibition (FTD-D) 206
test profile, early 209
frontotemporal lobar degeneration (FTLD) 207
FTD and AD, differences 207–8
functional brain development 151
functional magnetic resonance imaging (FMRI)
    studies 92, 140, 183, 186, 190
    effects 187
    encoding strategies 190
    event-related procedures 186
    levels-of-processing 186, 190

GABAergic interneurons 112, 114
GABAergic neurons 31, 41, 46
gamma oscillations 116
genetic manipulation, NMDAR 112
    long-term memory 112
    short-term memory 112
globus pallidus 44
GO-NOGO task 140
Goldman-Rakic 81. *See* working memory model
guided activation theory 77–9. *See*
    representational approach
    modulatory role, PFC 78

hedonic decision-making 146. *See* emotion bind-
    ing
    typical/atypical development 146
hemispheric encoding-retrieval asymmetry
    (HERA) model 183
hippocampal formation 30
Homo neanderthalensis 2
Homo sapiens sapiens 2
human evolution 1–4
human higher intellectual functions 10–11
    ability to mimic 11
    manual/facial gestures 11
    sign language 11
    vocalization 11, 12
Huntington's disease 201
    clinical characteristics 213
    dementia 213–4
    neuropathological characteristics 213
hybrid approach 70
hypothalamic autonomic centers 46

imitation behaviour 172
immunochemical analysis 111
impaired network behaviors 94
information processing 49
inhibitory control 138
   cognitive inhibition 139, 149
   executive inhibition 140
   neuroimaging correlates 140
   prefrontal grey matter thinning 141
   response inhibition 139, 140
   typical/atypical development 139
inhibitory neurons 46
intercalated masses (IM) 32, 46, 48, 49
interneuron-targeting calretinin-containing
    interneurons 113
ironic criticism 147, 148
irony 147, 148

Korsakoff's dementia 181

laminar microenvironment of connections 41–3
   excitatory/inhibitory interactions 41
laminar patterns of connections 40
language, evolution 9–10
   gestural mirror neuron system, humans 9
   human communication 10
    non-recursive ways 10
    recursive ways 10
    social abilities 10
   human sign language 9
   mother tongue language 10
large frontal lobes 5–7
   front-line brain imaging 6
   white matter 6
lateral hypothalamic area 47
lateral intraparietal cortex 33
lateral prefrontal areas 44
lateral prefrontal cortex 28–9
later-processing areas 34
left prefrontal function and semantic
    organization 178. See memory
limbic areas 128
limbic prefrontal areas 53
lobe atrophy 199
non-fluent aphasia (PNA) 209
localization/anti-localization approaches 163
long-term memory 29, 48, 52
Lund-Manchester research group 201, 202

medial prefrontal areas 27
medial prefrontal cortices 29–31
memory 178
   declarative memory 180
   episodic memory 180, 181
    dorsolateral prefrontal (DPFC) lesions 181
    impairments 181
    primate lesion studies 181
   hippocampal lesions, effects 180, 181
   long-term memory 178, 179
   procedural memory 180

   short-term memory 178, 179
   types 85
memory field 95, 113
metacognition 143. See mind binding
   typical/atypical development, 144
microcircuit neurodynamics 118
mind binding 143
mnemonic persistent neural activity 94–7, 102,
    115, 117
molecular markers 35
   inhibitory neurons 35
   calcium binding proteins (CBP) 35, 41
    calbindin 35
    parvalbumin 35
monosynaptic excitation 42
motor cortices 44
motor memory/(schemas) 80
Motor Neuron Disease with Dementia (MNDD)
    201–3
   clinical characteristics 211–2
MRI studies
   cross-sectional quantified 134
   longitudinal quantified 134
multimodal association cortex 128

neuroimaging/electrophysiological studies 74, 76
neuronal density 36–8, 54
NMDA/AMPA ratio 103, 111
   postsynaptic summation/saturation 111
   presynaptic short-term plasticity 111
   voltage dependence 111
NMDA, mRNA expression 111, 115
NMDA receptors 103, 115
   spike-frequency adaptation 103

oculomotor delayed response task 96
orbitofrontal area 31
orbitofrontal cortex 28, 33, 52, 128
orbitofrontal lesions 53
orbitomedial PFC neurons, role 81
orbital frontal syndrome 164
orientation selectivity 95

parvalbumin neurons 41, 42
phenylketonuria 135
perception 116
perisoma targeting parvalbumin-containing
    interneurons 113
PEMA-syndrome 209
Pick's disease (PiD) 202
positron emission tomography (PET) studies 182–4
   episodic retrieval 183
posterior orbitofrontal cortex 32, 46, 48
prefrontal areas, connectional association with
    basal ganglia 43–4
prefrontal cortex (PFC) 16, 21, 22, 69, 94, 106
   abilities 128
   behavior, synergistic action 48–50
   development 133–5
    magnetic resonance imaging (MRI) 134

myleogenesis 133
structural development 133
synaptic development 133
developmental issues 133
dopaminergic signaling
function, studies 129–31
    Broca 130
    Kennard 130
lesions 148–9
    developmental sociopathy 148
long-term representations 69, 70
memory representations 71
modality specificity of projections 24–8
neural machinery 71. See PFC neurons
neurons 73
principal pathways 21–54
processes 70
roles in memory 28–34
serial pathways 47
structure and evolution 70–2
topographic specificity of sensory cortical
    projections 28
prefrontal function processing resources
    138–41
prefrontal functional model 132–3
    assumptions 132
prefrontal microcircuitry 110–15
    degree of plasticity 112
prefrontal sectors in neurologic/psychiatric
    diseases 50–3
premotor cortices 44
progressive dynamic aphasia 208, 209
projections from visual cortices 25
processing approach 82
psychiatric diseases 53
pyramidal cells, local disinhibition 113

regional cerebral blood flow (CBF) 183
repetition priming 186
representation vs. processing 72–3. See processing
    approach
representational approach 70, 76, 78, 83
    action 71
reverberation 97, 103

schizophrenia 54, 94
    prefrontal dysfunction 115–17
schizophrenia/ADHD, evolutionary aspects
    13–15
    Homo sapiens 14
    maturation, delay 14
    social brain 14
    symptoms 15
selective complete white matter infarction (SIWI)
    214
semantic associative encoding 185
semantic dementia 202, 207.
    See also frontotemporal lobar degeneration
semantic encoding strategy 189, 192
semantic information encoding 182

semantic processing 185
schizophrenia, effect 187.
        See also schizophrenia
    brain function 189
    deep encoding 186
    encoding strategies 188
    patient overactivation 191
    patients, memory deficits 188
    residual retrieval problems 189
    'strategic memory' 188
    verbal episodic memory tasks 188
    verbal memory deficits 192
sensory association cortices 24
sensory modalities 24
sensory system, flow of information 34
serial position effect 179
social problem solving 145. See mind binding
    typical/atypical development 145
somatic marker hypothesis 79, 146
    ventromedial PFC, role 79
somatosensory association cortices 26
spatially tuned network activity pattern 98
specialization event 3
species-specific vocalization 33
stimulus selectivity/resistance 104–9, 117
    prefrontal neurons, spatial tuning 104
structured event complex (SEC) framework 76–7
    predictions 77
    representational form 75
supervisionary attentional system (SAS) 74
survival of the fittest 16
synaptic inhibition 99, 102
synaptic potentiation/depression 112

temporal organization model 80–1
    temporal integration 80
terminations, laminar pattern 42
theory of mind 143, 144, 150. See mind binding
    typical/atypical development 144, 145
time-binding 141
    autobiographical memory 141
        typical/atypical development 141
    planning 142
        typical/atypical development 142, 143
    prospective memory 142
        typical/atypical development 142
time travel/chronesthesia 141. See time-binding
traumatic brain injury (TBI) 136
    children/childhood 139, 143–5, 147, 149
typical/atypical development 128

utilization behaviour 172

vascular dementia (VaD) 201
    clinical characteristics 214
    frontal lobe features 214
    neuropathological characteristics 214
ventromedial area 128
visual association area 24

visual recognition, deficits 52
visuomotor functions 33
vocalization 45

Wood and Grafman, criteria 70
working memory 28, 48, 94, 95, 97, 98, 102, 109,
    111, 115, 117, 138, 149, 179

impairment 112
    spontaneous state 95
    stimulus-selective memory 95
working memory model 81–2
    sub-processes 75

Printed in the United States
By Bookmasters